ACSM's Resources for the
Personal Trainer

First Edition

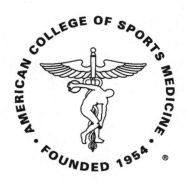

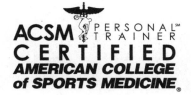

ACSM's Resources for the Personal Trainer

First Edition

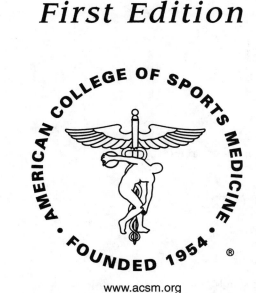

www.acsm.org

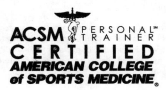

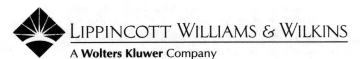

LIPPINCOTT WILLIAMS & WILKINS

A **Wolters Kluwer** Company

Philadelphia • Baltimore • New York • London
Buenos Aires • Hong Kong • Sydney • Tokyo

Acquisitions Editor: Peter Darcy
Co-managing Editor: Mike Niederpruem
Co-managing Editor: Julie Downing, PhD
Associate Editor: Chris Berger, MS
Associate Editor: Neal Pire, MA
Copy Editor: Kenneth O. Wilson
Marketing Manager: Christen Murphy
Designer: Jeff Richardson
ACSM Publication Committee Chair: Jeffery L Roitman, EdD, FACSM
ACSM Group Publisher: D. Mark Robertson

Copyright © 2005 American College of Sports Medicine

351 West Camden Street
Baltimore, Maryland 21201-2436 USA

530 Walnut Street
Philadelphia, Pennsylvania 19106-3621 USA

The publisher is not responsible (as a matter of product liability, negligence or otherwise) for any injury
resulting from any material contained herein. This publication contains information relating to general
principles of medical care which should not be construed as specific instructions for individual patients.
Manufacturers' product information and package inserts should be reviewed for current information,
including contraindications, dosages, and precautions.

Printed in the United States of America
First Edition, 2004

Library of Congress Cataloging-in-Publication Data

CIP data available from the Library of Congress

The publishers have made every effort to trace the copyright holders for borrowed material. If they have
inadvertently overlooked any, they will be pleased to make the necessary arrangements at the first
opportunity.

To purchase additional copies of this book, call our customer service department at (800) 638-3030 or fax
orders to (301) 824-7390. International customers should call (301) 714-2324.

To purchase additional copies of this book or for information concerning American College of Sports
Medicine certification and suggested preparatory materials, call (800) 486-5643.

050607
2 3 4 5 6 7 8 9 10

Acknowledgements

The editors thank the following individuals who contributed to this book by repurposing content, reviewing manuscripts, and providing editorial assistance.

Ken Baldwin, MEd
Chris Berger, MS
John Buzzerio, MS
Dierdra Bycura, MA
Veronica Clark, BS
Nikki Carosone, MS
Julie Downing, PhD
Lisa Duncan, BS
Robert Fields, BS
Tom Ford, BS
Steven Keteyian, PhD, FACSM
Tom McCann, BS
Michelle Miller, MS
Mike Niederpruem, MS
Neal Pire, MA
Michael Rankin, MS
Traci Rush, BA
Matt Saval, MS
Bill Soens, MS
Walt Thompson, PhD, FACSM
Nicole Wojno, MS

This publication was produced for the American College of Sports Medicine (ACSM) under the content oversight of the ACSM Committee on Certification and Registry Boards.

Table of Contents

ACSM's Resources for the Personal Trainer

Section I:
Introduction

The American College of Sports Medicine (ACSM) has been the leader in the field of exercise science since 1954. Membership is worldwide and because of rigid academic standards, ACSM continues to be the gold standard for certifications, publications (including Position Stands), and professional meetings. Upon successful certification, you will be part of a very prestigious group of trained exercise professionals. Thank you for choosing ACSM for your certification needs.

The information in this review manual is repurposed primarily from the following two ACSM publications. Information from any other source is listed separately at the end of each chapter. For a more detailed explanation of concepts, we encourage you to go directly to these two sources.

1) *ACSM's Guidelines for Exercise Testing and Prescription,* 6th Edition, Lippincott Williams & Wilkins Publishers, 2000.

2) *ACSM's Resource Manual for Guidelines For Exercise Testing and Prescription,* 4th Edition, Lippincott Williams & Wilkins Publishers, 2001.

It is not the intent of this review manual to be the one exclusive study tool and reading it does not guarantee passing the exam. The exam is challenging as it asks you to apply concepts from the review manual to real-life personal training situations.

ACSM's Guidelines for Exercise Testing and Prescription,
Sixth Edition

SENIOR EDITOR
BARRY A. FRANKLIN, PhD, FACSM
Director, Cardiac Rehabilitation and Exercise Laboratories
William Beaumont Hospital
Royal Oak, Michigan
Professor of Physiology
Wayne State University
Detroit, Michigan

ASSOCIATE EDITOR CLINICAL
MITCHELL H. WHALEY, PhD, FACSM
Associate Professor
School of Physical Education
Ball State University
Muncie, Indiana

ASSOCIATE EDITOR FITNESS
EDWARD T. HOWLEY, PhD, FACSM
Department of Exercise Science
University of Tennessee
Knoxville, Tennessee

AUTHORS
GARY J. BALADY, MD
KATHY A. BERRA, MSN, ANP
LAWRENCE A. GOLDING, PhD, FACSM
NEIL F. GORDON, MD, PhD, MPH, FACSM
DONALD A. MAHLER, MD, FACSM
JONATHAN N. MYERS, PhD, FACSM
LOIS M. SHELDAHL, PhD, FACSM

SPECIAL CONTRIBUTORS
I. MARTIN GRAIS, MD, FACC, FACP
DAVID L. HERBERT, Esq.
WILLIAM G. HERBERT, PhD, FACSM
DAVID P. SWAIN, PhD, FACSM
SHERI L. TOKARCZYK, MS, PA-C
ANDREW J. YOUNG, PhD, FACSM

*ACSM's Resource Manual for Guidelines for Exercise
Testing and Prescription,* **Fourth Edition**

SENIOR EDITOR
JEFFREY L. ROITMAN, EdD, FACSM
Director, Cardiac Rehabilitation
Research Medical Center
Kansas City, Missouri

SECTION EDITORS
EDWARD J. HAVER, MA FAACVPR
Director, Cardiac Rehabilitation Department
Charleston Area Medical Center
Charleston, West Virginia

MATT HERRIDGE, PhD
Cardiac Rehabilitation Department
Charleston Area Medical Center
Charleston, West Virginia

MOIRA KELSEY, RN, MS
Clinical Coordinator
Division of Thoracic and Cardiovascular Surgery
Ohio State University Medical Center
Columbus, Ohio

THOMAS P. LAFONTAINE, PhD
Manager
WELLAWARE Disease Prevention and Community
  Wellness Program
Boone Hospital Center
Columbia, Missouri

LYDIA MILLER, MS, RCEP
Co-Director of Cardiac Rehabilitation
Georgetown Hospital
Georgetown, Texas

MICHAEL WEGNER, PhD, FACSM
Medical Liason
KOS Pharmaceutical Inc.
Miami Lakes, Florida

MARK A. WILLIAMS, PhD, FACSM
Professor of Medicine
Division of Cardiology
Director, Cardiovascular Disease Prevention and
  Rehabilitation
Cardiac Center of Creighton University
Omaha, Nebraska

TRACY YORK, MS
Director of Operations
Lake Austin Spa Resort
Austin, Texas

Section II

- ✦ Bone, Skeletal Muscle, and Connective Tissue
- ✦ Anatomy of the Cardiovascular System
- ✦ Anatomy of the Respiratory System
- ✦ Biomechanical Principles
- ✦ Aerobic and Anaerobic Metabolism
- ✦ Normal, Acute Responses to Cardiovascular Exercise
- ✦ Normal, Chronic Physiological Adaptations Associated with Cardiovascular Exercise
- ✦ Normal, Acute Responses to Resistance Training
- ✦ Normal, Chronic Physiological Adaptations Associated with Resistance Training
- ✦ Physiologic Principles Related to Warm-up and Cool-down
- ✦ Muscle Fatigue
- ✦ Detraining

ACSM's Resources for the Personal Trainer

EXERCISE PHYSIOLOGY AND RELATED EXERCISE SCIENCE

A. Bone, Skeletal Muscle, and Connective Tissue

Beyond supporting soft tissue, protecting internal organs, and acting as an important source of nutrients and blood constituents, the bones are the rigid levers for locomotion. The skull, vertebral column, sternum, and ribs are considered the axial skeleton; the bones of the upper and lower limbs make up the appendicular skeleton. The major bones of the body are illustrated in Figure 2.1. An outer fibrous layer of connective tissue attaches the bone to muscles, deep fascia, and joint capsules. Just beneath the outer layer is a highly vascular inner layer that contains cells for the creation of new bone. The outer and inner layers that cover the bones constitute the periosteum.

The periosteum, continuous with tendons and adjacent articulated structures, anchors muscle to bone. Tendons are likewise continuous with the epimysium, the outer layer of connective tissue covering muscle. Individual skeletal muscles are composed of a varying number of muscle bundles referred to as fasciculi (an individual bundle is a fasciculus). Fasciculi are likewise covered and thus separated by perimysium. Individual muscle fibers are enveloped by the endomysium. Immediately beneath the endomysium is the thin, membranous sarcolemma, the cell membrane that encloses the cellular contents of the muscle fiber, nuclei, local stores of fat, glucose (in the form of glycogen), enzymes, contractile proteins, and other specialized structures such as the mitochondria. The major muscles of the body are illustrated in Figures 2.2 and 2.3.

Structure and Function of Joints in Movement

The effective interaction of bone and muscle to produce movement somewhat depends on joint function. Joints are the articulations between bones, and along with bones and ligaments, they constitute the articular system. Ligaments are tough, fibrous connective tissues that connect bone to bone, where as tendons connect muscle to bone. Joints are typically classified as fibrous,

Figure 2.1–Divisions of the skeletal system. (Courtesy of Tortora G, Anagnostakos N. Principles of Anatomy and Physiology. 6th ed. New York: Harper & Row, 1992; 163.)

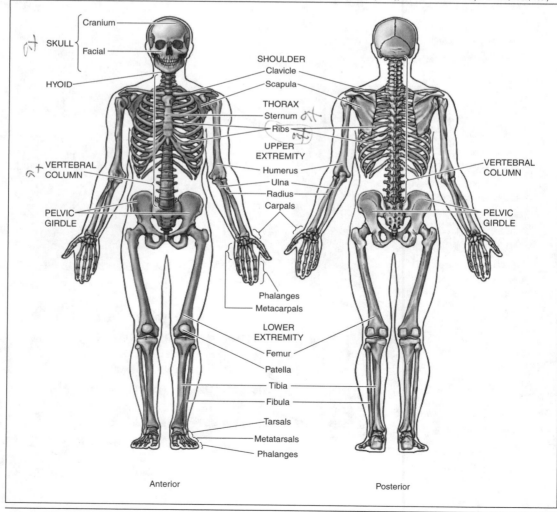

wherein bones are united by fibrous tissue, cartilaginous (cartilage or a fibrocartilaginous anchor), or synovial, in which a fibrous articular capsule and an inner synovial membrane lining enclose the joint cavity. The cavity is filled with synovial fluid, which provides constant lubrication during human movement to minimize the wearing effects of friction on the cartilaginous covering of the articulating bones.

Joints are typically well perfused by numerous arterial branches and are innervated by branches of the nerves supplying the adjacent muscle and overlying skin.

Proprioception is defined as the receipt of information from muscles and tendons that enables the brain to determine movements and position of the body and its parts. Proprioceptive feedback is an important joint sensation, as is pain, owing to the high density of sensory fibers in the joint capsule. This feedback has obvious importance in regulating human movement and in preventing injury.

The degree of movement within a joint is typically called the range of motion (ROM). ROM can be active (AROM), the range that can be reached by voluntary movement, or passive (PROM), the range that can be achieved by external means (e.g., an examiner or device). Joints are typically limited in range by the articulations of bones (as in the limitation of elbow extension by the olecranon process of the ulna), ligamentous arrangement, and soft tissue limitations, as occurs in elbow or knee flexion.

Movement at one joint may influence the extent of movement at adjacent joints, as a number of muscles and other soft tissue structures cross multiple joints. For example, finger flexion decreases in the presence of wrist flexion because muscles that flex both the wrist and fingers cross multiple joints. (Table 2.1 and Table 2.2)

Muscle Fiber Types

The human body has the ability to perform a wide range of physical tasks, combining varying composites of speed, power, and endurance. No single type of muscle fiber possesses the characteristics that would allow optimal performance across this continuum of physical challenges. Rather, muscle fibers possess certain characteristics that result in relative specialization. For example, certain muscle fibers are selectively recruited by the body for speed and power tasks of short duration, while others are recruited for

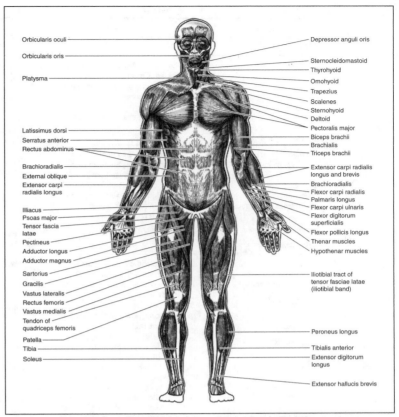

Figure 2.2 (above)–Posterior view of the superficial muscles. (Courtesy of Tortora G, Anagnostakos N. Principles of Anatomy and Physiology. 6th ed. New York: Harper & Row, 1992; 265.)

Figure 2.3 (below)–Anterior view of the superficial muscles. (Courtesy of Tortora G, Anagnostakos N. Principles of Anatomy and Physiology. 6th ed. New York: Harper & Row, 1992; 266.)

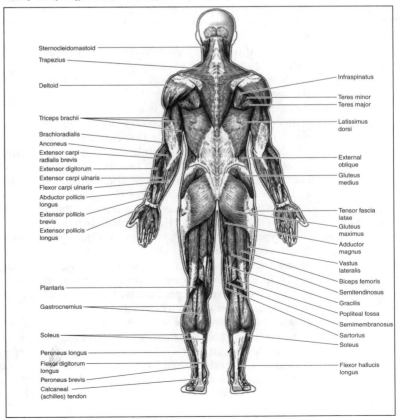

Table 2.1–Classification of Joints in the Human Body

JOINT CLASSIFICATION	FEATURES, EXAMPLES
FIBROUS	
Suture	Tight union unique to the skull
Syndesmosis	Interosseous membrane between bones (e.g., the union along the shafts of the radius and ulna, tibia and fibula)
Gomphosis	Unique joint at the tooth socket
CARTILAGINOUS	
Primary (synchondroses; hyaline cartilaginous)	Usually temporary to permit bone growth and typically fuse; some do not (e.g., at the sternum and rib [costal cartilage])
Secondary (symphyses; fibrocartilaginous)	Strong, slightly movable joints (e.g., intervertebral discs, pubic symphysis)
SYNOVIAL	
Plane	Gliding and sliding movements (e.g., acromioclavicular joint)
Hinge (ginglymus)	Uniaxial movements (e.g., elbow, knee extension and flexion)
Ellipsoidal (condyloid)	Biaxial joint (e.g., radiocarpal extension, flexion at the wrist)
Saddle	Unique joint that permits movements in all planes, including opposition (e.g., the carpometacarpal joint of the thumb)
Ball and socket	Multiaxial joints that permit movements in all directions (e.g., hip and shoulder joints)
Pivot	Uniaxial joints that permit rotation (e.g., humeroradial joint)

Table 2.2–Range of Motion of the Major Joints

JOINT	MOTION	AVERAGE RANGES (DEGREES)
Spinal		
Cervical	Flexion	0–60
	Extension	0–75
	Lateral flexion	0–45
	Rotation	0–80
Thoracic	Flexion	0–50
	Rotation	0–30
Lumbar	Flexion	0–60
	Extension	0–25
	Lateral flexion	0–25
Upper extremity		
Shoulder	Flexion	0–180
	Extension	0–50
	Abduction	0–180
	Adduction	0–50
	Internal rotation	0–90
	External rotation	0–90
Elbow	Flexion	0–140
Forearm	Supination	0–80
	Pronation	0–80
Wrist	Flexion	0–60
	Extension	0–60
	Ulnar deviation	0–30
	Radial deviation	0–20
Thumb	Abduction	0–60
	Flexion	
	Carpal–metacarpal	0–15
	Metacarpal–phalangeal	0–50
	Interphalangeal	0–50
	Extension	
	Carpal–metacarpal	0–20
	Metacarpal–phalangeal	0–5
	Interphalangeal	0–20
Fingers	Flexion	
	Metacarpal–phalangeal	0–90
	Proximal interphalangeal	0–100
	Distal interphalangeal	0–80
	Extension	
	Metacarpal–phalangeal	0–45
Lower extremity		
Hip	Flexion	0–100
	Extension	0–30
	Abduction	0–40
	Adduction	0–20
	Internal rotation	0–40
	External rotation	0–50
Knee	Flexion	0–150
Ankle	Dorsiflexion	0–20
	Plantar flexion	0–40
Subtalar	Inversion	0–30
	Eversion	0–20

endurance tasks of long duration and relatively low intensity. When the challenge requires elements of speed or power but also has an endurance component, yet another type of muscle fiber is recruited.

These different fiber types should not be thought of as mutually exclusive. In fact, intricate recruitment and switching occurs in muscle over the performance of many tasks, and fibers designed to be optimal for one type of task can contribute to the performance of another. The net result is a functioning muscle that can respond to a wide variety of tasks, and while the composition of the muscle may lend itself to performing best in endurance activities, it still can accomplish speed and power tasks to a lesser degree (1, 2).

Over the years there has been a fair amount of controversy about the classification of muscle fiber types (3). In addition, there are questions about whether these types can change in response to an intervention such as endurance training (4–7). In either case, there is general agreement that relative to exercise performance, two distinct fiber types—type I (slow twitch) and type II (fast twitch, with their proposed subdivisions)—have been identified and classified by contractile and metabolic characteristics such as the chemical breakdown of carbohydrate, fat, and protein for energy within the muscle cell (8, 9)

Type I Muscle Fibers

The characteristics of type I muscle fibers are consistent with muscle fibers that resist fatigue. Thus, type I fibers are selected for activities of low intensity and long duration. Within whole muscle, type I motor units contract but the units do not contract all at the same time; that is, in addition to their inherent fatigue resistance, endurance is prolonged by the constant switching that occurs to ensure freshly charged muscle as the exercise stimulus continues. Sedentary persons have approximately 50% type I fibers, and this distribution is generally equal throughout the major muscle groups of the body (10). In endurance athletes, the percentage of type I fibers is greater, but this is thought to be largely a genetic predisposition, despite some evidence suggesting that prolonged exercise training can alter fiber type (11, 12). Essentially, those most successful at endurance activities generally have a high proportion of type I fibers, and this is most likely due to genetic factors supplemented through appropriate exercise training. From a metabolic perspective, type I fibers are those frequently called aerobic, since the generation of energy for continued muscle contraction is met through the ongoing oxidation (chemical breakdown using oxygen) of available foodstuffs. Thus, with minimal accumulation of anaerobically (chemical breakdown without oxygen) produced metabolites, continued submaximal muscle contraction is favored in type I fibers.

Type II Muscle Fibers

At the opposite end of the continuum, those who achieve the greatest success in power and high-intensity speed tasks usually have a greater proportion of type II muscle fibers distributed through the major muscle groups. Since force generation is so important, type II fibers shorten and develop tension considerably faster than type I fibers (13). These fibers are typically thought of as type IIB fibers, the "classic" fast-twitch fiber. Metabolically, these fibers are the classic anaerobic fibers, because they rely on energy sources from within the muscle, not the fuels used by type I fibers. When an endurance component is introduced, such as in events lasting upward of several minutes (800–1500 m races, for example), a second type of fast-twitch fiber, type IIA, is recruited. The type IIA fibers represent a transition of sorts between the needs met by the type I and type IIB fibers. Metabolically, while type IIA fibers have the ability to generate a moderately large amount of force, they also have some aerobic capacity, although not as much as type I fibers. This is a logical and necessary bridge between the types of muscle fibers and the ability to meet the variety of physical tasks imposed. Reference to the existence of the type IIC fiber is necessary in a complete description of human muscle fiber types. The IIC fiber has been described as a rare and undifferentiated muscle fiber type that is probably involved in reinnervation of damaged skeletal muscle (14).

Anatomical Locations Definitions

The following are terms and their definitions related to anatomical location (15):

1. Anterior (ventral): refers to the front of the body
2. Anatomical position: the body is erect with feet together and the upper limbs hanging at the sides, palms of the hands facing forward, thumbs facing away from the body, and fingers extended. Typically, all anatomical references are made to the body in this position
3. Distal: farther away from any reference point
4. Inferior: away from the head

5. Lateral: away from the midline of the body
6. Medial: toward the midline of the body
7. Posterior (dorsal): refers to the back of the body
8. Proximal: closer to any point of reference
9. Superior: toward the head

Common Movement Terms Definitions

The following are terms and their definitions related to human movement (16):

1. Abduction: a movement away from the axis or midline of the body when in the anatomical position
2. Adduction: a movement toward the axis or midline of the body when in the anatomical position
3. Agonist: the prime mover—the muscle directly engaged in contraction as distinguished from muscles that are relaxing at the same time.
4. Antagonist: a muscle that has an action opposite that of the agonist and yields to the movement of the agonist
5. Circumduction: a movement in which the distal end of a bone inscribes a circle without the shaft rotating
6. Extension: a movement that increases the joint angle between two articulating bones
7. Flexion: a movement that decreases the joint angle between two articulating bones

Table 2.3–Major Movement of the Upper Extremity

REGION	ACTION(S)	PRINCIPAL MUSCLE(S)
Scapula	Fixation	Serratus anterior, pectoralis minor, trapezius, levator scapulae, rhomboids
Upper arm	Flexion	Anterior deltoid, pectoralis major (clavicular head)
	Extension	Latissimus dorsi, pectoralis major (sternocostal head)
	Abduction	Middle deltoid, supraspinatus
	Adduction	Latissimus dorsi, teres major, pectoralis major
	Medial (internal) rotation	Latissimus dorsi, teres major, subscapularis
	Lateral (external) rotation	Infraspinatus, teres minor
Lower arm	Flexion	Biceps brachii, brachialis, brachioradialis
	Extension	Triceps brachii, anconeus
	Supination	Supinator, biceps brachii
	Pronation	Pronator teres, pronator quadratus
Wrist	Flexion	Flexor carpi radialis, palmaris longus, flexor carpi ulnaris, flexor digitorum superficialis
	Extension	Extensor carpi radialis longus and brevis, extensor digitorum, extensor carpi ulnaris
	Adduction	Flexor and extensor carpi ulnaris
	Abduction	Extensor carpi radialis longus and brevis, flexor carpi radialis

Adapted with permission from Moore K, Agur A. Essential Clinical Anatomy. Baltimore: Williams & Wilkins, 1996.

Table 2.4–Major Movement of the Lower Extremity

Table 9.4. Major Movement of the Lower Extremity

REGION	ACTION(S)	PRINCIPAL MUSCLE(S)
Abdomen	Flexion and rotation of trunk	External and internal oblique
	Flexion	Rectus abdominis
Back	Laterally bend and rotate head	Splenius (capitus and cervicis), acting unilaterally
	Extension of head and neck	Splenius, acting bilaterally
	Extension of vertebral column	Erector spinae, acting bilaterally (flexion when contracting eccentrically)
	Lateral bending of vertebral column	Erector spinae, acting unilaterally
Thigh	Flexion at hip joint	Iliopsoas
	Extension	Gluteus maximus, hamstrings (semitendinosus, semimembranosus, long head of biceps femoris)
	Abduction and flexion	Tensor fasciae latae, sartorius
	Adduction and medial rotation	Gluteus medius and minimus
	Adduction	Adductor longus, brevis, magnus; gracilis
	Lateral rotation	Piriformis, obturator internis
Lower	Flexion	Hamstrings
Leg	Extension	Quadriceps femoris (rectus femoris; vastus lateralis, medialis, and intermedius)
Foot	Dorsiflexion	Tibialis anterior, extensor digitorum longus; extensor hallucis longus, peroneus tertius
	Plantarflexion	Gastrocnemius, soleus, tibialis posterior, flexor digitorum longus, flexor hallucis longus
	Eversion	Peroneus longus and brevis
	Inversion	Tibialis anterior and posterior

Adapted with permission from Moore K, Agur A. Essential Clinical Anatomy. Baltimore: Williams & Wilkins, 1996.

8. Hyperextension: a movement in the direction of extension that positions a joint angle beyond a normal degree of extension
9. Pronation: a movement that produces rotation on the axis of a bone. When applied specifically to the forearm, the palm of the hand faces down because the radius rotates on the ulna
10. Rotation: a movement of a segment that produces rotatory action around its own long axis
11. Supination: a movement that produces rotation on the axis of a bone. When applied specifically to the forearm, the palm of the hand faces up because the radius rotates on the ulna (Tables 2.3 & 2.4)

Muscle Actions

During static (isometric) contractions, the muscle or muscle group maintains a constant length as resistance is applied and no change in joint position occurs. Research has demonstrated that static training produces improvements in muscular strength. The strength gains, however, are limited to the specific joint angles at which the static contractions are performed (17, 19–21). As a result, static training may have limited value in enhancing functional strength. Functional strength is defined as performing work against resistance specifically in such a way that the strength gained directly benefits the execution of activities of daily life (ADLs) and movements associated with sports.

Static training has also been associated with acute elevations in blood pressure, perhaps due to increased intrathoracic pressure during static contractions. Despite the limitations, static training appears to play a positive role in physical rehabilitation. For example, it is effective for maintaining muscular strength and for preventing atrophy associated with the immobilization of a limb (e.g., application of a cast, splint, or brace) (17, 18, 20).

Dynamic (isotonic) resistance training is another common method. If movement of the joint occurs during contraction, it is dynamic. If force is sufficient to overcome resistance and the muscle shortens (e.g., the lifting phase of a biceps curl), the contraction is concentric. When resistance is greater than force and the muscle lengthens during contraction, it is eccentric (e.g., the lowering phase of the biceps curl).

Most dynamic resistance training includes both concentric and eccentric action. Significantly heavier loads can be moved eccentrically; in fact, in unfatigued muscle, the ratio of eccentric to concentric strength can be as high as 1.4:1 (17, 18). For example, maximal eccentric weight is 1.4 times the maximal concentric weight in the same muscle group/movement. Furthermore, at the onset of fatigue, the relative level of eccentric strength and eccentric–concentric ratio increases even more. Individuals who are eccentrically trained are subject to delayed-onset muscular soreness (DOMS) (22, 23). Eccentric training can, however, play an important role in preventing or rehabilitating certain musculoskeletal injuries. For example, eccentric training has been demonstrated to be effective for treating hamstring strains, tennis elbow, and patellofemoral pain syndrome (24, 25).

The other major type of resistance training, isokinetic exercise, entails constant-speed muscular contraction against accommodating resistance. The speed of movement is controlled, and the amount of resistance is proportional to the amount of force produced throughout the full range of motion. The theoretical advantage of isokinetic exercise is the development of maximal muscle tension throughout the range of motion. Research documents the effectiveness of isokinetic training (17, 20). Strength gains achieved during high-speed training (*i.e.,* contraction velocities of $180°·s^{-1}$ or faster) appear to carry over to all speeds less than that specific speed (26, 27). Improvement in strength at slow speeds of movement, however, has not been shown to carry over to faster speeds.

Planes of the Body

1. Median: the midline plane dividing the body into left and right halves.
2. Sagittal: the plane dividing the body into unequal left and right parts and parallel to the median plane. The term medial and lateral relate to this plane.
3. Frontal: the plane dividing the body into equal/unequal front and back parts. The terms anterior/posterior relate to this plane.
4. Transverse: The horizontal plane divides the body into upper (cranial or superior) and lower (caudal or inferior) parts (28).

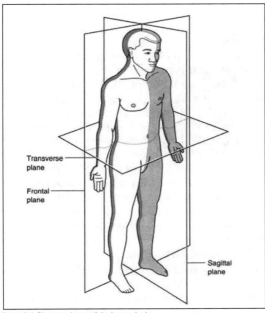

Figure 2.4–Planes and axes of the human body.

Muscle Sense Organs / Myotatic Stretch Reflex

Human movement can be initiated either voluntarily (with conscious thought) or involuntarily. Involuntary movements are often termed "reflexes" and are brought about by one or more sensory structures. Four proprioceptive sensory organ systems respond to a stretch stimulus (29, 30):

- Golgi tendon organs (GTO)
- Muscle spindles
- Pacinian corpuscles
- Ruffini end organs

These receptors are active during strong contraction or stretch. They inhibit or facilitate contraction with a coordinated effect to protect muscle from overcontraction or overstretch (30). The GTOs are located in muscle tendon, and when activated, they reflexively inhibit contraction and signal a stretched muscle to relax. Muscle spindles are sensory organs scattered throughout muscle tissue that reflexively activate muscle and concurrently inhibit the opposing, or antagonist, muscle. This response is known as the myotatic stretch reflex (30). If the stretch impulse is too great, muscle spindle input causes a protective contraction. Finally, Pacinian corpuscles and Ruffini end organs are located deeply in connective tissue and in tissues immediately surrounding the various joints of the body. These structures are stimulated by pressure from surrounding muscle and connective tissue when joints are moved. Extreme pressure results in pain perception and withdrawal from a harmful stretch stimulus such as heat (29, 30).

Neuromuscular Activation

Physical activity involves purposeful, voluntary movement on the part of the exerciser. The stimulus for voluntary muscle activation comes from the brain. The signal is relayed through the brainstem and spinal cord and transformed into a specific motor unit activation pattern. To perform a specific task, the required motor units meet specific demands for force production by activating associated muscle fibers (31, 32).

Motor Unit Activation

The functional unit of the neuromuscular system is the motor unit (33). It consists of the motor neuron and the muscle fibers it innervates. Motor units range in size from a few to several hundred muscle fibers. Muscle fibers from different motor units can be anatomically adjacent to each other, and therefore, a muscle fiber may be actively generating force while the adjacent fiber moves passively with no direct neural stimulation.

Several nomenclatures have been used to classify skeletal muscle fibers, including color (red or white), action speed (fast or slow twitch), oxidative or glycolytic enzyme content (fast glycolytic, fast oxidative glycolytic, or oxidative), combination schemes (fast glycolytic), and myosin adenosine triphosphatase (ATPase) content (type I, IIa, IIb).

When maximal force is required, all available motor units are activated. Another adaptive mechanism affected by heavy resistance training is the muscle force affected by different motor unit firing rates and/or frequencies.

Figure 2.5–Frontal section of the heart. The arrows indicate the path of blood flow through the heart. (Reprinted with permission from Spence AP. Mason EB, eds. Human Anatomy and Physiology. 4th ed. St Paul, MN: West, 1992;600.)

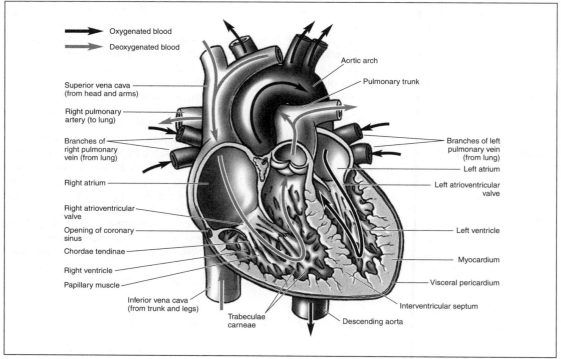

B. Anatomy of the Cardiovascular System

The cardiovascular system is a continuous closed arrangement including a pump (the heart) and more than 60,000 miles of conduits (blood vessels) (34). The primary function of the cardiovascular system is to provide an environment for the transport of nutrients and removal of waste products. The cardiovascular system assists with maintenance of normal function at rest and during exercise.

The cardiovascular system performs the following specific functions (35–37):

1. Transports oxygenated blood from the lungs to tissues and deoxygenated blood from the tissues to the lungs
2. Distributes nutrients (e.g., glucose, free fatty acids, amino acids) to cells
3. Removes metabolic wastes (e.g., carbon dioxide, urea, lactate) from the periphery for elimination or reuse
4. Regulates pH to control acidosis and alkalosis
5. Transports hormones and enzymes to regulate physiological function
6. Maintains fluid volume to prevent dehydration
7. Maintains body temperature by absorbing and redistributing heat

The following sections provide a brief overview of the basic structures and functions of the heart and blood vessels.

The Heart

The heart is positioned at an angle within the chest cavity. It is anterior to the vertebral column and posterior to the sternum. The lungs flank the heart on both sides and slightly overlap it. The heart has four chambers. The two superior chambers are the atria and the two inferior chambers are the ventricles. The external deep grooves of the heart (called sulci) define the boundaries of the four chambers of the heart (37, 38). The coronary sulcus separates the atria from the ventricles; the interventricular sulcus separates the left and right ventricles (LV, RV). The sulci also contain the major arteries and veins that provide circulation to the heart.

The heart has a base and an apex. The base consists mainly of the left atrium (LA), part of the right atrium (RA), and parts of the proximal portion of the large veins that enter the heart posteriorly. It is located superiorly and near the right sternal border at the level of second and third ribs. The apex of the heart is located inferiorly and to the left of the base at the level of the fifth intercostal space

The heart also has borders. The superior border consists of both atria and the bases of the pulmonary trunk and the aorta. The right border is formed by the RA. The left border consists of the LV and a small part of the LA. The inferior border is formed primarily by the RV and a portion of the LV at the apex.

The heart is rotated to the left in the chest so that the anterior portion of the heart forms the sternocostal surface, which consists mainly of the RA and RV. The diaphragmatic surface consists mainly of the LV where it slopes and rests on the diaphragm.

Tissue Coverings and Layers of the Heart

The heart is covered by a double-walled, loose-fitting membranous sac called the pericardium. The outer wall of the pericardium has both a fibrous (tough) layer and a serous (smooth) layer. The interior wall is the epicardium.

The thickest layer of tissue in the heart is the myocardium. The myocardium is cardiac muscle. Within the myocardium is a network of crisscrossing connective tissue fibers called the fibrous skeleton. This skeleton provides support for the myocardium and the valves of the heart and provides some separation between the atria and the ventricles.

Chambers, Valves, and Blood Flow of the Heart

The heart is two pumps in a single unit with four chambers, or cavities (Fig. 2.5). The right heart (RA and RV) and the left heart (LA and LV) make up the two pumps. The right side of the heart collects blood from the periphery and pumps it through the lungs (pulmonary circuit). The left side of the heart collects blood from the lungs and pumps it throughout the body (systemic circuit) (39–43).

The heart has four valves whose function is to maintain blood flow in one direction. The atrioventricular (AV) valves separate the atria from the ventricles. The semilunar valves separate the ventricles from the aorta and pulmonary artery trunk. The right AV valve has three cusps and is called the tricuspid valve, while the left AV valve has only two cusps and is called the bicuspid (or mitral) valve. The tricuspid valve controls the flow of blood from the RA to the RV, while the mitral valve controls blood between the LA and LV. The chordae tendineae and papillary muscles help open the AV valves and prevent them from swinging back into the atria, which would result in backward blood flow (44).

There are two semilunar valves in the heart, the pulmonic valve lies between the RV and the pulmonary artery. The aortic valve is between the LV and the aorta. The cusps of the semilunar valves prevent the backflow of blood from the arteries to the ventricles.

Blood flow through the heart is accomplished by the following sequence of events, beginning with the return of systemic blood to the RA:

1. Deoxygenated blood flows into the RA via the superior and inferior vena cava, the coronary sinus, and anterior cardiac veins.
2. The RA free wall contracts and blood moves through the tricuspid valve into the RV.
3. The RV free wall contracts, the tricuspid valve closes, and blood flows through the pulmonic valve into the pulmonary arteries and the branches of that system.
4. Blood enters the alveolar capillaries from the pulmonary arteries, where gas exchange occurs. Oxygen is absorbed and carbon dioxide is removed.
5. Blood flows back to the LA via the pulmonary veins.
6. The LA free wall contracts and blood flows through the mitral valve and into the LV.
7. The LV free wall contracts, the mitral valve closes, and blood flows through the aortic valve into the aorta and its branches, where it is distributed to the coronary circulation and the systemic circulation (44–47).

Cardiac muscle has properties that allow it to contract without a nervous system impulse. The components of the heart's conduction system include the sinoatrial (SA) node, the AV node, AV bundle (bundle of His), right and left bundle branches, and the Purkinje fibers.

The electrical impulse, which initiates cardiac contraction, begins at the SA node, or intrinsic pacemaker, of the heart. The electrical impulse is delayed at the AV node for approximately 0.13 s to allow the atria to contract and fill the ventricles. The impulse then moves rapidly through the bundle of His, through the right and left bundle branches, and through the network of Purkinje fibers in the myocardium of both ventricles. This rapid conduction allows the two ventricles to contract at approximately the same time.

The Blood Vessels

After blood flows from the heart, it enters the vascular system, which is composed of numerous blood vessels. The blood vessels form a closed system to deliver blood to the tissues; help promote the exchange of nutrients, metabolic wastes, hormones, and other substances with cells; and return blood to the heart.

Arteries carry blood away from the heart. Large arteries branch into smaller arteries and eventually to smaller arterioles. Arterioles branch into capillaries, which allow the exchange of blood with various tissues (e.g., digestive system, liver, kidneys). On the venous side of the circulation, capillaries converge into small venules, which converge to form larger vessels called veins. The largest veins return blood to the heart.

Arteries can be classified as elastic or muscular or as arterioles according to their size and function. Large arteries like the aorta and those of the pulmonary trunk are called elastic arteries. Smaller arteries distribute blood throughout the body. These arteries are called muscular arteries. Muscular arteries are less distensible than elastic arteries. Arterioles play a major role in regulating blood flow to the capillaries because of their ability to vasoconstrict (narrow the opening of the blood vessel) or vasodilate (widen the opening of the blood vessel).

Capillaries form dense networks that branch throughout all tissues. The average capillary is 1 mm in length and 0.01 mm in diameter. This is just large enough for a single red blood cell to pass through (3). Capillaries have extremely thin walls and are the site where the exchange of materials between blood and the interstitial fluid takes place.

Veins receive blood from the venules. In general, the veins are thinner and more compliant than arteries and act as blood reservoirs. The walls of some veins, such as those in the legs, contain one-way valves that help maintain venous return to the heart by preventing backward blood flow even under relatively low pressures.

Anatomical Sites for for Peripheral Pulses

Exercise professionals may measure peripheral (toward the outside) pulses to obtain an index of resting heart rate or aerobic exercise heart rate. Large, superficial (close to the surface) arteries are preferred for pulse determination, since they are easily palpable (easy to locate and feel). The two most common palpation sites are the common carotid and radial arteries.

Carotid Pulse

The right and left common carotid arteries are located on the anterior portion of the neck in the groove formed by the larynx (Adam's apple) and the sternocleidomastoid muscles (large muscles on the lateral sides of the neck) just below the mandible (lower jaw) (48). The carotid pulse is taken by placing the first two fingers in the groove and pressing gently inward. Take care when using this site, since baroreceptors in the carotid sinus may be sensitive to pressure and result in a reduc-

tion in heart rate in some individuals (49, 50). Baroreceptors are sensory nerve endings that are stimulated by changes in pressure and are found in the walls of the atria of the heart, vena cava, aortic arch, and carotid sinus. In extreme cases blood flow may be occluded to the point that light-headedness or fainting occurs. This is probably a concern mainly when taking the pulse immediately after exercise, less so at rest or during activity (51).

Radial Pulse

The radial artery is located deep on the lateral (thumb side) aspect of the forearm and becomes superficial near the distal head of the radius (48). Gently pressing the first two fingers over this distal region palpates the radial pulse. Figure 2.6 illustrates this location. Radial pulses may be difficult to obtain in individuals with large amounts of subcutaneous fat over the palpation site.

Brachial Pulse

The brachial artery is located through a groove formed between the triceps and biceps brachii muscles on the medial aspect (inside) of the arm anterior to the elbow. It should be palpated with the first two fingers in the medial part of this groove.

Other Pulse Sites

Pulses may be taken at any arterial site. Other arterial palpation sites include temporal (temple region of skull), popliteal (behind the knee), femoral (inguinal fold of groin), and dorsal pedis (top of foot). Lower extremity pulses may provide information regarding the adequacy of peripheral blood flow.

Taking Pulses

To obtain a pulse rate, the following can be done:
1. Locate a pulse with the index and long fingers of one hand.
2. Count the number of pulsations in a given period.
3. For the highest precision, if timing is initiated simultaneously with a pulsation, this first pulsation is counted as 0. If a second person is keeping time or if there is lag between the initiation of timing and the first pulsation that is felt, the first pulse is counted as 1.
4. To determine the pulse rate in beats per minute, multiply the number of pulse beats by the number of counting intervals in 1 min.

   10 s = 6 intervals (multiply pulse
              beats by six)
   15 s = 4 intervals
   20 s = 3 intervals
   30 s = 2 intervals

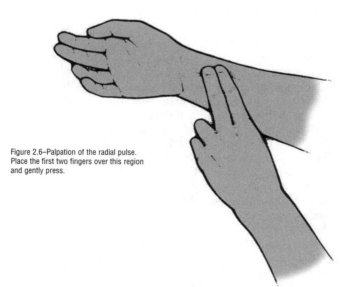

Figure 2.6–Palpation of the radial pulse. Place the first two fingers over this region and gently press.

The number of seconds a pulse is counted depends on the purpose of the pulse count and the degree of accuracy needed. For instance, during a 6-s pulse count, an error of one beat translates to an error of 10 beats per minute (bpm); during a 10-s count, a one-beat error equals a 6-bpm error; and during a 15-s count, a one-beat error means a 4-bpm error. At rest and during exercise, 15-s pulse counts are advisable, although it is difficult to obtain a pulse count during many forms of exercise. Therefore, the exerciser may have to stop and take a pulse immediately postexercise. Because heart rates decrease quickly after exercise, a 6-s or 10-s pulse count is suggested. Heart rate monitors are commonly used and can be useful in training, particularly for those desiring frequent, immediate feedback regarding exercise heart rate.

C. Anatomy of the Respiratory System

Control of Breathing

Respiratory muscles lack the ability to regulate their own contractions, therefore the control of breathing in an awake person results from the interplay of brainstem and other respiratory pathways (52). Automatic control structures are locat-

ed in the brainstem, and voluntary control structures are located in the cerebral cortex of the brain.

Distribution of Ventilation

Ventilation of the pulmonary system is accomplished in two major divisions, the upper and lower respiratory tracts, illustrated in figure 2.7.

Upper Respiratory Tract

The upper respiratory tract, which includes the nose, sinuses, pharynx, and larynx, acts as a conduction pathway for the movement of air into the lower respiratory tract. The function of these structures is to purify, warm, and humidify air before it reaches the gas exchange units. During normal quiet breathing, inspired air is heated to body temperature and the relative humidity is increased to more than 90% during passage through the nose. The pharynx is divided by the soft palate into the nasopharynx and the oropharynx. The epiglottis, located at the base of the tongue, protects the laryngeal opening during swallowing. The larynx contains the vocal cords, which contribute to speech and participate in coughing.

Receptors throughout the upper respiratory tract may initiate a cough response. Coughing is produced by closure of the vocal cords along with contraction of the expiratory muscles to create

Figure 2.7–The respiratory system consists of an upper respiratory tract (nose, pharynx, and larynx) and a lower respiratory tract (tracheobronchial tree and lungs)

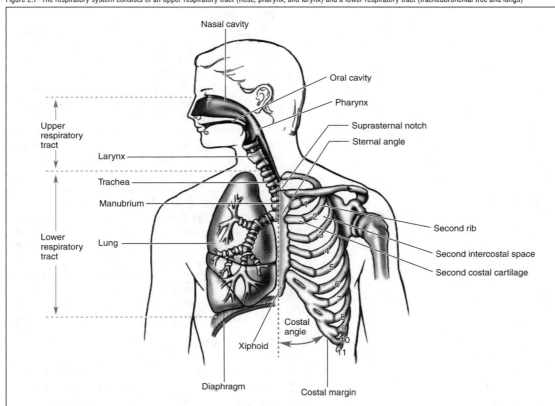

increased intrathoracic (within the chest cavity) pressures. With sudden opening of the vocal cords, the positive airway pressure forces into the atmosphere air carrying any mucus or particles from the tracheobronchial tree. A cough can move gas from the lung at rates up to $10 \text{ L} \cdot \text{s}^{-1}$ during the expulsion phase.

Lower Respiratory Tract

The lower respiratory tract begins in the trachea just below the larynx and includes the bronchi, bronchioles, and alveoli (Fig. 2.8). There are approximately 23 generations (divisions) of airways; the first 16 are conducting airways and the last 7 are respiratory airways ending blindly in approximately 300 million alveoli, which form the gas exchange surface. The structural components of the airways coincide with their functional properties. For example, the volume of the conducting zone is approximately 1 mL of air per pound of body weight and does not contribute to gas exchange, where as gas exchange areas occupy a proportionately greater volume in the lungs.

The trachea begins at the base of the neck and extends approximately 10–12 cm before it divides into the right and left main bronchi. It is anterior to the esophagus. The trachea consists of a series of anterior horseshoe-shaped cartilaginous rings and a posterior longitudinal muscle bundle.

The major bronchi contain cartilage that keeps the airway open as well as large numbers of mucus

glands that produce secretions in response to irritation, infection, and/or inflammation. In the large airway, irritant receptors initiate the cough reflex when stimulated. The right main bronchus divides into three lobar bronchi: upper, middle, and lower. The left main bronchus divides into two lobar bronchi, upper and lower. Fissures separate the two lobes with two layers of visceral pleura. The lobar bronchi divide into segmental bronchi and segments, 10 on the right and 10 on the left. Columnar cells lining the epithelium (inner lining) of the bronchi consist predominantly of ciliated cells that contain motile cilia, which move or beat in a coordinated manner to move the mucus layer toward the mouth ("mucociliary escalator"). The columnar epithelium is an important barrier for lung defense. Goblet cells interspersed among the ciliated cells secrete mucus.

Segmental bronchi divide further into the terminal bronchioles, which have a diameter of about 1 mm. Beyond the terminal bronchioles are respiratory bronchioles, alveolar ducts, and the alveoli. Air flows through the conducting airways, and at the level of the alveolar ducts and alveoli, movement of air or gas is by diffusion. Transition of the epithelium to squamous cells in alveoli is important to facilitate gas exchange.

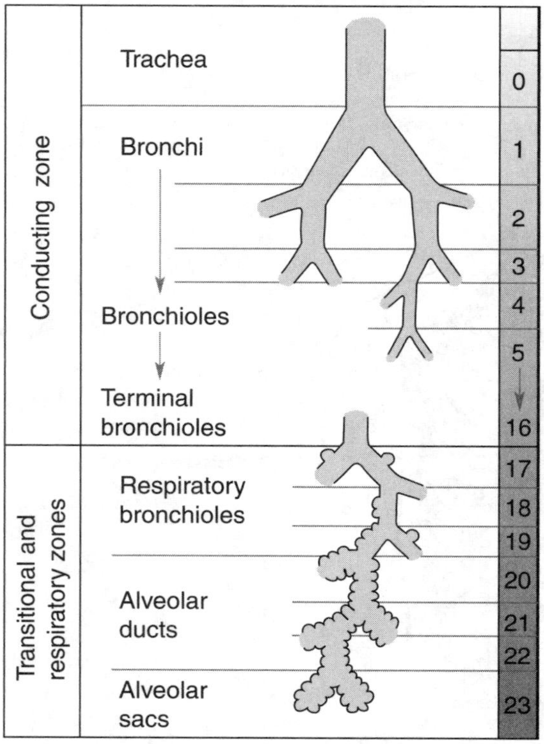

Ventilatory Pump

The ventilatory pump consists of the chest wall, the respiratory muscles, and the pleural space.

Chest Wall

The chest wall includes muscles of respiration (primarily intercostal muscles) and bones (spine, ribs, sternum). The ribs are hinged on the spine by ligaments and cartilage so that the ribs move upward and outward during inspiration and downward and inward during expiration. The hinging movement results in a change in thoracic volume. At rest and at the end of a normal expiration the elastic properties of the chest wall exert an outward (expansion) force, whereas the elastic properties of the lung structures exert an inward (recoil) force. Inspiration (airflow into the lungs) occurs by activation of the respiratory muscles, particularly the diaphragm, which creates a more negative pressure in the pleural space and the lungs than in the atmosphere. Air enters the lung until the intrapulmonary gas pressure equals atmospheric pressure. During expiration, when the respiratory muscles relax, air flows from the lung into the atmosphere because of the positive pressure generated by the elastic recoil of the lungs.

Respiratory Muscles

The muscles of respiration are the only skeletal muscles essential to life. The diaphragm, the major muscle of inspiration, is innervated by the phrenic nerve, which originates from the third to

Figure 2.8–Branching of the airways starting from the trachea to the alveolar sacs. There are approximately 23 generations of branching in the tracheobronchioal tree.

fifth cervical spinal segments. Spinal cord transection due to injury at or above this level compromises respiratory muscle function and consequently ventilation.

The diaphragm consists of a flattened centralized portion and vertical muscles called the costal portion. The diaphragm functions as a piston, with contraction and relaxation of the vertical muscle fibers. With contraction, the crural portion, or dome, moves downward and displaces the abdominal contents so that the abdomen moves outward, as does the chest wall. Expiration is normally passive under quiet breathing because of elastic recoil of the lung; it requires no work. However, during active breathing, when ventilatory requirements are increased (*e.g.,* during exercise), the muscles of expiration are recruited. The major muscles of expiration are the internal intercostals and the abdominal muscles (rectus abdominis, external and internal oblique, and transverse abdominis).

In clients with airflow obstruction (*e.g.,* acute bronchoconstriction in asthma or emphysema), hyperinflation of the lungs stretches the lung tissue and leads to additional elastic recoil, forcing the crural portion of the diaphragm downward and shortening the vertical muscle fibers. This impairs the diaphragm's ability to contract.

Pleura

The visceral (inner layer) and parietal (outer layer) pleura are thin membranes between the lung and the chest wall (53). The pleural space, which lies between the visceral and parietal pleura, contains a small amount of fluid. Because the pleural space is airtight and the chest wall and lung tissue pull against each other across the pleural space, negative pressure is produced at rest. During inspiration, both the visceral and parietal pleura expand outward and more negative pressure develops in the pleural space.

Air can enter the pleural space (*i.e.,* pneumothorax) by trauma to the chest wall (*e.g.,* a fractured rib with penetration of the parietal pleura). With a pneumothorax, the lungs collapse while the chest wall expands because of its intrinsic elastic properties. The parietal pleura contains abundant pain fibers, and irritation of this membrane by a pneumothorax or inflammation produces local chest pain exacerbated by motion of the pleura (e.g., deep inspiration).

Distribution of Blood Flow

The lungs receive blood from the pulmonary arteries, which contain systemic venous blood from the right ventricle and bronchial arteries, which contain oxygenated blood from the left ventricle. The pulmonary artery trunk emerges from the right ventricle and divides into right and left main pulmonary arteries anterior to the carina of the trachea. The pulmonary arteries divide into

branches corresponding to the divisions of the bronchial tree and supply the pulmonary arterioles. The pulmonary circulation is a low-pressure system with a normal mean pressure of approximately 15 mm Hg at rest. The majority of blood flow to the alveoli is derived from the pulmonary circulation, whereas the bronchial arteries supply the walls of the bronchi and bronchioles to the level of the alveoli. Pulmonary arterioles divide into pulmonary capillaries that form networks in the walls of the alveoli, where gas exchange occurs.

The pulmonary veins carry oxygenated blood from the pulmonary capillaries. These veins converge to form the main pulmonary veins, which empty into the left atrium. The pulmonary veins also receive blood from the bronchial circulation, which accounts for a right-to-left shunt that normally occurs in the lungs and includes up to 5% of cardiac output.

D. Biomechanical Principles

Biomechanics is the application of the principles of physics to the study of biological systems. A common focus of the discipline is the application of mechanics to human movement. While the human body is composed of a number of types of tissue, each one of these tissues is subjected to forces during motion. The forces to which these tissues are exposed are generally called loading, a collective term describing all external forces acting on the system.

Forces and Torques

For movement of a segment of the body to occur, force must be applied. A force is an interaction of two objects that produces a change in the state of motion of an object. A force may cause an object to move, to accelerate or decelerate, to change direction of movement, or to stop. The unit of force is the newton.

Newton's Laws of Motion

The three laws of motion put forth by Sir Isaac Newton (1642–1727) describe the interaction of forces on a body that result in movement.

The first law is the law of inertia, which states, "A body continues in its state of rest, or of uniform motion in a straight line, unless a force acts upon it." For human motion the mass (m) is a constant, which means that the velocity (v) does not change. To produce motion of an object that is at rest, a force must be applied. Likewise, to stop or alter a motion, a force must be applied to the object. The inertia of an object describes the resistance to motion and is directly related to the amount of matter (mass) of the object.

The second law, the law of acceleration, states, "A body acted on by an external force moves such that the force is equal to the time rate of change of linear momentum." However, mass is usually a constant, and the net force results in a change in velocity. Therefore, this law is probably more commonly expressed as "a force applied to an object causes an acceleration of the object that is proportional to the force and inversely proportional to the mass of the object."

Newton's third law, the law of action–reaction, states, "For every action there is an equal and opposite reaction." This law illustrates that forces never act in isolation but always in pairs. For example, during locomotion, the foot exerts a force each time it contacts the ground. The ground, however, exerts an equal and opposite force on the foot. The force that the ground exerts on the individual is referred to as the ground reaction force.

Forces Acting during Human Movement

Forces result from the interaction of biological systems and their environment. These forces have many classifications; those that are most often considered in the analysis of human movement are described next.

Body Weight

Gravity is the attractive force of the earth on an object, and the magnitude of this attraction is the body weight of the object. Since body weight is a force, it is measured in newtons. Body weight is proportional to mass because it is the product of the mass of the object and the acceleration due to gravity ($9.81 \text{ m} \cdot \text{s}^{-2}$).

Ground Reaction Force

Contact between the human body and another object (*e.g.,* catching a ball, carrying a suitcase, wearing ankle weights) results in the application of an external force on the human body, an example of Newton's law of action and reaction. A common external force is the ground reaction force, which is provided by the surface upon which the human moves. The ground reaction force changes in magnitude, direction, and point of application during the contact period with the surface and can be measured with a force platform. The ground reaction force can be resolved into several other components that have greater magnitude during running than during walking; the magnitude is also affected by the running speed (54). The ground reaction force is the net force acting at the center of an individual's mass; it reflects the force necessary to accelerate the total body center of mass.

Joint Reaction Force

In biomechanical analyses, a single segment is often examined isolated from other segments. In this case, the joint reaction force acting across a joint must be considered. According to Newton's third law, equal and opposite forces must act on each of the segments that constitute the joint. In most situations the magnitude of the joint reaction force is unknown but can be calculated given the appropriate data (55).

Friction

Friction is a force acting parallel to two surfaces in contact; it acts in the opposite direction of the motion or impending motion. Translational friction determines how much horizontal force is required to cause one surface to slide over the other surface. Rotational friction determines how much force must be applied as a torque to cause one surface to pivot on another. The translational and rotational components of friction are not independent parameters.

Elastic Force

Elastic forces are generated by the tendency of a deformed material to return to its original state. The amount that a material can be stretched depends on the nature of the material and the magnitude of the force that stretches it.

Muscle Force

The role of muscles in the human body is to exert forces on the skeleton that result in a desired segmental posture or motion. A muscle is attached to the skeleton at its origin and insertion so that it spans one or more joints. A muscle can generate only a pulling or tensile force, but it pulls on both segments to which it is attached. When a muscle produces force, it also produces torque, because its line of action forms a moment arm with the joint axis of rotation. The moment arm depends on the joint geometry and in general changes as a function of the joint angle. The muscle torque tends to cause both segments to rotate around the joint crossed by the muscle.

The amount of force that a muscle can exert depends on the excitation it receives from the neural system and on mechanical factors related to length and velocity. The force–velocity relationship dictates that the magnitude of force depends on the rate of length change or velocity (56). When a muscle shortens (concentric contraction), the force generated is less than that of an isometric contraction (no change in length; velocity = 0) for the same level of muscle excitation. As the velocity of shortening increases, the amount of force that can be generated decreases. During eccentric (muscle lengthening) contractions, the generated force is greater than that of an isometric contraction. The force–length relationship indicates the isometric force that a muscle can exert at different muscle lengths for the same level of excitation (57). At an intermediate optimal length the muscle can produce its greatest force, with reductions in force capability as the muscle attains shorter or longer lengths.

Muscles rarely work in isolation because there are multiple muscles crossing most joints. In many biomechanical analyses, it is assumed that the muscle torque acting across a joint is the net torque of all individual muscles crossing the joint. For example, if the total summed torque from all flexor muscles is greater than the total torque from all extensor muscles, the net torque is flexor.

Application to Human Movement

It has been suggested that there is an optimal window of loading that healthy individuals should maintain and that loading above this window increases the risk of injury (58). However, this window has not been defined, and it is difficult to estimate the load on the body for various activities (59). Nevertheless, the result of the loading on the body depends on three factors: 1) magnitude of the force, 2) rate at which the force is applied, and 3) repetition of load application. During normal activity, the magnitude of the force on tissue is within a range that will not cause tissue (e.g., bone) to fail, as in trauma, and in fact, this magnitude of force can be associated with positive effects, particularly when rate at which the force is applied is also considered (60). The greater the rate of loading, the more load can be withstood before failure.

The third factor is load repetition. Again, load repetition generally does not result in injury during normal activity, although it has been suggested that repeated impacts such as the collision of the foot with the ground during locomotion can result in microtrauma.

The human body has a number of mechanisms by which load is handled. These include structures such as the fat pads on the plantar surface of the foot, articular cartilage in the joints and bone, and soft tissue surrounding the bone. There are also particular motions of the segments that disperse shock. In the lower extremity, these include knee flexion, subtalar pronation, and ankle dorsiflexion. Under normal conditions these motions are effective. However, it has been suggested that structural abnormalities in conjunction with repeated activity patterns result in injury.

One particular source of loading on the body is the ground reaction force. The impact force resulting from the collision of the foot and the ground produces acceleration in the body that is transmitted throughout the skeletal system in the form of a shock wave. This shock wave travels through the skeletal system much as a sound wave travels through a solid object, taking about 10 ms to reach the head. As the wave travels through the body, it is absorbed by the body structures and by the kinematics of the body.

A number of factors influence the load on the body during locomotion. Increases in load can be seen in increased locomotor speed, in increased stride length at a constant speed, and in activities that produce high peak impact forces, such as running downhill. In downhill running, the center of mass of the runner falls a greater distance, resulting in a harder impact, and the lower extremity must absorb this added shock. The primary mechanism for absorbing this added impact is increased flexion of the knee during the initial portion of the support phase (61). Controlling this increased flexion are the quadriceps muscles of the anterior thigh. Although the quadriceps are knee extensors, they act eccentrically during this portion of support. Repeated eccentric activity over a prolonged period, such as with downhill running, has been related to myofibril and connective tissue damage. This damage has been linked to delayed-onset muscle soreness (62).

It would appear that altering kinematics may reduce the impact force to the system. As was suggested previously, increasing the degree of knee flexion is one possibility. However, there are trade-offs to this strategy. As an example, increasing the knee flexion angle at midstance (so-called Groucho running) indeed reduces the impact shock on the body; the shock transmission from the ankle to the head is decreased to less than 20% of its original value (63). However, the cost of such a strategy is an increased rate of energy use to the point that this style of running is responsible for a 50% increase in steady-state oxygen consumption.

The load on the human body may appear to be deleterious to the various tissues, but loading can also be beneficial. Bone has the ability to alter its size, shape, and structure to meet the demands of loads. Thus, bone can remodel itself in response to the level of the stress placed on it. For example, body weight and bone mass are positively correlated (64). Increasing body weight increases bone mass because the added weight constitutes an added mechanical stress on the bone. On the other hand, prolonged weightlessness, such as that of space travel, has been found to decrease bone mass (65). Similarly, when there is a partial or total immobilization of the lower extremity, the limb is not subjected to the normal mechanical stresses, and bone is absorbed.

E. Aerobic and Anaerobic Metabolism

The energy requirements of exercising human muscle may increase substantially in the transition from rest to maximal physical exertion. Because the available stores of adenosine triphosphate (ATP) are limited and capable of providing energy to maintain vigorous activity for only several seconds, ATP must be constantly resynthesized to provide continuous energy production. Therefore, exercising muscle must possess a large capacity for increasing metabolic rate to produce sufficient ATP so that increased activity can continue. Energy production relies heavily on the respiratory and cardiovascular systems for the delivery of oxygen and nutrients and for the removal of waste products to maintain the internal equilibrium of cells.

Adenosine Triphosphate (ATP)

Adenosine triphosphate (ATP) serves as the ideal energy-transfer agent that powers all of the cell's energy needs (66). The energy released through hydrolysis of the high-energy compound ATP to form adenosine diphosphate (ADP) and inorganic phosphate (Pi) powers skeletal muscle contractions. This reaction is catalyzed by the enzyme myosin ATPase:

$$ATP \xrightarrow{\text{(ATPase)}} ADP + Pi + energy$$

Figure 2.9–Relationship between glycolosis, the Krebs cycle, and the electron transport chain.

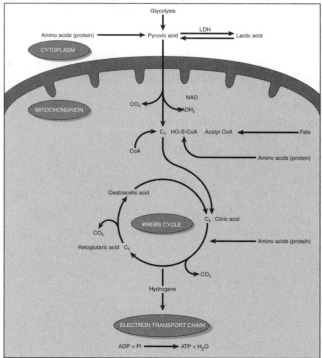

The amount of ATP directly available in muscle at any time is small, so it must be resynthesized continuously if exercise lasts for more than a few seconds. Muscle fibers contain the metabolic machinery to produce ATP by three pathways: creatine phosphate (CP), rapid glycolysis, and aerobic oxidation of nutrients to carbon dioxide and water.

Creatine Phosphate

The CP system transfers high-energy phosphate from CP to rephosphorylate ATP from ADP as follows:

$$ADP + CP \xrightarrow{\text{(Creatine kinase)}} ATP + C$$

This system is rapid because it involves only one enzymatic step (i.e., one chemical reaction); however, CP exists in finite quantities in cells, so the total amount of ATP that can be produced is limited. Oxygen is not involved in the rephosphorylation of ADP to ATP in this reaction, so the CP system is considered anaerobic (without oxygen).

Rapid Glycolysis

When glycolysis is rapid, it is capable of producing ATP without involvement of oxygen. Glycolysis, the degradation of carbohydrate (glycogen or glucose) to pyruvate or lactate, involves a series of enzymatically catalyzed steps. Although glycolysis does not use oxygen and is considered anaerobic, pyruvate can readily participate in aerobic production of ATP when oxygen is available in the cell. Therefore, in addition to being an anaerobic pathway capable of producing ATP without oxygen, glycolysis can also be considered the first step in the aerobic degradation of carbohydrate (67–70).

Aerobic Oxidation

The final metabolic pathway for ATP production combines two complex metabolic processes, the Krebs cycle and electron transport chain; it resides inside the mitochondria as illustrated in figure 2.9. Oxidative phosphorylation uses oxygen as the final hydrogen acceptor to form water and ATP. Unlike glycolysis, aerobic metabolism can use fat, protein, and carbohydrate as substrates to produce ATP.

Conceptually, the Krebs cycle can be considered a primer for oxidative phosphorylation. The primary function of the Krebs cycle is to remove hydrogens from four of the reactants involved in the cycle. The electrons from these hydrogens follow a chain of cytochromes (electron transport chain) in the mitochondria, and the energy released from this process is used to rephosphorylate ADP to form ATP. Oxygen is the final acceptor of hydrogen to form water, and this reaction is catalyzed by cytochrome oxidase (71).

Although not all ATP is formed aerobically, the amount of ATP yielded by anaerobic glycolysis is extremely small (66). Nevertheless, anaerobic mechanisms provide a rapid source of ATP, which is particularly important at the beginning of any exercise bout and during high-intensity activity that can only be sustained for a brief period. As duration of exercise increases, the relative contribution of anaerobic energy sources decreases (67).

The aerobic system requires adequate delivery and use of oxygen and uses glycogen, fats, and proteins as energy substrates. It can sustain high rates of ATP production for muscular energy over long periods of time. The relative contribution of anaerobic and aerobic metabolism depends on oxygen consumption (respiration), delivery (cardiovascular), and use (muscular extraction) at rates commensurate with the energy demands of activity.

The energy to perform most types of exercise does not come from a single source but from a combination of anaerobic and aerobic sources. The contribution of anaerobic sources (CP system and glycolysis) to exercise energy metabolism is inversely related to the duration and intensity of the activity. The shorter and more intense the activity, the greater the contribution of anaerobic energy production, whereas the longer the activity and the lower the intensity, the greater the contribution of aerobic energy production. Although proteins can be used as a fuel for aerobic exercise, carbohydrates and fats are the primary energy substrates during exercise in a healthy, well-fed individual. In general, carbohydrates are used as the primary fuel at the onset of exercise and during high-intensity work (72–74). However, during prolonged exercise of low to moderate intensity (longer than 30 min), a gradual shift from carbohydrate toward an increasing reliance on fat as a substrate occurs (74, 75).

Recovery From Exercise

Oxygen uptake remains elevated above resting levels for several minutes during recovery from exercise. This elevated postexercise oxygen consumption is referred to as Elevated Postexercise Oxygen Consumption (EPOC) (76). In general, postexercise metabolism is higher following high-intensity exercise than after light or moderate work. Furthermore, EPOC remains elevated longer after prolonged exercise than after shorter-term exertion.

F. Normal, Acute Response to Cardiovascular Exercise

Many mechanisms function collectively to support increased aerobic requirements of physical activity. The overall effect of changes in heart rate, stroke volume, cardiac output, blood flow, blood pressure, arteriovenous oxygen difference, and pulmonary ventilation is to oxygenate blood that is delivered to the active tissues.

As exercise intensity increases, oxygen consumption and carbon dioxide production by working muscles increase dramatically. The cardiorespiratory system is required to deliver oxygen to, and transport carbon dioxide from, these tissues in an attempt to maintain cellular homeostasis. The central nervous system responds by increasing neural ventilatory and cardiac drive, resulting in increased activity of cardiac and respiratory muscles. The lungs are largely passive, and the increased ventilatory and cardiac drives result in increasing blood and airflow and increased rate of transfer of oxygen and carbon dioxide across the gas-exchanging surfaces of the alveoli. However, limits to the degree to which increased airflow and blood flow can be supported can lead to pulmonary limitations to exercise either from mechanical ventilatory constraints or from compromised gas exchange. These limitations are generally not manifested in healthy individuals except in elite or older athletes.

Heart Rate

Heart rate (HR) increases in a linear fashion with the work rate and oxygen uptake during dynamic exercise. The magnitude of the HR response is related to age, body position, fitness, type of activity, presence of heart disease, medications, blood volume, and environmental factors such as temperature and humidity. In contrast to systolic blood pressure, which usually increases with age, maximum attainable HR decreases with age. The equation, max HR = 220 – age, provides an approximation of the maximum HR in healthy men and women, but the variance for any fixed age is considerable (standard deviation ~ ± 10 bpm) (77).

Stroke Volume

The stroke volume (SV) (volume of blood ejected per heart beat) is equal to the difference between end diastolic volume (EDV) and end systolic volume (ESV). During exercise, SV increases curvilinearly with the work rate until it reaches near maximal level equivalent to approximately 50% of aerobic capacity, increasing only slightly thereafter (78). At a higher HR, stroke volume may actually decrease because of the disproportionate shortening in diastolic filling time (77, 79).

Cardiac Output

The product of SV and HR determines cardiac output. Cardiac output in healthy adults increases linearly with increased work rate. However, maximum values of cardiac output depend on many factors, including age, posture, body size, presence of cardiovascular disease, and the level of physical conditioning. At exercise intensities up to 50% $\dot{V}O_2$, the increase in cardiac output is facilitated by increases in HR and SV (78). Thereafter, the increase results almost solely from the continued rise in HR.

Arteriovenous Oxygen Difference

Oxygen extraction by tissues reflects the difference between oxygen content of arterial blood (about 20 mL $O_2 \cdot 100$ mL$^{-1} \cdot$dL^{-1} at rest) and the oxygen content of venous blood (about 15 mL $O_2 \cdot$dL^{-1}), yielding a typical arteriovenous oxygen difference ($CaO_2 - CvO_2$) at rest of 5 mL $O_2 \cdot$dL^{-1}. This approximates a use coefficient of 25%. During exercise to exhaustion, the mixed venous oxygen content typically decreases to 5 mL$\cdot$dL^{-1} blood or lower, thus widening the arteriovenous oxygen difference from 5 to 15 mL$\cdot$dL^{-1} blood, corresponding to a use coefficient of 75% (78).

Blood Flow

At rest, 15–20% of the cardiac output is distributed to the skeletal muscles; the remainder goes to visceral organs, the heart, and the brain (80). However, during exercise as much as 85–90% of the cardiac output is selectively delivered to working muscle and shunted away from the skin and the splanchnic, hepatic, and renal vascular beds. Myocardial blood flow may increase four to five times with exercise, whereas blood supply to the brain is maintained at resting levels (81).

Blood Pressure

There is a linear increase in systolic blood pressure (SBP) with increasing levels of exercise. Maximal values typically reach 190–220 mm Hg (82). Nevertheless, maximal SBP should not be greater than 260 mm Hg (83). Diastolic blood pressure (DBP) may decrease slightly or remain unchanged; thus, pulse pressure (SBP minus DBP) generally increases in direct proportion to the intensity of exercise.

A SBP that fails to rise or falls with increasing work loads may signal a plateau or decrease in cardiac output, respectively (84). Exercise testing should be terminated in persons demonstrating exertional hypotension (SBP toward the end of a test decreasing below baseline standing level and/or SBP decreasing 20 mm Hg or more during exercise after an initial rise

Pulmonary Ventilation

Pulmonary ventilation (V_E), the volume of air exchanged per minute, generally approximates 6 L$\cdot$min^{-1} at rest in the average sedentary adult male. At maximal exercise, however, V_E often increases 15- to 25-fold over resting values. Pulmonary ventilation is perhaps regulated more by the requirement for carbon dioxide removal than by oxygen consumption and that ventilation is not normally a limiting factor to aerobic capacity (85, 86).

Maximal Oxygen Consumption

The most widely recognized measure of cardiopulmonary fitness is the aerobic capacity, or $\dot{V}O_{2max}$. This variable is defined physiologically as the highest rate of oxygen transport and use that can be achieved at maximal physical exertion. Oxygen consumption ($\dot{V}O_2$) may be expressed mathematically by a rearrangement of the Fick equation:

$$\dot{V}O_2 = HR \times SV \times (a - vO_2)$$

where: $\dot{V}O_2$ = oxygen consumption (mL$\cdot$kg$^{-1}\cdot$min^{-1})
HR = heart rate (bpm)
SV = stroke volume (mL$\cdot$beat^{-1})
($a - vO_2$) = arteriovenous oxygen difference

Thus, it is apparent that both central (i.e., cardiac output) and peripheral (i.e., arteriovenous oxygen difference) regulatory mechanisms affect the magnitude of body oxygen consumption.

$\dot{V}O_{2max}$ may be expressed on an absolute or relative basis. Absolute $\dot{V}O_{2max}$ usually uses the units of liters per minute, reflecting total body energy output and caloric expenditure (i.e., 1 L ~ 5 kcal). Relative $\dot{V}O_{2max}$ divides the absolute $\dot{V}O_{2max}$ value by body weight in kilograms (typically mL$\cdot$kg$^{-1}\cdot$min^{-1}). Because large persons usually have larger absolute oxygen consumption by virtue of larger muscle mass, the latter expression allows for a more equitable comparison between individuals of different body mass. When expressed as milliliters of oxygen per kilogram of body weight per minute or METs, this variable is widely considered the single best index of physical work capacity or cardiorespiratory fitness (87). In terms of cardiovascular fitness, the bigger the $\dot{V}O_{2max}$, the better.

G. Normal, Chronic Physiological Adaptations Associated with Cardiovascular Exercise

Physical inactivity is now classified as a major contributing risk factor for heart disease, with an overall weight for preventive value similar to elevated blood cholesterol, cigarette smoking, and hypertension (88). Moreover, longitudinal studies have shown that higher levels of aerobic fitness are associated with a lower mortality from heart disease even after statistical adjustments for age, coronary risk factors, and family history of heart disease (89). These findings and other recent reports in persons with and without heart disease have confirmed an inverse association between aerobic capacity and cardiovascular mortality (90–95).

Endurance exercise training increases functional capacity and provides relief of symptoms in a majority of clients with coronary artery disease (CAD). This is particularly important since most clients with clinically manifest CAD have a subnormal functional capacity (50–70% age, gender-predicted) and some may be limited by symptoms at relatively low levels of exertion. Improvement in function appears to be mediated by increased central and/or peripheral oxygen transport and supply, while relief of angina pectoris may result from increased myocardial oxygen supply, decreased oxygen demand, or both.

Most exercise studies on healthy subjects demonstrate 20% ± 10% increases in aerobic capacity ($\dot{V}O_{2max}$), with the greatest relative improvements among the most unfit (96). Because a fixed submaximal work rate has a relatively constant aerobic requirement, the physically trained individual works at a lower percentage of $\dot{V}O_{2max}$, with greater reserve after exercise training. Enhanced oxygen transport, particularly increased maximal stroke volume and cardiac output, has traditionally been regarded as the primary mechanism underlying the increase in $\dot{V}O_{2max}$ with training.

The effects of chronic exercise training on the autonomic nervous system act to reduce myocardial demands at rest and during exercise. Exercise bradycardia may be attributed to an intracardiac mechanism (an effect directly on the myocardium, *e.g.,* increased stroke volume during submaximal work) or an extracardiac mechanism (*e.g.,* alterations in trained skeletal muscle) or both. The result is reduced heart rate and systolic blood pressure at rest and at any fixed oxygen uptake or submaximal work rate.

The increased oxidative capacity of trained skeletal muscle appears to offer a distinct hemodynamic advantage. Lactic acid production and muscle blood flow are decreased at a fixed external work load, whereas submaximal cardiac output and oxygen uptake are unchanged or slightly reduced. As a result, there are compensatory increases in arteriovenous oxygen difference (a–vO_2) at submaximal and maximal exercise.

Respiratory Changes

Several respiratory adaptations result from physical conditioning regimens. Although ventilation generally does not limit exercise in apparently healthy individuals, the limits of ventilation may be reached at $\dot{V}O_{2max}$ in elite athletes (97). Ventilation increases linearly with $\dot{V}O_{2max}$ up to about 50% $\dot{V}O_{2max}$, after which the increase is proportionately greater than the increase in work rate or $\dot{V}O_{2max}$ (97, 98). Physically trained persons demonstrate larger lung volumes and diffusion capacity at rest and during exercise than their sedentary counterparts. For responses to aerobic conditioning in untrained individuals see table 2.5.

Ventilation is either unaffected or only modestly affected by cardiorespiratory training. Maximal ventilatory capacity may be increased by exercise training, but it is unclear that this provides any advantage other than increased buffering capacity for lactate. Submaximal ventilation is probably not affected, but it may be decreased in some circumstances because a decrease in the production of lactate coincides with a decrease in the need to buffer lactate which results in decreased ventilation.

Cardiovascular Adaptations

Heart Rate

The heart rate response plays a critical role in the delivery of oxygen to working skeletal muscle. Heart rate is the number of times the heart beats per minute and resting heart rate decreases by approximately 10–15 bpm as a result of cardiovascular training (103).

Stroke Volume

The stroke volume is the amount of blood pumped per beat. Stroke volume will increase both at rest and during exercise up to a point, as a result of long term cardiovascular training.

Cardiac Output

Cardiac output is heart rate multiplied by stroke volume, and provides an estimate of the amount of blood pumped per minute. Cardiac output will increase during exercise but will not change significantly at rest in cardiovascularly trained individuals.

Table 2.5–Physiological Responses to Aerobic Conditioning in Untrained Individuals

Variable[a]	Unit of Measure	Response
$\dot{V}O_{2max}$	mL/kg/min	↑
Resting heart rate	beats/min	↓
Exercise heart rate (submax)	beats/minute	↓
Maximum heart rate	beats/min	↔ (or slight ↓)
A-vDO$_2$	mL O$_2$/100 mL blood	↑
Maximum minute ventilation	Liters/minute	↑
Stroke volume	mL/beat	↑
Cardiac output	Liters/min	↑
Blood volume (resting)	Liters	↑
Systolic blood pressure	mm Hg	↔ (or slight ↑)
Blood lactate	mL/100 mL blood	↑
Oxidative capacity skeletal muscle	multiple variables[b]	↑

[a] At maximum exercise unless otherwise specified.
[b] Represents increases in skeletal muscle mitochondrial number and size, capillary density, and/or oxidative enzymes.
↑, increase
↓, decrease
↔, no change

Table 2.6–Benefits of Increasing Cardiorespiratory Activities and/or Improved Cardiorespiratory Fitness

Decreased fatigue in daily activities
Improved work, recreational, and sports performance
Improved cardiorespiratory function
    Increased maximal oxygen uptake
    Increased maximal cardiac output and stroke volume
    Increased capillary density in skeletal muscle
    Increased mitochondrial density
    Increased lactate threshold
    Lower heart rate and blood pressure at a fixed submaximal work rate
    Lower myocardial oxygen demand at a fixed submaximal work rate
    Lower minute ventilation at a fixed submaximal work rate
Decreased risk of the following:
    Mortality from all causes
    Coronary artery disease
    Cancer (colon, perhaps breast and prostate)
    Hypertension
    Non–insulin-dependent diabetes mellitus
    Osteoporosis
    Anxiety
    Depression
Improved blood lipid profile
    Decreased triglycerides
    Increased high density lipoprotein cholesterol
    Decreased postprandial lipemia
Improved immune function
Improved glucose tolerance and insulin sensitivity
Improved body composition
Enhanced sense of well-being

Many of the health benefits accrue from physical activities that may have relatively little effect on increasing cardiorespiratory fitness (2, 8-10).

Arteriovenous Oxygen Difference

The difference between arterial and venous content of oxygen in blood reflects the ability of skeletal muscle tissue to extract oxygen (105, 106). This difference increases with chronic cardiovascular training, particularly near maximal exertion.

Systolic and Diastolic Blood Pressure

Both resting systolic blood pressure (pressure against the artery wall during the beat of the heart) and diastolic blood pressure (pressure against the artery wall in between the heart beats) may decrease (if elevated consistently prior to starting regular cardiovascular training) with chronic cardiovascular training. Resting lactate levels remain relatively unchanged with long term cardiovascular training (104).

Blood Lactate

Lactic acid (lactate) is a byproduct of anaerobic glycolysis. As a result of proper cardiovascular training, less lactic acid will be produced at submaximal workloads during exercise (97, 105).

Gender-Specific Improvement

The salutary effects of chronic endurance training in men are well documented (Table 2.6). Numerous studies now provide ample data on $\dot{V}O_{2max}$, cardiovascular hemodynamics, body composition, and blood lipids as well as changes with physical conditioning of middle-aged and older women. The results demonstrate that women with and without CAD respond to aerobic training in much the same way as men when subjected to comparable programs in terms of frequency, intensity, and duration of exercise (99, 100). Improvement is negatively correlated with age,

habitual physical activity, and initial $\dot{V}O_{2max}$ (which is generally lower in women than men) and positively correlated with conditioning frequency, intensity, and duration (101).

There are, however, large differences between individuals in the effects of physical conditioning independent of age, initial capacity, or conditioning program. These individual variations in response to aerobic exercise training may be due to childhood patterns of activity, state of conditioning at the initiation of the program, or degree of physiological aging. Body compositional differences in trainability may also play an important role with respect to the results of physical conditioning. Obese women demonstrate lower aerobic capacity (per kilogram body weight), altered cardiovascular hemodynamics, and elevated serum lipids compared to leaner women (102). This initial varied profile may serve to modify the outcome of an aerobic conditioning program with respect to the magnitude of quantitative change.

Program Variation/Periodization for Cardiovascular Training

Periodization is an advanced training technique that divides the season or annual calendar into cycles or phases (Figure 2.10). These phases focus adaptive development so the athlete approaches peak performance at the most advantageous time in the competitive schedule while varying exercise mode, intensity, and volume to diminish the possibility of overtraining. Exercise programming for sport and specific activities is clearly based on the concept of fitting the details

Figure 2.10–Interrelationships of volume, intensity, and technique for periodicity training.

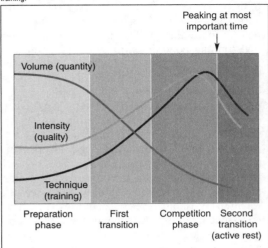

above rest (with or without a Valsalva maneuver) and is significantly greater than during the concentric phase of a repetition (106). The Valsalva maneuver is a potentially unsafe technique used by weight lifters to be able to overcome greater resistances. The technique involves holding one's breath while lifting and in doing so, both blood pressure and heart rate increase dramatically, possibly to dangerously high levels. This technique should be avoided for safety reasons.

During both the concentric and eccentric phases of a repetition, cardiac output may be increased. Cardiac output during squat exercise may increase to approximately 20 L during the eccentric phase but be only 15 L during the concentric phase. However, during exercise involving smaller muscle mass (e.g., knee extension), cardiac output may be elevated above rest only during the eccentric phase. The differing response between eccentric and concentric phases may result in no overall change from rest in mean cardiac output and stroke volume during exercise involving a small muscle mass. Heart rate is not significantly different between the concentric and eccentric phases. Because stroke volume is significantly greater during the eccentric than the concentric phase of a repetition, the higher cardiac output during the eccentric phase is due to increased stroke volume.

of training to the specific perfornace demands of the sport or activity. People become fit through programs that fit them. Designing cardiovascular training programs tailored to the goals, needs, and limitations of each exerciser is a central skill of the exercise professional.

H. Normal, Acute Responses to Resistance Training

Heart Rate and Blood Pressure

Heart rate and blood pressure increase during dynamic resistance exercise using machines, free weights, or isokinetic devices. Peak blood pressure response is higher during weight training in which a concentric and an eccentric phase occur than during isokinetic exercise (106). Peak blood pressure and heart rate normally occur during the last several repetitions of a set to voluntary concentric failure. Blood pressures are higher during sets at submaximal resistance to voluntary failure than at 1 RM. In dynamic resistance exercise, blood pressure but not heart rate rises during the concentric as compared to the eccentric portion of a repetition. In addition, blood pressure increases with active muscle mass, but the increase is not linear (106).

Stroke Volume and Cardiac Output

Stroke volume is not significantly elevated above resting during the concentric phase of resistance training exercise with or without a Valsalva maneuver. However, during the eccentric phase, stroke volume is significantly increased

I. Normal, Chronic Physiological Adaptations Associated with Resistance Training

Both acute and chronic physiological changes occur with resistance exercise. An acute response usually results in an immediate change, whereas a chronic change is a function of the response to a repeated exercise stimulus. The term *adaptation* refers to the physiological process by which adaptation to physical training occurs. Ultimately, the adaptation to training determines whether resistance training is effective and whether a higher level of physiological function and/or performance is possible. Since resistance exercise protocols can be differentially configured to present a variety of demands, training adaptations appear to be specific to the type of protocol used. The specificity is related to the particular pattern of neuromuscular activation required to perform a resistance exercise. In turn, this neuromuscular stimulation activates a variety of other systems (e.g., endocrine, cardiovascular) that act to support the adaptive changes in the neuromuscular system. The sequence of adaptation events is initiated with the first exercise session and follows a time course specific to the individual and the type of protocol used. Studies of chronic adaptations to resistance training have come primarily from training programs of less than four-month duration.

Muscle Enlargement

Hypertrophy

One of the most prominent adaptations to a properly designed and implemented resistance training program is muscle growth. Increased muscle size has been primarily attributed to muscle fiber hypertrophy (increased size of individual fibers) (107). Only fibers activated during training are subject to this adaptation response. The mechanisms of muscle enlargement are unclear, but it is a complex phenomenon of many combined factors that affects the genetic machinery. Initial increases in water content, changes in the type of muscle proteins, and eventual increases in contractile proteins are supported and signaled by a host of influences, from hormones to nutrition. Clearly, resistance exercise disrupts or damages certain muscle fibers, which later undergo repair and remodeling. This process may well involve many regulatory mechanisms (*e.g.,* hormonal and metabolic) interacting with the training status as well as the availability of protein.

Increased muscle size is generally attributed to hypertrophy of existing muscle fibers. Muscle fiber hypertrophy is thought to occur through remodeling of protein within the cell and increased size and number of myofibrils. Furthermore, increases in the number of contractile filaments (actin and myosin) and sarcomeres contribute to increased muscle fiber size and ultimately intact muscle.

Hyperplasia

It has been suggested that increased muscle size may also be due to muscle fiber hyperplasia (increased number of muscle fibers). Hyperplasia following resistance training has not been demonstrated in humans because of methodological difficulties (*e.g.,* unavailability of whole muscle for examination), but it has been shown in response to various exercise protocols in both birds and mammals (107, 109). Though no clear evidence supports hyperplasia in humans, some findings indicate that it may occur.

While hyperplasia in humans may not be the primary adaptational response of muscle fibers, it may be an adaptation to resistance training that occurs when some fibers reach a theoretical upper limit in cell size. Intensive long-term training may make some type II muscle fibers primary candidates for such adaptation. If hyperplasia does occur, it probably accounts for only a small portion (5–10%) of the increase in muscle size.

Muscle Fiber Transformation

A continuum of muscle fiber types exists, and transformation (e.g., type IIB to type IIA) within a particular subtype is a common adaptation to resistance training (110). It is doubtful that in normal training conditions, muscle fibers transform from type II to type I. However, some change along the continuum within a fiber type clearly occurs.

The shift from type IIB to type IIA reverses during detraining. Furthermore, it appears that when resistance training is restarted, the conversion from type IIB to type IIA is quicker relative to starting in an untrained state. Thus, type IIB fibers appear not to be a recruited pool of fibers that improve in oxidative ability when recruited for high threshold types of activities (i.e., heavy resistance exercise). In general, the proportion of type I muscle fibers remain unchanged with resistance training. The extent that this muscle fiber remodeling contributes to muscle strength is unknown; however, gradual increases in number and size of myofibrils and perhaps the fast fiber type conversions of type IIB to IIA may contribute to force production. Thus, while nervous system alterations likely account for the most dramatic effects in strength and power changes early in training, many other changes that occur in the remodeling of muscle fibers may influence when hypertrophy reaches a critical threshold. Therefore, the quality of the protein type being generated because of the influence of resistance training is an important aspect of muscular development.

Connective Tissue

Physical activity also increases the size and strength of ligaments, tendons, and bone. To prevent injury, ligaments, tendons, and bones must adapt to support the greater forces generated by skeletal muscles. Bone tends to adapt more slowly (6–12 months for changes in bone density) than muscle (111). Both the attachment site of a ligament or tendon and the muscle–tendinous junction are frequent sites of injury. Research on laboratory animals demonstrates that with endurance training, the amount of force necessary to cause separation at these areas increases (112). It is probable that resistance training produces similar results.

The sheath of connective tissue that surrounds the entire muscle (epimysium), groups of muscle fibers (perimysium), and individual muscle fibers (endomysium) may also adapt to resistance training. These sheaths form the framework that supports an overload. Hypertrophy induced in the muscle of laboratory animals also causes an increase in the collagen content of the sheaths. Surprisingly, bodybuilders do not differ from age-matched control subjects in the relative amount of connective tissue in the biceps brachii. Thus, connective tissue sheaths appear to increase at the same rate as muscle tissue. Furthermore, resistance training has been demonstrated to increase the thickness of hyaline cartilage on the articular surfaces of bone. One major function of hyaline cartilage is to absorb shocks between the bony surfaces of a joint. Increasing the thickness of this cartilage may facilitate improved shock absorption.

Energy Substrates

The final source of energy for muscular activity is ATP that is ultimately derived from intramuscular phosphagens (phosphocreatine and ATP), carbohydrate (muscle glycogen and blood glucose), and lipids (plasma fatty acids and intramuscular triglycerides). In humans, it has been demonstrated that strength training increases resting intramuscular concentrations of phosphocreatine and ATP. However, this finding is not supported by other studies, even when significant amounts of muscle fiber hypertrophy occur (113). Recent evidence that creatine supplementation expands the total creatine content of muscle by about 20–30%, even in trained individuals, appears to support the concept that training induces only small changes even though stores can be improved by supplementation.

Five months of resistance training may increase intramuscular glycogen stores. However, muscle glycogen content does not change during resistance training (113). The aerobic energy system uses glycogen from hepatic and intramuscular sources, triglycerides from intramuscular and adipose tissue sources, and some protein to produce ATP; endurance training also enhances intramuscular storage and mobilization of triglycerides. Whether resistance training induces similar adaptations is equivocal, since increased triglyceride use has been observed in the triceps but not in the quadriceps after training. Thus, there may be differences in the response of different muscle groups with respect to triglyceride storage and mobilization.

Although dietary practices and type of program may affect triglyceride concentrations, it is possible that because most resistance training programs are anaerobic, intramuscular concentrations of triglycerides are minimally affected by resistance training.

Neural Adaptations with Resistance Training

Following resistance training, the correlation between increases in strength and changes in whole muscle cross-sectional area, limb circumference, and muscle fiber cross-sectional area is low, indicating that other factors are responsible for gains in strength (108). This is true especially

during the initial weeks of training. On the basis of this type of evidence, it has been concluded that neural factors profoundly influence muscular force production. Such neural factors are related to the following processes:

- Increased neural drive to muscle
- Increased synchronization of motor units
- Increased activation of the contractile apparatus
- Inhibition of protective mechanisms of the muscle (*i.e.*, Golgi tendon organs)

Evidence suggests that the amount of muscle required to be activated following resistance training is less than that required to perform the same exercise protocol prior to training. This reduction in the amount of muscle needed to move a given resistance post training demonstrates that unless resistance progressively increases, less muscle is activated as muscular strength increases (114–116).

Since less neural drive is required to produce a given submaximal force after training, either activation of muscle improves or muscle fibers develop a more efficient recruitment pattern. Since no improvement in activation of muscle after training has been demonstrated, some suggest that more efficient recruitment order may play an important role in increased force production in trained muscle. Furthermore, some evidence suggests that these neural adaptations are specific to certain muscle fibers and therefore may contribute to increased force output in some but not all muscles.

After the initial neural adaptations, muscle hypertrophy becomes the most important factor in increased strength, especially for younger men. Eventually muscle hypertrophy also reaches a plateau. Whole-muscle image systems (*e.g.*, magnetic resonance imaging and computed tomography) have confirmed that fiber changes do not necessarily reflect the magnitude of change in whole muscle. Whole muscle must be frequently stimulated at several angles of movement to activate all available tissue over the cross-sectional area. Nevertheless, strength and power gains derived from the progressively and properly loaded and activated musculature appear to be bounded by a genetic upper limit of neuromuscular adaptation. Although neural adaptations account for much of the strength increase early in a resistance training program, strength and power improvement in advanced resistance trained athletes (*i.e.*, Olympic weight lifters) may also be due to neural factors (116).

Cardiovasular Adaptations

Cardiovascular adaptations, as with other adaptations to resistance training, are affected by training volume and intensity. Cardiovascular adaptations are due to the training stimulus on the cardiovascular system and thus are different from muscular adaptations to resistance training. In general, the differences are due to the large volume of blood pumped at a relatively low pressure during endurance exercise, and a relatively small volume of blood at a high pressure during resistance training.

Heart Rate and Blood Pressure

Strength-trained athletes have average or lower than average resting heart rates (118). Short-term resistance training studies result in either significant (5–12%) or no significant decrease in resting heart rate (119). Decreased resting heart rate due to physical training is attributed to a combination of decreased sympathetic and increased parasympathetic stimulation to the heart. Short-term training studies of men also demonstrate no change or slightly decreased resting systolic and diastolic blood pressures (118, 119). Decreased resting blood pressure is probably due to decreased body fat, decreased body salt, and alterations in the sympathetic drive to the heart. Despite evidence to the contrary, there is a common misconception that resistance training results in hypertension. Hypertension, when it occurs in resistance-trained athletes, is most likely related to genetic hypertension, chronic overtraining, use of steroids, large increases in muscle mass, or increases in total body weight (119).

Stroke Volume

Highly resistance-trained men have normal or above normal absolute resting stroke volumes. However, relative to body surface area or lean body mass, resting stroke volume of highly resistance-trained men is not significantly different from normal. Greater than normal absolute stroke volume is due to a significantly greater left ventricular diastolic diameter, indicating increased ventricular filling and a normal ejection fraction. A long training period and/or a high training volume are probably required to increase absolute resting stroke volume (118).

Peak Oxygen Consumption

Heavy resistance training may induce small increases (5–10%) in peak oxygen consumption ($\dot{V}O_{2peak}$), in contrast to the 15–20% increases in $\dot{V}O_{2peak}$ that occur with traditional endurance training. Again, the volume of work appears to be critical for stimulating an adaptational response in aerobic power. For example, circuit weight training (e.g., 12–15 repetition sets at 40–60% of 1 RM) with short rest periods (15–30 s) has been shown to increase $\dot{V}O_{2peak}$ marginally (5–10%). The $\dot{V}O_{2peak}$ of competitive Olympic weight lifters, power lifters, and bodybuilders ranges from 41 to 55 mL·kg^{-1}·min^{-1} (117). The mechanism by which resistance training induces small increases in $\dot{V}O_{2peak}$ may be related to a true aerobic training effect. It is possible that certain training programs

Table 2.7–Physiological Adaptations Associated with Chronic Resistance Training in Humans

VARIABLE	DIRECTIONAL CHANGE IN ADAPTATION
Performance	
Muscle strength and endurance	Increases
Aerobic power	No change
Maximal rate of force development	Increases
Vertical jump	Increases
Anaerobic power	Increases
Sprint speed	Improves
Muscle fibers	
Fiber size	Increases
Capillary volume density	No change or decreases
Mitochondrial volume density	Decreases
Myosin heavy chains	
Fast	Increases
Slow	No change or decreases
Enzyme activity	
Creatine phosphokinase	Increases
Myokinase	Increases
Phosphofructokinase	Increases
Metabolic energy stores	
Stored ATP	Increases
Stored creatine phosphate	Increases
Stored glycogen	Increases
Intramuscular triglycerides	May increase
Connective tissue	
Ligament strength	? (theoretically increases)
Tendon strength	? (theoretically increases)
Collagen content	? (theoretically increases)
Bone density	? (theoretically increases)
Body composition	
Percent body fat	Decreases
Fat-free mass	Increases
Neuroendocrine	
Growth hormone (acute exercise)	Increases
Growth hormone (chronic)	No change or decreases
Testosterone (acute and chronic)	Increases
Cortisol (acute)	Increases
Cortisol (chronic)	No change
Cardiovascular	
Heart rate	No change or decreases
Heart size	Increases
Blood pressure	Decreases
Max VO_2	No change
Serum lipids	
Total Cholesterol	Decreases
HDL	Increases
LDL	Decreases or no change
Triglycerides	Decreases
Neuromuscular	
Activation of synergistic muscles	Increases
Inhibition of antagonistic muscles	Increases
Neural protective mechanisms	Decreases
Motor neuron excitability	Increases

(e.g., circuit training and Olympic weight training) may reach a minimum threshold for improving $\dot{V}O_{2peak}$ (Table 2.7).

Body Composition

Body composition changes occur in short-term resistance training programs (6–24 wk) (120). In general, strength training decreases body fat and increases body mass and fat-free mass in both men and women using dynamic, constant external resistance, variable resistance, and isokinetic training with programs involving a variety of combinations of exercises, sets, and repetitions.

Table 2.8–The Effects of Resistance Training on Morphology, Biochemistry, Neural Function, Body Composition, and Performance

	EFFECT		
	INCREASE	DECREASE	NO CHANGE
Morphological factors			
Size of type II (fast-twitch) muscle fibers	X		
Number of muscle fibers			X
Relative amount of muscle fibers			X
Number and size of myofibrils			X
Amount of contractile proteins	X		
Size and strength of connective tissue (e.g., tendons, ligaments, fascia)	X		
Bone mass and bone density	X		
Biochemical factors			
CP and ATP concentration	X		
Mitochondrial density		X	
Myokinase activity	X		
Neural factors			
Discharge frequency of motor neurons	X		
Motor unit recruitment	X		
Synchrony of recruitment	X		
Neural inhibitions		X	
Motor skill performance	X		
Body compositional factors			
Total body weight			X
Lean body weight	X		
Fat weight		X	
Percent body fat		X	
Performance factors			
Speed, power, balance, agility, and flexibility	X		

Because of the variation in the numbers of sets, repetitions, and exercises, and relatively small body composition changes, it is impossible to reach definitive conclusions regarding the optimal program for decreasing percent fat and increasing fat-free mass. The largest increases in fat-free mass are slightly greater than 3 kg (6.6 lb) in 10 wk of training. This is equivalent to a fat-free mass increase of about 0.66 lb·wk^{-1}. Though some coaches desire huge gains in body mass for athletes during the off-season, this may not be possible if the added body mass is to be muscle mass (Table 2.8).

Program Variation/Periodization for Resistance Training

Variation in the volume and intensity of training, or periodization, is important for optimal strength gain (121, 123). Much of the early research focused on the concept that there is an optimal combination of sets and repetitions that induce increased strength. Such an optimal combination probably does not exist; instead, variations in resistance, number of sets, and number of repetitions is associated with greater strength gains. The most popular term for changing acute program variables is periodization. Periodization is planned variation in acute program variables.

Selye's general adaptation syndrome underlies the concept of periodization. This theory proposes three phases of adaptation during acute stress (i.e.,

resistance exercise): 1) shock, 2) adaptation, and 3) staleness. The first stage, shock, occurs after the initiation of a novel stimulus (resistance exercise or new resistance), resulting in development of syndromes of maladaptation (e.g., soreness) and a resultant performance decrement. The second phase, adaptation, occurs during repeated training exposure to the stimulus and results in increased performance. In the third phase, adaptation has occurred and the same stimulus does not produce further adaptation. Performance may reach a plateau in this phase, and for further adaptation to occur, a change in stimulus or rest must be imposed.

Programs that do not provide sufficient variation and rest result in a classic plateau of training or perhaps decreased performance (overtraining). Periodization can help avoid staleness and/or overtraining by allowing for adequate rest so that the exercise stimulus–response is maintained. Thus, variation in exercise stimulus is an important factor for consistent improvements in performance capacity.

The classic form of periodization breaks the training program into specific times. The longest period is the macrocycle, about a year. The macrocycle can be divided into mesocycles, generally 3–4 months each. A mesocycle may be further divided into a microcycle of approximately 2–6 wk. Each training phase has a specific goal and is a planned part of the total program. This type of training was originally designed for track and field and weight lifting to assist competitors in peaking. Furthermore, only large muscle groups were normally periodized. Others have learned the benefits of such training and have adapted periodization for use in various sports and fitness activities. There are two models for periodization of training, the Classic Periodization Model and the Nonlinear Periodization Model.

Classic Periodization Model

The goals of a program determine the number of training cycle phases, and it is thought that several shorter cycles are better than one long cycle; therefore, the length of each phase typically ranges from two to four weeks. This example program contains only one set and repetition scheme; other schemes depend on the target training goal. Training frequency is typically three times per week. In this example the primary training goals are strength and power and associated muscle hypertrophy, which develops with such loadings.

GENERAL PRE-PREPARATION PHASE. At least 6–8 wk are required for general conditioning to allow tolerance of strength training. Proper techniques should be emphasized with little or no resistance. Intensity allowing 12–15 repetitions, low volume (one or two sets), and limited number of exercises is ideal for this phase. Exercises may be added as proper technique is demonstrated.

Exercises for the large muscle groups are generally periodized, and small muscle groups are exercised at a slightly higher intensity (8–10 RM), but they can also be periodized. A length of 2–4 wk is used for all of the following cycles. *Note: RM is an abbreviation for repetition maximum or in other words, the most resistance or weight one can successfully overcome or lift for a pre-determined number of repetitions (Table 2.9).*

PREPARATION PHASE. This is the first phase of a formal training cycle. The number of exercises and initial tolerance should be established in the previous cycle. The intensity allows 12–15 repetitions in 3–4 sets with a 1–2 min rest between sets and exercises. This is a high-volume, low-intensity stimulus.

STRENGTH PHASE. Resistance work allows 3–5 repetitions in 2–3 sets with 2–2.5 min rest periods between sets and exercises. Technique is emphasized along with progression of resistance.

POWER PHASE. This phase uses resistance allowing 1–4 repetitions at 30–60% of 1 RM in 5–6 sets with 3–4 min rest periods between sets and exercises. The key is optimizing the rest for a maximal effort in all power exercise training. Again, technique is emphasized along with progression. Plyometric exercise or alternative resistance modalities such as isokinetics, pneumatics, and hydraulics can be added to the program for speed specificity at this point.

TRANSITION PHASE. The transition phase is used for active rest (*i.e.*, performing endurance rather than resistance exercise). This phase can range from a few days to a couple of weeks, depending on the program and the amount of prior training.

Nonlinear Periodization Model

Nonlinear, or undulating, models for periodization are becoming more common. This model is nonlinear because it has larger resistance changes than those commonly used in linear models. The nonlinear model varies exercise within 1–2 wk periods among light, moderate, heavy, and even very heavy resistance for appropriate exercises (*e.g.*, core exercises). It begins with a general pre-preparation phase identical to that previously discussed. Then, for example, it uses 8–10 RM (moderate resistance) on the first training day of the week, 3–5 RM (heavy) on the next day, and 12–15 RM (light) on the third day for 12 wk. The 12-wk cycle is followed by a short active rest or transition phase and repeated. This model may be most appropriate for some team and individual sports where peaking is not practical because many competitions may take place in a season. A higher volume of training can be performed when light and moderate resistances are used and both training intensity and volume vary dramatically on a daily basis.

Muscular Strength and Endurance

The fitness characteristics of muscular performance typically targeted by a resistance training program include the following:

- Local muscular endurance, or the ability of a muscle or muscle group to perform repeated muscle actions against a submaximal resistance.
- Muscle strength, or the ability of a muscle or muscle group to produce maximal force at a given velocity of movement.

Within the concept of muscle strength, power should also be considered:

$$power = \frac{force \times distance}{time} = \frac{work}{time}$$

The ability to engage and produce force early in the activation pattern (rate of force production) is becoming recognized as an important feature of the acute functional ability of muscle (122, 123). Although maximum strength may be the same, the rate of force development to maximum is faster in some individuals than in others. The ability to engage the muscle rapidly seems to be important not only for sports performance but also for daily challenges, such as reacting to loss of balance, climbing stairs, and picking up a bag of groceries and putting it on a shelf (121).

Table 2.9–Estimating 1RM from a "n-RM"

Estimating 1RM from a "n-RM"

To estimate a person's 1RM after you've determined a "n RM" (where n=10, for example), you can use a regression equation attributed to Brzycki (1993).

1 RM = weight lifted during n RM / (1.0278 - .0278(n))

Alternatively,

1 RM = weight lifted during n RM * (1 + (0.033(n))

The formula permits one to "assess muscular strength in a safe, efficient manner ... [without requiring] clients to attempt maximum lifts " (Brzycki, 2000). Brzycki's equation predicts the 1 RM in a bench press more accurately than competing formulas, as long as its estimate is based on ten or fewer repetitions (Mayhew, Prinster, Ware, Zimmer, Arabas, & Bemben, 1995).

Brzycki's equation also estimates loads for a "nRM" as a percentage of the 1RM:

The estimated load for a is _____ percent of a 1RM	10RM	8RM	6RM	5RM	4RM
	75	80.5	86	89	91.7

Brzycki, M. (1993). Strength testing - Predicting a one-rep max from a reps-to-fatigue. Journal of Physical Education, Recreation and Dance 64 (1), 88-90.
Brzycki, M. (June, 2000). Assessing strength. Fitness Management.
Mayhew, J.L., Prinster, J.L., Ware, J.S., Zimmer, D.L., Arabas, J.R., & Bemben, M.G. (1995). Muscular endurance repetitions to predict bench press strength in men of different training levels. Journal of Sports Medicine & Physical Fitness. 35(2), 108-13.

J. Physiologic Principles Related to Warm-up and Cool-down

A disproportionate number of cardiovascular complications have been reported during the warm-up and cool-down phases of cardiac exercise training (125). A progressive warm-up that includes both musculoskeletal (*e.g.,* stretching, flexibility exercises) and cardiorespiratory activities may prevent musculoskeletal injuries (124) and decrease the occurrence of ECG and wall motion abnormalities that are suggestive of myocardial ischemia and/or ventricular irritability. Abnormalities that may be provoked by sudden strenuous exertion (126, 127). A cool-down enhances venous return during recovery, reducing the possibility of postexercise hypotension and related symptoms. Flexibility exercises can be done as part of the warm-up, cool-down, or both. In contrast, intermittent mild-to-moderate intensity activity can generally be performed without a warm-up or cool-down.

K. Muscle Fatigue

The nature and extent of muscle fatigue clearly depend on the type, duration, and intensity of exercise, the fiber type composition of the muscle, individual fitness level, and environmental factors. For example, fatigue experienced in high-intensity, short-duration exercise depends on factors differing from those precipitating fatigue in endurance activity. Similarly, fatigue during tasks involving heavily loaded contractions (*e.g.,* weight lifting) probably differs from that produced during relatively unloaded movement (running and swimming). Finally, the often debilitating fatigue that accompanies viral or bacterial infections, recovery from injury or surgery, chronic fatigue syndrome, depression, sleep deprivation, and jet lag probably has little to do with the muscles themselves and likely involves factors within the central nervous system (CNS).

Muscle fatigue is defined as the loss of force or power output in response to voluntary effort leading to reduced performance. This definition illustrates the likelihood that both central and peripheral factors may be involved. Central fatigue is the progressive reduction in voluntary drive to motor neurons during exercise, whereas peripheral fatigue is the loss of force and power that is independent of neural drive. This chapter focuses primarily on muscle fatigue resulting from two general types of activity: short-duration, high-intensity and endurance exercise. However, it should be noted and remembered that muscle fatigue is a common phenomenon that confronts daily activities in ways that may be unrelated to athletic participation (128–132).

Short-Duration, High-Intensity Exercise

Fatigue during short-duration, high-intensity exercise may result from impairment anywhere along the chain of command from upper brain areas to contractile proteins. Although the preponderance of evidence suggests that a dysfunction within the muscle itself is the most likely cause of fatigue under these circumstances, central deficits in motor drive may also occur.

Peripheral Mechanisms

It is clear that the primary sites of fatigue are within the muscle and do not generally involve peripheral nerves or the neuromuscular junction (NMJ). The observation that fatigued muscles generate the same tension whether stimulated directly or by the motor nerve argues against NMJ fatigue.

High-intensity exercise involves an energy demand that exceeds maximal aerobic power and thus requires a high level of anaerobic metabolism. Consequently, the levels of high-energy phosphates, adenosine triphosphate (ATP), and creatine phosphate (CP) decrease, and levels of inorganic phosphate (Pi), ADP, lactate, and the H^+ ion increase as fatigue develops. All of these changes are possible fatigue-inducing agents, and each has been studied extensively (131, 132, 133).

Adequate tissue ATP levels must be maintained to avoid fatigue because this substrate supplies the immediate source of energy for force generation. CP levels decrease with contractile activity, and some suggest that low muscle CP levels may induce fatigue (135). The declines in CP concentration and tension during contractile activity, however, follow different time courses, making a causal relationship unlikely (134). The evidence suggests that fatigue produced by other factors reduces the ATP use rate before ATP becomes limiting. ADP, Pi, and H^+ ions increase during intense contractile activity and may cause fatigue by direct inhibition of hydrolysis of ATP (136–138).

A major source of H^+ production during intense muscular activity is anaerobic production of lactic acid. Although lactic acid has long been implicated as a source of fatigue, the general consensus is that fatigue results from elevated H^+ (139).

Endurance Exercise

Numerous factors have been linked to fatigue resulting from prolonged endurance activity, including depletion of muscle and liver glycogen, decreases in blood glucose, dehydration, and increases in body temperature. Undoubtedly each of these factors contributes to fatigue to a varying degree, the relative importance depending on environmental conditions and the nature of the activity.

Glycogen Depletion

It has long been suggested that the rate of carbohydrate use depends on the intensity of work. This belief was based on the observation that the respiratory exchange ratio (RER), also known as the respiratory quotient (RQ) increases from rest to exercise. RER must be measured in the lab and is defined as the ratio of carbon dioxide exhaled to oxygen consumed. When this ratio is closer to 1.0, the subject is using primarily carbohydrate energy (glycogen) for fuel. When the ratio is closer to 0.7, the subject is using primarily fat for energy. A mixed energy usage by the subject would be suggested by an RER close to 0.85.

Early theories have been confirmed by direct measurements of glycogen use at different work intensities (133, 140). The rate of body carbohydrate usage depends not only on intensity but also on the state of fitness. At a fixed workload, trained individuals have a lower RER, deplete glycogen more slowly, and can work longer than untrained individuals (140). High-carbohydrate diets and ingestion of carbohydrate drinks during exercise can further delay fatigue by increasing the availability and oxidation of carbohydrates (141). These observations support the hypothesis that depletion of carbohydrate stores causes muscular fatigue during endurance activity. However, the exact mechanism is not known. Low muscle glycogen concentration may reduce nicotinic acid dehydrogenase (NADH) production and electron transport, drain intermediates of the Krebs cycle, and/or reduce fat oxidation, the effects of which would be to inhibit ATP production and cause fatigue (132, 142).

Practical Application

It is clear that the adaptation to exercise training may reduce fatigue. The principles of specificity suggest that fatigue suppression applies to the specific intensities, durations, and modes of exercise regularly used in the training program, although some crossover effects may be possible. Training may somehow affect the basis of these components of fatigue. While the exact mechanisms may not be entirely clear, regular, specific exercise training reduces the onset and the effects of fatigue on the activities. In endurance exercise a number of factors are involved, including glycogen depletion which can be delayed by ingesting carbohydrates both before and during exercise. In this case, training may contribute by enhancing intracellular metabolic machinery, thus increasing cellular ability to use nutrients and produce energy. While other mechanisms also contribute to fatigue in endurance activity, the practical applica-

tion of those mechanisms is at this point unclear.

Muscle Soreness

Muscle soreness may occur after an acute resistance training session. The exact mechanisms of muscle soreness remain speculative. Soreness is typically observed after excessively intense resistance training. It is most dramatic in relatively inexperienced or novice weight lifters. However, experienced weight lifters have soreness with novel exercise or excessive progression of intensity.

Several investigations demonstrate that eccentric exercise precipitates delayed-onset muscle soreness (DOMS). Eccentric contractions may damage the basic ultrastructure of the muscle cell. The focal point of the damage is the Z-disk, a structural component that anchors the contractile protein actin.

The loss of structural integrity of the Z-disks may be the stimulus leading to the associated symptoms. The appearance of DOMS ranges from 24 to 48 h after exercise and may last up to 10 days. Symptoms of DOMS include local muscular stiffness, tenderness, local edema, limited range of motion due to edema, and pain, which varies from low-grade ache to severe pain. Severity and location of discomfort specifically relate to the muscles used. The reason for increased soreness associated with eccentric training is unclear. However, one bout of eccentric exercise appears to result in protection from excessive soreness from another bout for up to 5–6 wk in untrained or novice individuals. Thus, a slow progression in intensity is critical to limit soreness. It appears that excessive soreness develops from using resistance greater than the concentric 1 RM.

Overtraining

Exercise programs that do not provide sufficient variation and rest results in a classic plateau of training or perhaps decreased performance (overtraining). Periodization can help avoid staleness and/or overtraining by allowing for adequate rest so that the exercise stimulus-response is maintained. Variation in exercise stimulus is an important facto for consistent improvements in performance capacity (143, 144). An elevated morning pulse rate, inability to reach maximum heart rate, muscle aching or injury, chronic fatigue, lack of motivation, mood altering, and decreased performance are all possible indicators of overtraining. A reasonable guideline for resistance training is to avoid increases in repetitions or volume of training more than 2.5–5% at one time. For cardiovascular training, avoid increasing volume by more than 10% per week.

L. Detraining

The effects of regular exercise training show the remarkable ability of the human body to respond to the stimuli of regular exercise. After several weeks of training, the specific systems of the body (*e.g.,* cardiovascular, muscular, nervous) that are stressed display physiological adaptations that improve tolerance for the type of exercise encountered in training. The level of adaptation and the magnitude of improvement in exercise tolerance are proportional to the potency of the physical training stimuli.

Although physical training promotes a variety of physiological adaptations, long periods of inactivity (*i.e.,* detraining) are associated with a reversal of many adaptations. The reversibility concept holds that when physical training is stopped or reduced, the bodily systems readjust in accordance with the diminished physiological stimuli. The focus of the following section is on the time course of loss of the adaptations to endurance training and the possibility that certain adaptations persist to some extent when training is stopped. Because endurance exercise training generally improves cardiovascular function and promotes metabolic adaptations within the exercising skeletal musculature, the reversibility of these specific adaptations is considered.

Cardiovascular Detraining

Maximal Oxygen Uptake

Endurance training induces increases in maximal oxygen uptake ($\dot{V}O_{2max}$), cardiac output, and stroke volume (145, 146). When sedentary people participate in a 6–10 wk low-intensity training program, $\dot{V}O_{2max}$ increases by 6–10%, and it appears that $\dot{V}O_{2max}$ sometimes remains at this level for 2–3 wk after cessation of low-intensity training (147, 148). However, more prolonged detraining (8–10 wk) has been reported to result in a complete return of $\dot{V}O_{2max}$ to pretraining levels (149). Moderate endurance training increases $\dot{V}O_{2max}$ by 10–20%, yet $\dot{V}O_{2max}$ may decline to pretraining levels when training is stopped (150–153). $\dot{V}O_{2max}$ values decline rapidly during the first month of inactivity, and a slower decline to untrained levels occurs during the second and third months of detraining (150–153). Therefore, the available evidence suggests that increases in $\dot{V}O_{2max}$ produced by endurance training involving exercise of low to moderate intensities and durations are totally reversed after several months of detraining and adoption of a totally sedentary lifestyle.

Stroke Volume and Heart Size

Prolonged and intensive endurance training promotes increased heart mass, whereas detraining results in decreased heart mass (145, 154, 155). However, it is not clear whether training-induced increases in ventricular volume and myocardial wall thickness regress totally with inactivity. Athletes who become sedentary have larger hearts and higher $\dot{V}O_{2max}$ than those of people who have never trained (156).

One of the most striking effects of detraining in endurance-trained individuals is the rapid decline in stroke volume. In studies of rats, it seems that endurance training programs promote significant increases in heart mass that are completely reversed after 3–7 wk of detraining (155, 157). Endurance-trained athletes and professional soccer players also lose heart mass after 3–8 wk of detraining.

Blood Volume

It appears that rapid detraining-induced reduction of stroke volume during exercise in the upright position is related to decreased blood volume (158). Intensive exercise training usually results in blood volume increasing by approximately 500 mL through the expansion of plasma volume (159, 160). This adaptation is gained after only a few bouts of exercise and is quickly reversed when training ceases (158–161). The decline in stroke volume and the increase in heart rate during submaximal exercise, which normally accompany several weeks of detraining, can be reversed, returning to near trained levels when the blood volume expands to a level similar to that of trained subjects (158).

Heart Rate during Maximal and Submaximal Exercise

Maximal heart rate increases markedly with detraining, reflecting an attempt (cardiovascular compensation) to offset the large reductions in blood volume and stroke volume.

Muscle Capillarization

Endurance training promotes increased capillarization of the exercising musculature, which theoretically both prolongs the transit time of blood flow through the muscle and reduces diffusion distances, improving the availability of oxygen and nutrients to the muscle. This also allows for better removal of metabolic waste products. Moderate endurance training of several months' duration increases muscle capillarization by 20–30% above pretraining levels (152, 164). However, it appears that 8 wk of detraining can fully or partially reverse these increases in capillarization (152, 165). More prolonged and intensive training increases muscle capillary density by 40–50% from untrained levels (164), and this high degree of capillarization can be maintained at trained levels for periods of a month or more of detraining.

Muscular Adaptations that Persist with Detraining

The detrained responses in the skeletal musculature of highly trained people, who regularly engaged in intensive exercise for several years, apparently differ from those who have trained for only a few months. No loss of increased muscle capillarization for at least three months occurs with cessation of prolonged intensive training, although such a loss does occur when moderate training is stopped. Cessation of moderate training results in a complete reversal of training-induced increases in mitochondrial enzyme activity, whereas only a partial decline, and therefore a persistent elevation of mitochondrial activity above untrained levels, occurs with cessation of exercise after prolonged intensive endurance training (163).

It is likely that the relatively high $\dot{V}O_{2max}$ observed in these detrained athletes is partially due to genetics. It was also observed that these detrained subjects displayed the ability to exercise at a relatively high percentage of $\dot{V}O_{2max}$, before becoming fatigued or undergoing an increase in blood lactate concentration (162). The ability to exercise at a high percentage of $\dot{V}O_{2max}$ in a detrained state reflects maintenance of muscular adaptations (i.e., high capillary density and mitochondria in fast-twitch muscle fibers).

Reduced Training Rather than Detraining

Detraining is the total cessation of exercise training and therefore removal of the stimuli to maintain adaptations. Detraining produces more marked effects than reduced training, which may more effectively maintain cardiovascular and metabolic adaptations. Indeed, it has been demonstrated that $\dot{V}O_{2max}$ and heart size can be maintained at trained levels when training frequency is reduced from 6 to 1–2 $d \cdot wk^{-1}$, provided that the intensity is sufficiently high (85–100%) $\dot{V}O_{2max}$ (166, 167).

Deconditioning and Bed Rest: Induced Effects on Bone Health

Just as physical training induces an integrated adaptive response (physiological adaptation), so too does cessation of active training (detraining) or the more restricted activity of bed rest. The magnitude of decrement observed in both muscle and bone depends on the training status prior to detraining or bed rest and on the severity and duration of reduced activity relative to habitual activity. The atrophy of skeletal muscle by the end of a 6-wk period of casting (*e.g.*, after orthopaedic injury) is obvious; unseen but no less insidious is the effect of immobilization on bone mass and calcium metabolism. Similar effects on bone, including measurable changes in bone mineral density (BMD), are observed at multiple anatomical sites during strict bed rest (168, 169).

Changes with Detraining

Relatively few longitudinal studies yield information on whether gains in bone mass achieved with training are lost with subsequent detraining. Dalsky et al. (171) demonstrated complete reversal of training-induced increases in lumbar spine BMD in postmenopausal women who trained vigorously for 22 months. After an additional eight months of sedentary living, spine BMD returned to baseline levels. Simply reducing the weekly hours of weight-bearing exercise may produce significant decrements in mineral content of lumbar spine trabecular bone in active men and women over age 50 (172). In young women, gains in lower limb BMD acquired after one year of unilateral resistance training are essentially lost within three months of detraining (173). A study of detraining in rats suggested that bones of young or male animals may be more resistant to bone loss with detraining than old or female animals (174).

Practical Implications

It is doubtful that changes in bone mass of bed-rested subjects have any immediate effect on functional work capacity, as do decrements in muscle strength and endurance upon return to normal weight-bearing activity. A greater concern is increased risk of bone fracture, particularly after muscle strength is regained and resumed activity imposes higher forces on relatively weak osteopenic bone. There also is a possibility of increase in risk of clinically relevant osteoporosis later in life.

Deconditioning and Bed Rest: Musculoskeletal Response

Decreased muscle activity can result from detraining, bed rest, casting, use of crutches, paralysis, aging, or even the microgravity of space flight. The effects of reduced muscular activity are not confined to diseased or disabled populations, but can also affect elite or weekend athletes.

Consequences of Reduced Use (Unloading) On Skeletal Muscle

Regardless of the method of unloading, the predominant adaptive response to decreased use is skeletal muscle atrophy (186, 187). Atrophy is the process whereby muscle size is reduced, almost exclusively because of reductions in the contractile proteins actin and myosin (188). Reduction in muscle size may occur through reduced cross-sectional area of individual fibers, a decrease in fiber number, or both. In unloading of a few weeks to a month, a decrease in fiber cross-sectional area is responsible.

The atrophic response to detraining appears to occur at least as slowly as the hypertrophic response to training (about 1% per week) (170–173). Thus, the atrophic response to resistance training cessation appears to be slower than to that of unloading in previously sedentary individuals. Therefore, with respect to muscle atrophy, detraining in exercising individuals is less deleterious than in bedridden, previously sedentary individuals. A short period of detraining may not be especially detrimental, but a patient on bed rest should attempt to walk as early as possible. Nonetheless, fiber atrophy results in lower total mitochondrial content, so unloading compromises absolute muscular endurance (178, 180).

Unloading reduces muscular strength, regardless of the type of action or movement performed or the method of strength expression (174–185, 189). Strength reduction is nearly linearly related to the duration of unloading and extent of muscle atrophy for the first few weeks. The magnitude of strength reduction is also specific to muscle group, with weight-bearing muscles most affected.

Retraining

Short-term retraining after detraining appears to return muscle strength and size to those of the previously trained state (173). However, it appears that there is less deconditioning than expected during detraining and more rapid adaptation after resuming training than expected.

SECTION II REFERENCES

1. Coggan AR, Spina RJ, King DS, et al. Skeletal muscle adaptations to endurance training in 60- to 70-yr-old men and women. J Appl Physiol 72:1780–1786, 1992.
2. Jansson E, Kaijser L. Muscle adaptation to extreme endurance training in man. Acta Physiol Scand 100:315, 1977.
3. Armstrong RB. Muscle fiber recruitment patterns and their metabolic correlates. In: Horton ES, Terjunk RL, eds. Exercise, Nutrition and Energy Metabolism. New York: Macmillan, 1988.
4. Gollnick P, Armstrong R, Sembrowich W, et al. Glycogen depletion pattern in human skeletal muscle fiber after heavy exercise. J Appl Physiol 34:615–618, 1973.
5. Chi MMY, Hintz CS, Coyle EF, et al. Effects of detraining on enzymes of energy metabolism in individual human muscle fibers. Am J Physiol 244 (Cell Physiology 13):C276–C287, 1983.
6. Jacobs I, Esbjornsson M, Slyvan C, et al. Sprint training effects on muscle myoglobin, enzymes, fiber types, and blood lactate. Med Sci Sports Exerc 19:368–374, 1987.
7. Jansson E, Sjodin B, Tesch P. Changes in muscle fiber type distribution in man after physical training. Acta Physiol Scand 104:235–237, 1978.
8. Brooke MH, Kaiser KK. Muscle fiber types: How many and what kind? Arch Neurol 23:369–379, 1970.
9. Edstrom L, Nystrom B. Histochemical types and sizes of fibers of normal human muscles. Acta Neurol Scand 45:269–279, 1969.
10. Fox EL, Bowers RW, Foss ML. The Physiological Basis of Physical Education and Athletics. 4th ed. Dubuque: WC Brown, 1989:106–107.
11. Burke F, Cerny F, Costill D, Fink W. Characteristics of skeletal muscle in competitive cyclists. Med Sci Sports Exerc 9:109–112, 1977.
12. Costill D, Daniels J, Evans W, et al. Skeletal muscle enzymes and fiber composition in male and female track athletes. J Appl Physiol 40:149–154, 1976.
13. Vrbova G. Influence of activity on some characteristic properties of slow and fast mammalian muscles. Exerc Sport Sci Rev 7:181–213, 1979.
14. Komi PV, Karlsson J. Skeletal muscle fiber types, enzyme activities and physical performance in young males and females. Acta Physiol Scand 103:210, 1978.
15. Spence AP, Reading MA: Basic Human Anatomy. 3rd ed. Redwood, CA: Benjamin/Cummings, 1991.
16. Cooper JM, Adrian M, Glassow RB. Kinesiology. St. Louis: Mosby, 1982.
17. Fleck SJ, Kraemer WJ. Designing Resistance Training Programs. 2nd ed. Champaign, IL: Human Kinetics, 1997.
18. DiNubile NA. Strength training. Clin Sports Med 10:33, 1991.
19. Graves JE, Pollock ML, Jones AE, et al. Specificity of limited range of motion of variable resistance training. Med Sci Sports Exerc 21:84, 1989.
20. Knapik JJ, Mawdsley RH, Ramos NU. Angular specificity and test mode specificity of isometric and isokinetic strength training. J Orthop Sports Phys Ther 5:58, 1983.
21. Gardner G. Specificity of strength changes of the exercised and nonexercised limb following isometric training. Res Q 34:98, 1963.
22. Byrnes W. Muscle soreness following resistance exercise with and without eccentric contractions. Res Q 56:283, 1985.
23. Talag TS. Residual muscular soreness influenced by concentric, eccentric, and static contractions. Res Q 44:458, 1973.
24. Stanish WD, Rubinovich RM, Curwin S. Eccentric exercise in chronic tendinitis. Clin Orthop 208:65, 1986.
25. Fleck SJ, Falkel JE. Value of resistance training for the reduction of sports injuries. Sports Med 3:61, 1986.
26. Coyle E et al. Specificity of power improvements through slow and fast isokinetic training. J Appl Physiol 51:1437, 1981.
27. Lesme G, Costill D, Coyle E, et al. Muscle strength and power changes during maximal isokinetic training. Med Sci Sports Exerc 10:266, 1978.
28. Kapit W Elson L: The Anatomy Coloring Book, Harper Colling Publishers, 1977.
29. McNaught M, Callender L. Illustrated Physiology. 3rd ed. New York: Churchill Livingstone, 1975:241–245.
30. Per-Olof A, Rodahl K. Textbook of Work Physiology. 2nd ed. St Louis: McGraw Hill, 1977:72–79.
31. Edgerton VR, Roy RR, Gregor RJ, et al. Muscle fiber activation and recruitment. In: Knuttgen HG, Vogel JA, Poortmans S, eds. Biochemistry of Exercise. Champaign, IL: Human Kinetics, 1983:31–49.
32. Faulkner J, Claflin D, McCully K. Power output of fast and slow fibers from human skeletal muscles. In: Jones N, McCartney N, McComas A, eds. Human Muscle Power. Champaign, IL: Human Kinetics, 1986:81–90.
33. Noth J. Motor units. In: Komi PV, ed. Strength and Power in Sport. Oxford, UK: Blackwell Scientific, 1992:21–28.
34. McArdle WD, Katch FI, Katch VL. Essentials of Exercise Physiology. 2nd ed. Baltimore: Lippincott Williams & Wilkins, 1999.
35. Martini F. Fundamentals of Anatomy and Physiology. 3rd ed. Englewood Cliffs, NJ: Prentice-Hall, 1995.
36. Marieb EN. Human Anatomy and Physiology. 3rd ed. Redwood City, CA: Benjamin/Cummings, 1998.
37. Spence AP, Mason EB. Human Anatomy and Physiology. 4th ed. St Paul, MN: West, 1992.
38. Williams PL, Warwick R, Dyson M, Bannister LH, eds. Gray's Anatomy. 38th ed. London: Churchill Livingstone, 1995.
39. Brooks GA, Fahey TD, White TP, Baldwin K. Human Bioenergetics and Its Applications. 3rd ed. Mountain View, CA: Mayfield, 1999.
40. deVries HA, Housh T. Physiology of Exercise for Physical Education, Athletics, and Exercise Science. 5th ed. Madison, WI: WCB Brown and Benchmark, 1994.
41. Fox EL, Bowers RW, Foss ML. The Physiological Basis of Physical Education and Athletics. 5th ed. Madison, WI: WCB Brown and Benchmark, 1993.
42. McArdle WD, Katch FI, Katch VL. Exercise Physiology, Energy, Nutrition, and Human Performance. 4th ed. Baltimore: Williams & Wilkins, 1996.
43. Powers SK, Howley ET. Exercise Physiology: Theory and Application to Fitness and Performance. 3rd ed. Madison, WI: Brown & Benchmark, 1997.
44. Hall-Craggs ECB. Anatomy as a Basis for Clinical Medicine. Baltimore: Williams & Wilkins, 1995.
45. Williams MA. Cardiovascular and respiratory anatomy and physiology: Responses to exercise. In: Baechle TR, ed. Essentials of Strength Training and Conditioning, 2nd ed. Champaign, IL: Human Kinetics, 2000.

46. Montgomery RL. Basic Anatomy for the Health Professions. Baltimore: Urban & Schwarzenberg, 1980.

47. Thibodeau GA, Patton KT, Anthony. CP Anatomy and Physiology. 4th ed. St. Louis: Mosby, 2000.

48. Spence AP, Reading MA: Basic Human Anatomy. 3rd ed. Redwood, CA: Benjamin/Cummings, 1991.

49. White JR. EKG changes using carotid artery for heart rate monitoring. Med Sci Sports 9:88, 1977.

50. Boone T, Frentz KL, Boyd NR. Carotid palpation at two exercise intensities. Med Sci Sports Exerc 17:705, 1985.

51. Gardner GW, Danks DI, Scharfsienin L. Use of carotid pulse for heart rate monitoring. Med Sci Sports 11:111, 1979.

52. Berger AJ. Control of breathing. In: Murray JF, Nadel JA, eds. Textbook of Respiratory Medicine, vol 1. 2nd ed. Philadelphia: Saunders, 1994:199–218.

53. Light RW. Pleural Diseases. 2nd ed. Philadelphia: Lea & Febiger, 1990:1–7.

54. Munro CF, Miller DI, Fuglevand AJ. Ground reaction forces in running: A reexamination. J Biomech 20:147–155, 1987.

55. Winter DA. Moments of force and mechanical power in jogging. J Biomech 16:91–97, 1983.

56. Hill AV. The heat of shortening and the dynamic constants of muscle. Proc R Soc 126:136–195, 1938.

57. Gordon AM, Huxley AF, Julian JF. The variation in isometric tension with sarcomere length in vertebrate muscle fibres. J Physiol 184:170–192, 1966.

58. Nigg BM, Cole GK, Bruggeman GP. Impact forces during heel–toe running. J Appl Biomech 11:407–432, 1995.

59. Forwood MR, Burr DB. Physical activity and bone mass: Exercise in futility? Bone Min 21:89–112, 1993.

60. Nordin M, Frankel VH. Basic Biomechanics of the Musculoskeletal System. 2nd ed. Philadelphia: Lea & Febiger, 1989.

61. Buczek FL, Cavanagh PR. Stance phase knee and ankle kinematics and kinetics during level and downhill running. Med Sci Sports Exerc 22:669–677, 1990.

62. Schwane JA, Johnson SR, Vandenakker CB, Armstrong RB. Delayed-onset muscular soreness and plasma CPK and LDH activities after downhill running. Med Sci Sports Exerc 15:51–56, 1983.

63. McMahon TA, Valiant G, Frederick EC. Groucho running. J Appl Physiol 62:2326–2337, 1987.

64. Exner GU, Prader A, Elasser U, et al. Bone densitometry using computed tomography: 1. Selected determination of trabecular bone density and other bone mineral parameters. Normal values in children and adults. Br J Radiol 52:14–23, 1979.

65. Rambaut PC, Johnston RS. Prolonged weightlessness and calcium loss in man. Acta Astronautica 6:1113–1122, 1979.

66. McArdle WD, Katch FI, Katch VL. Exercise Physiology, Energy, Nutrition, and Human Performance. 4th ed. Baltimore: Williams & Wilkins, 1996.

67. Graham T. Mechanisms of blood lactate increase during exercise. Physiologist 27:299, 1984.

68. Katz A, Sahlin K. Oxygen in regulation of glycolysis and lactate production in human skeletal muscle. Exerc Sport Sci Rev 18:1, 1990.

69. Richardsen RS, Noyszewsky EA, Leogh JS, Wagner PD. Lactate efflux from exercising human skeletal muscle: Role of intracellular PO_2. J Appl Physiol 85:627, 1998.

70. Stainsby W, Brooks C. Control of lactic acid metabolism in contracting skeletal muscles during exercise. Exerc Sport Sci Rev 18:29, 1990.

71. Senior A. ATP synthesis by oxidative phosphorylation. Physiol Rev 68:177, 1988.

72. Gollnick P, Riedy M, Quintinskie J, Bertocci L. Differences in metabolic potential of skeletal muscle fibres and their significance for metabolic control. J Exp Biol 115:191, 1985.

73. Gollnick P. Metabolism of substrates: Energy substrate metabolism during exercise and as modified by training. Fed Proc 44:353, 1985.

74. Newsholme E. The control of fuel utilization by muscle during exercise and starvation. Diabetes 28(Suppl 1):1, 1979.

75. Powers S, Riley W, Howley E. Comparison of fat metabolism between trained men and women during prolonged aerobic work. Res Q Exerc Sport 51:427, 1980.

76. Gaesser G, Brooks C. Metabolic bases of excess post-exercise oxygen consumption: A review. Med Sci Sports Exerc 16:29, 1984.

77. Dehn MM, Mullins CB. Physiologic effects and importance of exercise in patients with coronary artery disease. J Cardiovasc Med 2:365–387, 1977.

78. Mitchell JH, Blomqvist G. Maximal oxygen uptake. N Engl J Med 284:1018–1022, 1971.

79. Ferguson RJ, Faulkner JA, Julius S, et al. Comparison of cardiac output determined by CO_2 rebreathing and dye-dilution methods. J Appl Physiol 25:450–454, 1968.

80. Rowell I.B. Circulation. Med Sci Sports 1:15–22, 1969.

81. Zobi EG, Talmers FN, Christensen RC, et al. Effect of exercise on the cerebral circulation and metabolism. J Appl Physiol 20:1289–1293, 1965.

82. Naughton J, Haider R. Methods of exercise testing. In: Naughton JP, Hellerstein HK, Mohler IC, eds. Exercise Testing and Exercise Training in Coronary Heart Disease. New York: Academic, 1973:79.

83. ACSM. Guidelines for Exercise Testing and Prescription. 5th ed. Baltimore: Williams & Wilkins, 1995:97.

84. Comess KA. Fenster PE. Clinical implications of the blood pressure response to exercise. Cardiology 68:233–244, 1981.

85. Davis JA, Vodak P, Wilmore JH, et al. Anaerobic threshold and maximal aerobic power for three modes of exercise. J Appl Physiol 41:544–550, 1976.

86. Costill DL. Physiology of marathon running. JAMA 221:1024–1029, 1972.

87. Buskirk E, Taylor HL. Maximal oxygen intake and its relation to body composition, with special reference to chronic physical activity and obesity. J Appl Physiol 2:72–78, 1957.

88. Fletcher GF, Balady G, Blair SN, et al. Statement on exercise: Benefits and recommendations for physical activity programs for all Americans. Circulation 94:857–862, 1996.

89. Blair SN, Kohl HW III, Paffenbarger RS, et al. Physical fitness and all-cause mortality: A prospective study of healthy men and women. JAMA 262:2395–2401, 1989.

90. Vanhees L. Fagard R. Thijs L, et al. Prognostic significance of peak exercise capacity in patients with coronary artery disease. J Am Coll Cardiol 23:358–363, 1994.

91. Blair SN, Kohl HW III, Barlow CE, et al. Changes in physical fitness and all-cause mortality: A prospective study of healthy and unhealthy men. JAMA 273:1093–1098, 1995.

92. Blair SN, Kampert JB, Kohl HW III, et al. Influences of cardiorespiratory fitness and other precursors on cardiovascular disease and all-cause mortality in men and women. JAMA 276:205–210, 1996.

93. Barlow CE, Kohl HW III, Gibbons LW, et al. Physical fitness, mortality and obesity. Int J Obes 19:S41–S44, 1995.

94. Paffenbarger RS, Hyde RT, Wing AL, et al. The association of changes in physical-activity level and other lifestyle characteristics with mortality among men. N Engl J Med 328:538–545, 1993.

95. Sandvik I, Erikssen J, Thaulow E, et al. Physical fitness as a predictor of mortality among healthy, middle-aged Norwegian men. N Engl J Med 328:533–537, 1993.

96. Pate RR, Pratt M, Blair SN, et al. Physical activity and public health: A recommendation from the Centers for Disease Control and Prevention and the American College of Sports Medicine. JAMA 273:402–407, 1995.

97. Beck KC, Johnson BD. Pulmonary adaptations to dynamic exercise. In: Durstine JL, ed. Resource Manual for Guidelines for Exercise Testing and Prescription. 2nd ed. Baltimore: Williams & Wilkins, 1993.

98. Durstine JL, Pate RR, Branch JD. Cardiorespiratory responses to acute exercise. In: Durstine JL, ed. Resource Manual for Guidelines for Exercise Testing and Prescription. 2nd ed. Baltimore: Williams & Wilkins, 1993.

99. Ades PA, Waldmann ML, Polk DM, et al. Referral patterns and exercise response in the rehabilitation of female coronary patients aged ≥62 years. Am J Cardiol 69:1422–1425, 1992.

100. Getchell LH, Moore JC. Physical training: Comparative responses of middle-aged adults. Arch Phys Med Rehab 56:250–254, 1975.

101. Franklin BA, Bonzheim K, Berg T. Gender differences in rehabilitation. In: Julian DG, Wenger NK, eds. Women and Heart Disease. London: Martin Dunitz, 1997:151–171.

102. Franklin B, Buskirk E, Hodgson J, et al. Effects of physical conditioning on cardiorespiratory function, body composition and serum lipids in relatively normal-weight and obese middle-aged women. Int J Obes 3:97–109, 1979.

103. Frick M, Elovainio R, Somer T. The mechanism of bradycardia evoked by physical training. Cariologia 51:46–54, 1967.

104. Astrand PO, Rodahl K. Textbook of Work Physiology: Physiological Bases of Exercise. 4th ed. New York: McGraw-Hill, 1986.

105. Rerych, SK, Sholz PM, Sabiston DC, et al. Effects of exercise training on left ventricular function in normal subjects: A longitudinal study by radionuclide angiography. Am J Cardiol 45:244–252, 1980.

106. Fleck SJ. Cardiovascular response to strength training. In: Komi P, ed. Strength and Power in Sports: The Encyclopaedia of Sports Medicine. Oxford, UK: Blackwell Scientific, 1992:305–315.

107. MacDougal JD. Hypertrophy or hyperplasia. In: Komi P, ed. Strength and Power in Sports: The Encyclopaedia of Sports Medicine. Oxford, UK: Blackwell Scientific, 1992:230–238.

108. Staron RS, Karapondo DL, Kraemer WJ, et al. Skeletal muscle adaptations during the early phase of heavy-resistance training in men and women. J Appl Physiol 76:1247–1255, 1994.

109. Antonio J, Gonyea WJ. Muscle fiber splitting in stretch-enlarged avian muscle. Med Sci Sports Exerc 26:973–977, 1994.

110. Staron RS. Correlation between myofibrillar ATPase activity and myosin heavy chain composition in single human muscle fibers. Histochem 96:21–24, 1991.

111. Conroy BP, Kraemer WJ, Maresh CM. Bone mineral density in elite junior weight lifters. Med Sci Sports Exerc 25:1103–1109, 1993.

112. Tipton CM, Matthes RD, Maynard JA, et al. The influence of physical activity on ligaments and tendons. Med Sci Sports 7:165–175, 1975.

113. Tesch PA, Thorsson A, Colliander EB. Effects of eccentric and concentric resistance training on skeletal muscle substrates, enzyme activities and capillary supply. Acta Physiol Scand 140:575–580, 1990.

114. Häkkinen K. Neuromuscular adaptation during strength training, again, detraining and immobilization. Crit Rev Phys Rehab Med 6:161–198, 1994.

115. Häkkinen K. Neuromuscular and hormonal adaptations during strength and power training: A review. J Sports Med 29:9–26, 1989.

116. Häkkinen K, Parkarinen A, Alen M, et al. Neuromuscular and hormonal adaptations in athletes to strength training in two years. J Appl Physiol 65:2406–2412, 1988.

117. Kraemer WJ. Endocrine responses to resistance exercise. Med Sci Sports Exerc 20(Suppl):S152–S157, 1988.

118. Fleck SJ. Cardiovascular adaptations to resistance training. Med Sci Sports Exerc 20:S146–S151, 1988.

119. Fleck SJ. Cardiovascular response to strength training. In: Komi PV, ed. The Encyclopaedia of Sports Medicine: Strength and Power in Sport. Oxford, UK: Blackwell Scientific, 1992:305–315.

120. Kraemer WJ, Fleck SJ. Designing Resistance Training Programs. 2nd ed. Champaign, IL: Human Kinetics, 1987:153–157.

121. Fleck SJ, Kraemer WJ. Designing Resistance Training Programs. 2nd ed. Champaign, IL: Human Kinetics, 1997.

122. Newton RU, Kraemer WJ. Developing explosive muscular power: Implications for a mixed methods training strategy. J Strength Cond 16:20, 1994.

123. Kraemer WJ, Koziris LP. Muscle strength training: Techniques and considerations. Phys Ther Pract 2:54–68, 1992.

124. Pollock ML, Gaesser GA, Butcher JD. The recommended quantity and quality of exercise for developing andmaintaining cardiorespiratory and muscular fitness, and flexibility in healthy adults. Med Sci Sports Exerc 1998;30:975–991.

125. Haskell WL. Cardiovascular complications during exercise training of cardiac patients. Circulation 1978;57:920–924.

126. Barnard RJ, MacAlpin R, Kattus AA, et al. Ischemic response to sudden strenuous exercise in healthy men. Circulation 1973;48:936–942.

127. Foster C, Anholm JD, Hellman CK, et al. Left ventricular function during sudden strenuous exercise. Circulation 1981;63:592–596.

128. Bigland-Ritchie B, Rice CL, Garland SJ, et al. Task-dependent factors in fatigue of human voluntary contractions. In: Gandevia SC, Enoka RM, McComas AJ, et al, eds. Fatigue: Neural and Muscular Mechanisms. New York: Plenum, 1995:361–380.

129. Davis JM, Bailey SP. Possible mechanisms of central nervous system fatigue during exercise. Med Sci Sports Exerc 29:45–57, 1997.

130. Enoka RM, Stuart DG. Neurobiology of muscle fatigue. J Appl Physiol 72:1631–1648, 1992.

131. Fitts RH. Cellular mechanisms of muscle fatigue. Physiol Rev 74:49, 1994.

132. Fitts RH. Cellular, molecular, and metabolic basis of muscle fatigue. In: Rowell LB, Shephard JT. eds. Handbook of Physiology: Section 12: Regulation and Integration of Multiple Systems. New York: Oxford University, 1996.

133. Bergstrom J. Muscle electrolytes in man. Scand J Clin Lab Invest 14(Suppl 68), 1962.

134. Fitts RH, Holloszy JO. Lactate and contractile force in frog muscle during development of fatigue and recovery. Am J Physiol 231:430, 1976.

135. Sahlin K, Edstrom L, Sjoholm H. Force, relaxation and energy metabolism of rat soleus muscle during anaerobic contraction. Acta Physiol Scand 129:1, 1987.

136. Cooke R, Franko K, Luciana GB, et al. The inhibition of rabbit skeletal muscle contraction by hydrogen ions and phosphate. J Physiol 395:77, 1988.

137. Godt RE, Nosek TM. Changes of intracellular milieu with fatigue or hypoxia depress contraction of skinned rabbit skeletal and cardiac muscle. J Physiol 412:155, 1989.

138. Nosek TM, Fender KY, Godt RE. It is deprotonated inorganic phosphate that depresses force in skinned skeletal muscle fibers. Science 236:191, 1987.

139. Hill AV. The absolute value of the isometric heat coefficient T1/H in a muscle twitch, and the effect of stimulation and fatigue. Proc R Soc Lond B Biol Sci 103:163, 1928.

140. Saltin B, Karlsson J. Muscle glycogen utilization during work of different intensities. In: Pernow P, Saltin B, eds. Muscle Metabolism During Exercise. New York: Plenum, 1971.

141. Wagenmakers AJ, Bechers EJ, Brouns F, et al. Carbohydrate supplementation, glycogen depletion, and amino acid metabolism during exercise. Am J Physiol 260:E883–890, 1991.

142. Davis JM, Bailey SP, Woods JA, et al. Effects of carbohydrate feedings on plasma free-tryptophan and branched-chain amino acids during prolonged cycling. Eur J Appl Physiol 65:513–519, 1992.

143. Fleck SJ, Kraemer WJ. Designing Resistance Training Programs. 2nd ed. Champaign, IL: Human Kinetics, 1997.

144. Kraemer WJ, Koziris LP. Muscle strength training: Techniques and considerations. Phys Ther Pract 2:54–68, 1992.

145. Blomqvist CG, Saltin B. Cardiovascular adaptations to physical training. Annu Rev Physiol 45:169–189, 1983.

146. Rowell LB. Human cardiovascular adjustments to exercise and thermal stress. Physiol Rev, 54: 75–159, 1974.

147. Henriksson J, Reitman JS. Time course of changes in human skeletal muscle succinate dehydrogenase and cytochrome oxidase activities and maximal oxygen uptake with physical activity and inactivity. Acta Physiol Scand 99:91–97, 1977.

148. Moore RL, Thacker EM, Kelley GA, et al. Effect of training/detraining on submaximal exercise responses in humans. J Appl Physiol 63:1719–1724, 1987.

149. Orlander J, Kiessling KH, Karlsson J, Ekblom B. Low intensity training, inactivity and resumed training in sedentary men. Acta Physiol Scand 101:351–362, 1977.

150. Fringer MN, Stull GA. Changes in cardiorespiratory parameters during periods of training and detraining in young adult females. Med Sci Sports 6:20–25, 1974.

151. Fox EL, Bartels RL, Billings CE, et al. Frequency and duration of interval training programs and changes in aerobic power. J Appl Physiol 38:481–484, 1975.

152. Klausen K, Andersen LB, Pelle I. Adaptive changes in work capacity, skeletal muscle capillarization and enzyme levels during training and detraining. Acta Physiol Scand 113:9–16, 1981.

153. Drinkwater BL, Horvath SM. Detraining effects on young women. Med Sci Sports Exerc 4:91–95, 1972.

154. Ehsani AA, Hagberg JM, Hickson RC. Rapid changes in left ventricular dimensions and mass in response to physical conditioning and deconditioning. Am J Cardiol 42:52–56, 1978.

155. Hickson RC, Hammons GT, Holloszy JO. Development and regression of exercise-induced cardiac hypertrophy in rats. Am J Physiol 236:H268–H272, 1979.

156. Saltin B, Grimby GG. Physiological analysis of middle-aged and old former athletes: Comparison with still active athletes of the same ages. Circulation 38:1104–1115, 1968.

157. Craig BW, Martin G, Betts J, et al. The influence of training-detraining upon the heart, muscle and adipose tissue of female rats. Mech Ageing Dev 57:49–61, 1991.

158. Coyle EF, Hemmert MK, Coggan AR. Effects of detraining on cardiovascular responses to exercise: Role of blood volume. J Appl Physiol 60:95–99, 1986.

159. Convertino VA, Brock PJ, Keil LC, et al. Exercise training-induced hypervolemia: Role of plasma albumin, renin, and vasopressin. J Appl Physiol 48:665–669, 1980.

160. Green HJ, Thomson JA, Ball ME, et al. Alterations in blood volume following short-term supramaximal exercise. J Appl Physiol 56:145–149, 1984.

161. Shoemaker JK, Green HJ, Ball-Burnett M, Grant S. Relationships between fluid and electrolyte hormones and plasma volume during exercise with training and detraining. Med Sci Sports Exerc 30:497–505, 1998.

162. Coyle EF, Martin WH, Bloomfield SA, et al. Effects of detraining on responses to submaximal exercise. J Appl Physiol 59:853–859, 1985.

164. Ingjer F. Capillary supply and mitochondrial content of different skeletal muscle fiber types in untrained and endurance-trained men: A histochemical and ultrastructural study. Eur J Appl Physiol 40:197–209, 1979.

165. Schantz PG. Plasticity of human skeletal muscle with specific reference to effects of physical training on enzyme levels of the NADH shuttles and phenotypic expression of slow and fast myofibrillar proteins. Acta Physiol Scand Suppl 558:1–62, 1986.

166. Hickson RC, Foster C, Pollock ML, et al. Reduced training intensities and loss of aerobic power, endurance and cardiac growth. J Appl Physiol 58:492–499, 1985.

167. Madsen K et al. Effects of detraining on endurance capacity and metabolic changes during prolonged exhaustive exercise. J Appl Physiol 75:1444–1451, 1993.

168. Bloomfield SA. Changes in musculoskeletal structure and function with prolonged bed rest. Med Sci Sports Exerc 29:197, 1997.

169. Uebelhart D, Demiaux-Domenech B, Roth M, et al. Bone metabolism in spinal cord injured individuals and in others who have prolonged immobilization: A review. Paraplegia 33:669, 1995.

170. Hather BM, Bruce M, Tesh PA, et al. Influence of eccentric actions on skeletal muscle adaptations to resistance training. Acta Physiol Scand 143:177, 1991.

171. Narici MV, Roi GS, Landoni L, et al. Changes in force, cross-sectional area and neural activation during strength training and detraining of the human quadriceps. Eur J Appl Physiol 59:310, 1989.

172. Houston ME, Froese EA, Valeriote P, et al. Muscle performance, morphology and metabolic capacity during strength training and detraining: A one leg model. Eur J Appl Physiol 51:25, 1983.

173. Staron RS, Leonardi MJ, Karapondo DL, et al. Strength and skeletal muscle adaptations in heavy-resistance-trained women after detraining and retraining. J Appl Physiol 70:631, 1991.

174. Dudley GA, Duvoisin MR, Convertino VA, et al. Alterations of the in vivo torque-velocity relationship of human skeletal muscle following 30 days exposure to simulated microgravity. Aviat Space Environ Med 60:659, 1989.

175. Gogia PP, Schneider VS, LeBlanc AD, et al. Bed rest effect on extremity muscle torque in healthy men. Arch Phys Med Rehabil 69:1030, 1988.

176. LeBlanc A, Gogia P, Schneider V, et al. Calf muscle area and strength changes after five weeks of horizontal bed rest. Am J Sports Med 16:624, 1988.

177. Berg HE, Larsson L, Tesch PA. Lower limb skeletal muscle function after 6 weeks of bedrest. J Appl Physiol 82:182–188, 1996.

178. Duchateau J. Bed rest induces neural and contractile adaptations in triceps surae. Med Sci Sports Exerc 27:1581, 1995.

179. Berg HE, Dudley GA, Haggmark T, et al. Effects of lower limb unloading on skeletal muscle mass and function in humans. J Appl Physiol 70:1882, 1991.

180. Berg HE, Dudley GA, Hather BM, et al. Work capacity and metabolic and morphologic characteristics of the human quadriceps muscle in response to unloading. Clin Physiol 13:337, 1993.

181. Berg HE, Tesch PA. Changes in muscle function in response to 10 days of lower limb unloading in humans. Acta Physiol Scand 157:63–70, 1996.

182. Adams GR, Hather BM, Dudley GA. Effect of short-term unweighting on human skeletal muscle strength and size. Aviat Space Environ Med 65:1116, 1994.

183. Dudley GA, Duvoisin MR, Adams GR, et al. Adaptations to unilateral lower limb suspension in humans. Aviat Space Environ Med 63:678, 1992.

184. Hather BM, Adams GR, Tesch PA, et al. Skeletal muscle responses to lower limb suspension in humans. J Appl Physiol 72:1493, 1992.

185. Ploutz-Snyder LL, Tesch PA, Crittenden DJ, et al. Effect of unweighting on skeletal muscle use during exercise. J Appl Physiol 79:168, 1995.

186. Hillegass EA, Dudley GA. Surface electrical stimulation of skeletal muscle after spinal cord injury. Spinal Cord 37:251–257, 1999.

187. Castro MJ, Apple DF Jr, Hillegass EA, Dudley GA. Influence of complete spinal cord injury on skeletal muscle morphology within six months of injury. Eur J Appl Physiol 80:373–378, 1999.

188. Manfredi TG, Fielding RA, O'Reilly KP, et al. Plasma creatine kinase activity and exercise-induced muscle damage in older men. Med Sci Sports Exerc 23:1028, 1991.

189. Koryak Y. Contractile properties of the human triceps surae muscle during simulated weightlessness. Eur J Appl Physiol 70:344, 1995.

Section III

- ✦ Cardiorespiratory Endurance
- ✦ Muscular Strength and Endurance
- ✦ Exercise Recommendations for Flexibility and Range of Motion
- ✦ Specificity of Exercise Training and Testing
- ✦ Medical Complications of Exercise

ACSM's Resources for the Personal Trainer

EXERCISE PRESCRIPTION AND PROGRAMMING

A. General Principles of Fitness

Physical activity is defined as any bodily movement produced by muscles that results in caloric expenditure. Exercise is defined as body movement done to improve one or more components of fitness. The focus of this section is exercise programming to increase cardiorespiratory (CR) fitness; however, health benefits associated with general physical activity are also discussed (1, 2).

Cardiorespiratory activities are those that cause an increase in oxygen uptake by skeletal muscle. These activities, performed on a regular basis, increase CR fitness and lead to numerous health benefits (1, 2). However, CR exercise and activity performed incorrectly may result in serious complications. Thus, it is important to understand both the principles of exercise programming and the actual approach to CR conditioning to meet the goals of the individual.

Principles of Exercise Adaptation

An assumption in exercise programming is that fitness improvement occurs as a result of continual exercise. This assumption is based on a number of principles. The most important of these is the principle of adaptation, which states that if a body system is stressed by a training stimulus on a regular basis, the capacity of this body system usually expands. Adaptation also depends on two correlated principles, threshold and overload. To obtain a positive change, the body system capacity must be challenged beyond a minimal level called the training threshold. If training stimulus exceeds this threshold, it is a training overload, and the process of positive physiological change usually occurs. As the capacity of the body expands, the initial training stimulus may be called subthreshold, and the workload must increase (via progression) to maintain overload. The concept of progression also includes the practice of using modest levels of work during the initial sessions of an exercise program.

Medical Clearance and Supervision

Exercise training may not be suitable for everyone. Some clients limited by disease may be unable to benefit from exercise. In this small group of people with unstable disease, exercise programming may be fatal, injurious, or simply not beneficial. The *ACSM Guidelines for Exercise Testing and Prescription* (3) lists contraindications to exercise training and testing. Medical clearance is used to rule out these conditions prior to the start of an exercise program.

For individuals without known contraindica-tions to exercise training, various levels of screening related to health and fitness preferences are required. These topics are covered in the *ACSM Guidelines* and are discussed briefly here (3). The recommended level of screening prior to beginning or increasing an exercise program depends on the individual risk and the intensity of the planned activity (3). For individuals planning to participate in low- to moderate-intensity activities, the Physical Activity Readiness Questionnaire (PAR-Q) should be the minimum level of screening. A "yes" answer to any question on the PAR-Q indicates the need for a physician's referral before the client begins or increases physical activity. The PAR-Q can be found in the *ACSM Guidelines* along with specific recommendations for screening (3).

Supervised exercise programs are recommended for those with poor health status (3). Beyond health and functional status, whether a person exercises under supervision depends primarily on goals and personal preference.

Types of Fitness

The principle of specificity implies that fitness is a diverse group of related adaptations that may be differentially developed. Physical fitness has been defined as a set of attributes that people possess or achieve that relates to the ability to perform physical activity (1). The components of physical fitness that lead to increased vigor in daily life and help protect against disease are called the health-related aspects of fitness (3). They are CR endurance, muscular strength and endurance, flexibility, and body composition.

Cardiorespiratory or aerobic fitness refers to the numerous and related improvements that enhance $\dot{V}O_{2max}$ and/or aerobic work capacity. Clearly, CR conditioning is the primary goal of exercise programs for endurance athletes. It is also a primary goal in cardiac rehabilitation programs and thus helps compensate for impaired heart function (4). Finally, this type of conditioning is also associated with health benefits in the general population (2, 3, 4–8).

Components of an Exercise Session

Typical components of an exercise session are warm-up, exercise stimulus, and cool-down. An appropriate warm-up can improve performance and decrease risk of cardiac disease events (9, 10). Cool-down has these benefits as well as clearing metabolic waste from skeletal muscle (9). Warm-up and cool-down are periods of adjustment from rest to exercise and exercise to rest, respectively. Thus, the most important types of warm-up and cool-down are activities similar to the exercise stimulus activity, performed at approximately 50% of the exercise stimulus intensity (9). Older individuals and those at increased risk of cardiac disease event benefit from longer periods of warm-up and cool-down (10). Warm-up and cool-down may take 5–15 min, depending on the age and risk of the individual. Stretching to increase flexibility is appropriate but should not substitute for activity that increases metabolism. The conditioning stimulus may contain a period of aerobic conditioning, muscle conditioning, or both. It may be as short as 20 min or longer than an hour, depending on the exercises selected (3, 5).

Conditioning for Health Versus Fitness

There are some unresolved issues concerning the amount of CR exercise necessary to achieve a positive response to exercise stimulus. In recent years it has become clear that the physical activity required to achieve health benefits is less than that needed to attain a high level of CR fitness (2, 6–8, 11–13, 15). For example, Blair et al. (13) recently demonstrated that activity sufficient to cause a small improvement in CR fitness may have significant health benefits. This research, combined with the low physical activity level of the United States population, has stimulated recommendations for levels of activity less than previously suggested for the general public (2, 6, 15). A recent joint statement from the Centers for Disease Control and Prevention (CDC) and the American College of Sports Medicine (ACSM) concludes that "every US adult should accumulate 30 minutes or more of moderate-intensity physical activity on most, preferably all, days of the week" (2). Consistent with this recommendation is the report of the Surgeon General (8), which recommends moderate exercise energy expenditures, roughly equal to 1000 kcal·wk^{-1} or 150 kcal·d^{-1}. This recommendation differs from previous recommendations by acknowledging the health benefits of moderate-intensity activities, by recognizing that benefits accrue from intermittent regular activity as well as regular continuous exercise, and by stressing the effectiveness of higher-frequency activities. An example of activity meeting the CDC–ACSM criteria would be brisk walking over uneven ground at three to four mph, three times a day for 10–15 min each session, 5–7 d·wk^{-1}. Using stairs instead of elevators is an additional means of engaging in intermittent moderate exercise.

Reports of additional health benefits obtained by higher-intensity exercise do not contradict this recommendation (14). Thus, the CDC–ACSM recommendation complements but does not replace recommendations based on the evidence supporting the type of exercise needed to improve CR fitness (5).

B. Muscular Strength and Endurance

Until recently, resistance training was primarily performed by certain athletes and by individuals desiring to enhance physique. Today resistance training has become an integral part of the exercise program for an array of individuals including those interested in fitness, competitive athletes, children, older adults, and cardiac rehabilitation patients (16–26).

Much of the increased popularity of resistance training can be attributed to successful education efforts regarding the number of positive benefits associated with it. Commonly cited reasons to engage in resistance training include:
- Prevent and/or rehabilitate injury
- Change body composition
- Prevent or treat osteoporosis
- Enhance athletic performance
- Manage stress

Given the increasing body of knowledge concerning the benefits of resistance training, it is not surprising that several professional organizations and numerous members of both the exercise science and medical communities recommend that individuals of all ages and both genders participate in medically sound resistance training programs. This section addresses the principles and guidelines needed to develop safe and effective resistance training programs for healthy adults and certain special populations.

Resistance Training Program Considerations

Resistance training is an important component of a comprehensive fitness program. A resistance training program should be based on several factors, including health and fitness status, goals of the participant, proper application of the principles of training, and the training environment.

Health and Fitness Status

Participants should complete a health and medical questionnaire before starting a resistance training program. As stated previously, the PAR-Q is one of the most widely used (25) and simple yet valid forms used for screening individuals prior to beginning an exercise program.

A muscular fitness test should also be considered for anyone who is to begin resistance training. Such tests help determine initial level of muscular fitness, which can affect the magnitude and rate of improvement (27). Generally, muscularly fit individuals do not improve as much or as quickly as untrained individuals. This can be important when establishing goals or in evaluating the effectiveness of training.

Goals

Once preexercise screening and testing are complete, it is important to develop realistic goals and objectives. Unrealistic expectations can lead to discouragement, poor adherence, and injury. An understanding of the physiological adaptations is important, because it enhances the likelihood that training is based on appropriate expectations. Table 3.1 summarizes the effects of resistance training on morphological, biochemical, neural, anthropometric, and performance factors (28).

Principles of Training

Overload and specificity are principles of resistance training, that relate to the ability to adapt to stress. Adherence to these principles is necessary to provide consistent improvement in muscular fitness.

Overload occurs when a greater than normal physical demand is placed on muscles or muscle groups. The amount of overload required depends on the level of muscular fitness. For example, a football player requires a different level of overload from that of a sedentary person. To produce strength and endurance gains, resistance training should progressively overload the muscular system, which can be done by:

- Increasing the resistance or weight
- Increasing the repetitions
- Increasing the sets
- Decreasing the rest period between sets or exercises

Table 3.1—The Effects of Resistance Training on Morphology, Biochemistry, Neural Function, Body Composition, and Performance

	EFFECT		
	INCREASE	DECREASE	NO CHANGE
Morphological factors			
Size of type II (fast-twitch) muscle fibers	X		
Number of muscle fibers			X
Relative amount of muscle fibers			X
Number and size of myofibrils			X
Amount of contractile proteins	X		
Size and strength of connective tissue (e.g., tendons, ligaments, fascia)	X		
Bone mass and bone density	X		
Biochemical factors			
CP and ATP concentration	X		
Mitochondrial density		X	
Myokinase activity	X		
Neural factors			
Discharge frequency of motor neurons	X		
Motor unit recruitment	X		
Synchrony of recruitment	X		
Neural inhibitions		X	
Motor skill performance	X		
Body compositional factors			
Total body weight			X
Lean body weight	X		
Fat weight		X	
Percent body fat		X	
Performance factors			
Speed, power, balance, agility, and flexibility	X		

As a muscle or muscle group adapts, a progressive overload is required to continue improvement. A training intensity of approximately 40–60% of one repetition maximum (1 RM) appears to be sufficient for the development of muscular strength in most normally active individuals. While intensities of 80–100% have been shown to produce the most rapid gains in muscular strength (29), the greater the increase in training load, the more careful a participant must be to avoid overtraining.

Specificity relates to the nature of changes that occur in an individual as a result of training. These adaptations are specific and occur only in the overloaded muscle groups or muscles. The concept of specificity has other applications when applied to resistance training. Sports require specific movement patterns, which a properly designed program should consider. Although an appropriately designed resistance training program should include exercises for all of the major muscle groups, it can be modified to address the unique demands of a particular sport or activity (24, 30). The program for a baseball pitcher, for example, should emphasize the rotator cuff, the shoulder girdle, and the upper extremities more than a soccer player's program, which focuses on the lower extremities and includes exercises to develop strength and endurance for the gluteals, quadriceps, hamstrings, abductors, adductors, and gastrocnemius.

One of the most controversial issues of specificity is the debate over how to develop muscular strength versus muscular endurance. Muscular strength is the ability to generate force at a given speed (velocity) of movement, while muscular endurance is the ability to persist in physical activity or resist muscular fatigue (19, 24). Generally, strength is developed with more resistance and fewer repetitions, while endurance requires low to moderate resistance and more repetitions (24, 28, 29). Both strength and endurance are developed to some extent regardless of the program, because the two components exist on a continuum. However, one component may be emphasized, depending on the specific program.

Strength gains also depend on the mode of resistance training (static, dynamic, isokinetic), the type of contraction (concentric, eccentric), the speed of contraction, and the joint position (24, 29).

Types of Resistance Training Equipment

A variety of equipment can accommodate various types of training and various training goals. Almost any type of resistance equipment enables individuals to meet training goals provided that it allows an overload and that appropriate guidelines are followed. Individuals should select equipment that is accessible and consistent with personal needs and interests. Table 3.2 compares three common types of equipment on selected criteria.

Table 3.2–Comparative Overview of Various Types of Resistance Training Equipment

	FREE WEIGHTS (BARBELLS, DUMBBELLS)	MULTISTATION MACHINES	SELECTORIZED MACHINES
Cost	Low	Somewhat high	High
Functionality	Excellent	Limited	Limited
Learning curve	Limited	Excellent	Excellent
Muscle isolation	Variable	Excellent	Excellent
Rehabilitation	Excellent	Excellent	Excellent
Safety	Relatively safe	Very safe	Very safe
Space efficiency	Variable	Excellent	Variable
Time efficiency	Variable	Excellent	Excellent
Variety	Excellent	Limited	Limited
Versatility	Excellent	Limited	Limited

Guidelines for Developing Muscular Fitness

As with any exercise prescription, instructions regarding intensity, duration, and frequency; guidelines for rate of progression; and precautions are important. This information should be based on health and fitness status and personal goals and interests.

Muscular fitness can be developed through either static (isometric) or dynamic (isotonic and isokinetic) exercises. Dynamic resistance is recommended for most adults who want basic resistance training. Furthermore, because the primary objective of resistance training should be to develop total body muscular fitness in a safe and time-efficient manner, individuals should be encouraged to perform eight to ten different exercises to condition major muscle groups.

Appropriate resistance training for healthy adults should be based on the following guidelines and principles:
- Use a brief warm-up prior to performing resistance exercise.
- Adhere to proper techniques for performing each exercise.
- Perform at least one set of 8–12 repetitions of each exercise to the point of volitional fatigue (8–12 RM). There is no single formula regarding the number of sets and repetitions that provide optimal gains in muscular fitness for all individuals.
- Increase the resistance when a predetermined number of repetitions (typically 8–12) can be completed using proper form. Increases in resistance should be made gradually (e.g., increments of approximately 5%).
- Exercise at least twice a week. Recovery time (rest) is an important component of muscular growth and strength development, and most individuals require approximately 48 hours to recover from a typical resistance training session. When training at very low loads (i.e., in certain therapeutic settings), more frequent training sessions may be tolerated.
- Perform both the lifting (concentric phase) and lowering (eccentric phase) portions in a controlled manner. Performing quick, jerky movements during resistance training can compromise safety and effectiveness.
- Perform each exercise through a functional range of motion. This helps ensure that joint mobility is maintained and, in some instances, enhanced.
- Maintain a normal breathing pattern; breath holding may induce excessive elevations in blood pressure.
- When possible, exercise with a training partner who provides feedback, assistance, and encouragement. Spotting is recommended whenever possible, especially during overhead exercises. Multiple spotters may be appropriate when handling very heavy loads.

Spotting

The cPT's primary responsibility is the safety of the client. Spotting is a hands-on technique that the cPT can use while training a client to ensure safe and effective execution of a resistance training exercise. While spotting, the cPT should be alert to all changes throughout the range and path of motion of a given exercise in order to be able to assist the client if and when necessary due to fatigue or break in technique. To ensure safe effective spotting, the cPT should clearly communicate with the lifter throughout each exercise, pointing out technique observations and cueing accordingly so that the client can correct his/her own technique.

The cPT should position him/herself close to the client when spotting. During barbell exercises over the lifter's head or face, the spotter (cPT) should keep his/her hands in a mixed/alternated grip position near, but not touching, the bar. When spotting similar dumbbell exercises, the spotter's hands should be held close to but not touching the client's wrists. The cPT should always be prepared to take and rack the barbell or dumbbells from the client at the point of fatigue.

When spotting during a "ground based" or standing exercise like a squat, lunge, or step-up, the spotter (cPT) should stand close to the client with his/her hands close to the client's hips, waist, or torso.

Resistance Training For Special Populations

Resistance training is useful for many special populations. For example, though modification is necessary, children can safely train and benefit from the positive effects (18). Resistance training has also been demonstrated to be beneficial for various age-related medical conditions and in certain types of cardiovascular disease (19, 29). Not surprisingly, there are no age or gender restrictions for resistance training. Research documents that women reap similar benefits as men and under normal circumstances do not develop large muscles (30). Furthermore, resistance training can be safely incorporated into an exercise regimen for pregnant women. In fact, the improved level of muscular fitness attendant on sound resistance training may decrease the severity and/or incidence of orthopedic discomfort (19, 30).

Children

In the past, the prevailing attitude among much of the medical community was that preadolescent children should not engage in resistance training because of concerns related to a lack of physical maturity. Collectively, these concerns appear to have focused on three issues:

- Whether resistance training places excess stress on the musculoskeletal systems of preadolescents
- Whether resistance training provides demonstrable benefits for children
- How resistance training programs for children should be designed to maximize benefits and minimize risks

At least three major organizations have developed position papers making formal recommendations regarding children and resistance training (16, 17, 31). Research has demonstrated that resistance training for children, when properly performed, can be productive and beneficial (*i.e.*, benefits outweigh risks) (16–18, 31). Unfortunately, despite the benefits, resistance training for children carries some risk. One concern is the potential that inappropriate training may damage a developing skeletal system and the supportive tissues (17, 18). Lifting excessively heavy weights may significantly increase risk of growth cartilage injury. However, growth cartilage injuries associated with properly designed and supervised resistance training are rare. The risk of injury in resistance training in children is quite low if a proper lifting technique is used and only appropriate demands are placed on the child.

There are no minimum age standards for resistance training in children. Several factors should be considered before beginning resistance training in children:

- Ability to accept and follow instructions
- Desire to participate
- Basic motor skills and ability to perform exercises safely

Resistance training may be more appropriate for some children than others, depending on the aforementioned factors. Once the decision has been made, however, all programs for children must adhere to certain guidelines and principles:

- All children have developing musculoskeletal systems.
- Proper training technique for all exercises is required.

Table 3.3–Example of Suggested Exercise Order

	Push	Pull
Legs	Leg press	Leg curl
Chest, back	Bench press	Seated row
Shoulder, back	Military press	Lat pull-down
Arms	Triceps extension	Biceps curl
Trunk	Back extension	Abdominal curl

- All exercises should be performed in a controlled manner, and fast, jerky ballistic movement must be avoided.
- Resistance must be matched to the child's needs and structural limitations. Excessive resistance can damage developing skeletal and joint structures. Each set of an exercise should consist of 8–12 repetitions. Adolescents should not exercise to the point of volitional muscular fatigue.
- Overload initially by increasing the number of repetitions, subsequently by increasing the resistance.
- The selection of exercises should include at least one for each major muscle group (*e.g.*, gluteals, quadriceps, hamstrings, pectorals, latissimus dorsi, deltoids, erector spinae, and abdominals). Perform one or two sets of 8–10 different exercises.
- Perform two resistance training sessions per week with at least one rest day between sessions. Lower training volume reduces stress and allows for other forms of physical activity.
- Perform full-range multijoint exercises (*e.g.*, leg press, lat pull-down), as opposed to single-joint exercises (*e.g.*, leg extension, biceps curl), because such exercises facilitate development of functional strength.
- Appropriately trained personnel capable of providing proper strength training instruction must closely supervise all resistance training.
- Achieve muscular balance in each session by alternating pairs of muscle groups (*i.e.*, perform a pull exercise for each push exercise) (Table 3.3).

Seniors

Impaired muscular function has been linked to impaired functional ability in older adults. Difficulty in rising from a seated position, poor walking, and poor balance are common functional disabilities in older adults. The long-range implication of lack of strength is limited independence. Appropriate resistance training may enhance overall function and well-being in older adults.

Resistance training may assist in effective management of osteoarthritis (32). Functional ability can be improved if surrounding muscles and unaffected joints share stress with affected joints. Stronger muscles absorb more of the attendant stress on a joint, thereby reducing stress on affected joint surfaces.

Evidence indicates that resistance training slows bone loss and can increase bone density (25, 27). Osteoporosis is characterized by decreased bone mineral content (decreased density) and may be improved by resistance training. Furthermore, training-induced improvements in muscular strength and balance may prevent falls that cause many fractures among elderly women with osteoporosis.

Resistance preserves muscle tissue during aging and may contribute to weight control by maintaining an increased metabolic rate. In addition, most daily activities require some muscular fitness. With appropriate resistance training, older adults improve the likelihood that they can maintain appropriate levels of muscular fitness and improved daily function.

Regardless of which specific resistance training protocol is adopted, several guidelines for resistance training in older adults should be followed:
- Design the program to develop sufficient muscular fitness to enhance ability to live independently.
- Closely supervise and monitor initial sessions with trained personnel who are sensitive to the special needs and capabilities of older adults.
- Use minimum levels of resistance during the first 8 wk to allow for adaptation of connective tissue elements.
- Instruct and use proper technique for performing all exercises.
- Instruct all older participants to maintain normal breathing patterns while exercising.
- Overload by increasing number of repetitions at first and only subsequently by increasing resistance.
- Use a resistance that can be comfortably lifted for at least six repetitions per set. Heavy resistance is dangerous and may damage skeletal and joint structure.
- Weights should be lifted and lowered in a slow, controlled manner. No ballistic movements should be allowed (to prevent orthopaedic trauma to joint structures).
- Perform all exercises in a pain-free range of motion, that is, the maximum range of motion that does not elicit pain or discomfort. As positive adaptations occur, individuals may gradually increase range of motion and improve flexibility.
- Perform multijoint exercises (as opposed to single-joint exercises) that tend to assist in the development of functional muscular fitness.

The use of machines offers several advantages:
- They require less skill to use.
- They generally provide more support for the back by stabilizing body position.
- They enable participants to start with lower levels of resistance (depending on the specific type of equipment).
- They typically enable increased resistance level through smaller increments (not true for all resistance training machines).
- They allow greater control of the exercise range of motion.
- They generally provide a more time-efficient workout.

Do not overtrain. Two resistance training sessions per week is the minimum number required to produce positive physiological adaptation. While more frequent training may elicit larger strength gains, additional improvement is relatively small.

Resistance training must be avoided during periods of active pain or inflammation in older adults with arthritis; exercise during these periods may exacerbate the inflammation.

The resistance training program should be performed on a regular basis throughout the year. Research demonstrates that cessation of resistance training results in rapid, significant loss of strength (24). When resuming after a layoff, begin with resistance levels equivalent to or less than 50% of the intensity prior to discontinuing. As adaptation occurs, slowly and progressively increase resistance.

Pregnant Women

Many women hesitate to continue resistance training during pregnancy because of the seemingly inconsistent and diverse opinions on the subject. In the past 10 years, however, specific advice for pregnant women interested in resistance training has been published (19, 30). Limited data indicate that appropriate resistance training poses little risk to either the mother or the fetus and may be beneficial. For example, proper resistance training provides a pregnant woman with an enhanced level of muscular fitness, which may help compensate for the postural adjustments typical of pregnancy that are often associated with low back pain. The activities of daily living may be performed with greater relative ease with an enhanced level of muscular fitness.

However, experts are relatively quick to note that resistance training is not advisable for all pregnant women. The following recommendations regarding resistance training and pregnancy are appropriate:
- Women with any of the American College of Obstetrics and Gynecology (ACOG) contraindications for aerobic exercise during pregnancy should not participate in resistance training (Table 3.4) (19, 25).
- Women who have never participated in resistance training should not begin during pregnancy.
- Ballistic exercises should be strictly avoided, since pregnancy is associated with joint and

connective tissue laxity, which may increase susceptibility to injury.

- Women should be encouraged to breathe normally during resistance training, because oxygen delivery to the placenta may be reduced during breath holding.
- Heavy resistance should be avoided, since it may expose the joints, connective tissue, and skeletal structures of an expectant woman to excessive forces. An exercise set consisting of at least 12–15 repetitions without undue fatigue generally ensures that the resistance is appropriate.
- As training advances, overload initially by increasing number of repetitions and only subsequently by increasing resistance.
- Resistance training on machines is usually preferred over free weights because machines require less skill and can be more easily controlled.
- If a specific exercise causes pain or discomfort, it should be discontinued and an alternative exercise used. The following warning signs or complications require consultation with a physician:
- Vaginal bleeding
- Abdominal pain or cramping
- Ruptured membranes
- Elevated blood pressure or heart rate
- Lack of fetal movement

Limited research demonstrates that resistance training can be an integral part of a balanced exercise prescription during pregnancy. It appears that resistance training may assist in management of many of the rigors of pregnancy. Research also suggests that resistance training may not be appropriate for all pregnant women. Until more data are available, medical advice and a physician's recommendation should be obtained prior to resistance training during pregnancy. In addition, exercise prescription for resistance training during pregnancy should be individualized. As a rule, exercise

Table 3.4–Contraindications for Exercising During Pregnancy

1. Pregnancy-induced hypertension
2. Preterm rupture of membrane
3. Preterm labor during previous or current pregnancy
4. Incompetent cervix
5. Persistent second- or third-trimester bleeding
6. Intrauterine growth retardation

Table 3.5–The Benefits of Increased Flexibility

Reduced muscle tension and increased relaxation
Ease of movement
Improved coordination through greater ease of movement
Increased range of motion
Injury prevention
Improvement and development of body awareness
Improved circulation and air exchange
Decreased muscle viscosity, causing contractions to be easier and smoother
Decreased soreness associated with other exercise

professionals designing resistance training programs for pregnant women should be conservative in the approach to manipulating variables.

C. Exercise Recommendations for Flexibility and Range of Motion

Flexibility is the ability to adapt to new and/or changing requirements to the range of motion (ROM), which occurs at a single joint or series of joints (33, 34). Increased flexibility improves fluidity, ease, coordination, and responsiveness of movement.

Who should and should not stretch?

Everyone can learn to stretch, regardless of age or initial flexibility. Including methods that are easy and gentle and adapting the program to individual needs is important for all ages. Children benefit from stretching as much as adults and high levels of fitness are not required to begin a stretching program.

Some individuals have naturally loose ligaments and connective tissue therefore may connective tissue may allow for excessive ROM. These hypermobile individuals should not be allowed to stretch into the extremes of ROM because joint stability should be maintained as much as possible.

During pregnancy a hormone called Relaxin softens the ligaments and connective tissue, especially of the pelvis. Excessive stretching during pregnancy is not recommended. It can lead to hypermobility of the low back, sacroiliac region, and other areas during and after pregnancy. The benefits of flexibility training are listed in Table 3.5. The contraindications and precautions for stretching and flexibility training are shown in Tables 3.6 and 3.7, respectively (38–40).

When To Stretch

Individual preference determines appropriate time of day for flexibility exercise. Spontaneous stretching, done properly anywhere, is effective and desirable. Stretching before and after physical activity should be part of warm-up and cool-down. Warm-up with light activity, such as walking, before stretching is recommended. Warm muscle tissue accepts stretch easier than cold. Stretching is indicated after sitting or standing for long periods, especially during or after a long drive. Stretching can prevent discomfort from sedentary periods.

Table 3.6–Contraindications For Flexibility Testing

Motion limited by bony block at a joint interface
Recent unhealed fracture
Infection and acute inflammation affecting the joint or surrounding tissues
Sharp pain associated with stretch or uncontrolled muscle cramping when attempting to stretch
Local hematoma as a result of an overstretch injury
Contracture (desired functional shortening) requiring stability to a joint capsule or ligament contracture that is intentional to improve function, particularly in clients with paralysis or severe muscle weakness (e.g., tenodesis of finger flexors to allow grasp in an individual with quadriplegia)

Table 3.7–Precautions for Flexibility Training

Stretch a joint through limits of normal ROM only.
Do not stretch at healed fracture sites for about 8–12 weeks post fracture, after which gentle stretching may be initiated.
In individuals with known or suspected osteoporosis, stretch with particular caution (e.g., men older than 80 years and women older than 65 years, older persons with spinal cord injury).
Avoid aggressive stretching of tissues that have been immobilized (e.g., cast or splinted). Tissues become dehydrated and lose tensile strength during immobilization.
Mild soreness should take no longer than 24 hours to resolve after stretching. If more recovery time is necessary, the stretching force was excessive.
Use active comfortable ROM to stretch edematous joints or soft tissue.
Do not overstretch weak muscles. Shortening in these muscles may contribute to joint support that muscles can no longer actively provide. Combine strength and stretching exercise so that gains in mobility coincide with gains in strength and stability.
Be aware that physical performance may vary from day to day.
Set individual goals.

Frequency And Duration Of Training Devoted To Flexibility

There is wide opinion about the most effective frequency and duration for flexibility training. Beaulieu (41) states that a stretch may be held for 10–15 s initially and gradually increased to 45–60 s over 4–5 wk. Anderson (38) suggests beginning with an easy stretch for 10–30 s followed by a "developmental" stretch for an additional 10–30 s. Moffatt (42) recommends maintaining stretching posture for about 8–12 s. In contrast, Feldenkrais suggests taking three or four exercises and repeating those exercises slowly three or four times for a total of 30 min of exercise (43). Yoga practitioners dedicate 30–45 min each day to stretching (44, 45). The American College of Sports Medicine proposes that a stretch should last for 10–30 s (46).

Connective tissue deformation and neuroinhibitory effects require 30–90 s to effect tissue change and a relaxation response (35, 36, 37). Beaulieu (41) states that stretching should be done for 10–20 min, two or three times per week. DeVries found that stretching for 30 min twice a week improves flexibility within 5 wk (47, 48). Feldenkrais and yoga practitioners recommend daily stretching because of the relaxation benefits (43, 44).

How To Stretch

The guidelines in Table 3.8 are synthesized recommendations from Anderson (38, 49), Krusen et al. (50), Kuland (51), Morris (34), Hittleman (45), and Bersin et al. (43). It is helpful to have an exer-

Table 3.8–Guidelines for Proper Stretching

Determine posture or position to be used. Ensure proper position and alignment prior to the stretch.
Emphasize proper breathing. Inhale through the nose and exhale through pursed lips during the stretch. One may stretch with the eyes closed to increase concentration and awareness.
Hold end points progressively for 30–90 seconds and take another deep breath.
Exhale and feel the muscle being stretched, relaxed, and softened so that further ROM is achieved.
Discomfort may increase slightly, but continue to focus on breathing.
Repeat the inhale–exhale–stretch cycle until the end of the available range for the day.
Do not bounce or spring while stretching.
Do not force a stretch while holding the breath.
Increased stretching range during exhalation encourages full body relaxation.
Slowly reposition from the stretch posture and allow muscles to recover at natural resting length.

cise professional observe clients during the initiation of a stretch to ensure proper alignment. Incorrect stretching can be ineffective and may be damaging. Proper alignment is defined as good biomechanical relation of each joint to the adjacent joints.

Techniques Used To Gain Flexibility

Static Stretching

A static stretch is slow and sustained to increase motion at a particular joint when one segment is manipulated relative to another (34, 50). The advantages of static stretching include the following (47, 51–54):

- Decreased possibility of exceeding normal range of motion
- Lower energy requirements
- Less muscle soreness
- The types of static stretching include passive, active assistive, active, and proprioceptive neuromuscular facilitation (PNF).

Passive Stretching

Passive stretch requires assistance from another person or a device. Optimal passive stretch requires relaxation of all voluntary and reflex muscular resistance, which is often hard to achieve. Trust that the partner will not go too far or too fast is essential (46). Types of passive stretching include (55):

1. *Manual Passive Stretching* is hands-on technique where the cPT applies the force and controls the direction, speed, intensity, and duration of the stretch to the soft tissues; tissues elongated beyond resting length.
2. *Prolonged Mechanical Stretching* uses a low-intensity external force applied over a long period of time with mechanical equipment; applied through positioning, weighted traction or pulley system, etc.
3. *Cyclic Mechanical Stretching* uses a device to apply intermittent stretch loads followed by brief periods of rest; for exam-

ple, 10-s stretch followed by 10-s rest. Cyclic mechanical stretching is usually done for prolonged periods 15–30 min.

4. *Passive Self Stretching* occurs when the client performs the exercises himself; may use body weight or assistive device (towel, stretching rope or strap, cane)

Active Assistive Stretching

In active assistive stretching the muscle or joint being stretched may require assistance moving through the ROM because of weakness. The stretch requires the assistance of a partner and has the same limitations as passive stretching (46).

Active Stretching

During active stretching a muscle or joint is actively moved through the ROM. This technique requires greater energy than passive or static stretching. It may elicit a stretch reflex and thereby cause the stretch to be improperly performed (46).

Proprioceptive Neuromuscular Facilitation (PNF)

Types of PNF techniques for stretching include the contract–relax (hold–relax) stretch and the contract–relax–contract (hold–relax–contract) stretch (56). For contract–relax PNF, a muscle is contracted, relaxed, then further stretched into the available ROM during this brief relaxation phase. The same procedure is used for contract–relax–contract, but subsequent contraction of the antagonist gains additional ROM. The disadvantages are the difficulty in teaching proper technique to clients, and that it is best accomplished with a partner. The end result is similar to that of passive and active assistive stretching (46). Hutton (57) compared static, contract–relax and contract–relax–contract in increasing hamstring length and demonstrated contract–relax–contract to be most effective but difficult to teach and more uncomfortable to perform. Etnyre (58) compared static stretch to contract–relax PNF and contract–relax–antagonist contract PNF stretching and found the two PNF techniques to be more effective in both men and women for increasing hip and shoulder extension ROM. PNF stretching techniques require training and should only be practiced by those qualified to do so.

Dynamic, Phasic, or Ballistic Stretching

Dynamic, phasic, or ballistic activities refer to rapid movements requiring jerking and often bouncing movements (34). The disadvantages of this type of stretching outweigh the advantages. Ballistic movements predispose to muscle strain injury. Ballistic movements are used to simulate sport-specific, preactivity warm-up. Static stretching and plyometrics are recommended as safer options for warm-up flexibility. Studies conclude that static stretching is safer, requires less energy, and may reduce muscle soreness associated with other exercise (47, 48, 57, 59, 60).

Flexibility Exercises

Specific examples of positions and postures for flexibility exercises are shown in Figures 3.1 to 3.6. These specific exercises address positions for almost every joint. Stretching techniques using props and partners are included for variety in relation to individual needs. Refer to Table 3.8 and Figure 3.6 and follow illustrated and written directions for safe execution of these exercises. Also, individual exercises or some combination of these exercises may be contraindicated in a variety of populations.

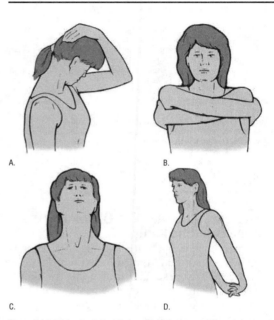

A.   B.

C.   D.

Figures 3.1 A-D (above) – A. Neck flexion with gentle pressure. This technique can be used with side bending and a combination of side bending, flexion, and rotation. Use caution with complaints of dizziness, and avoid extension and rotation postures of the neck. B. Hugging and shoulder protraction stretch. Reach across the body with both arms and grasp the shoulders. Inhale deeply, focusing the sensation of stretch between the scapulae. C. Next extension stretch. Neck extension with jaw thrust to increase stretch on the anterior neck and jaw musculature. Precaution: avoid complaints of dizziness. D. Anterior chest stretch. Shoulder extension, internal rotation, and scapular retraction with full elbow extension and hands interlocked.

Figures 3.2 A-D (below and top of next page) – A. Triceps and inferior capsule stretch. Full shoulder abduction. Elbow is fully flexed and gentle overpressure is applied pulling toward the midline. Precaution: Avoid overstressing the neck anteriorly in this posture. B. Latissimus dorsi stretch. Begin on hands and knees. The hands stay firmly planted and the person rocks backward on hips, resting buttocks on calves. Proper position localizes stretch to low back and shoulder girdle. C. Thigh, abdomen, and chest stretch. Begin kneeling and reach posteriorly, extending both arms and spine, bearing weight fully on hands. Press abdomen and hips anteriorly to localize stretch to chest, abdomen, and thighs. D. Anterior chest and torso, mild rotation stretch. Begin on hands and knees. Reach up with one arm in extension and abduction. Allow the torso and head to rotate up, looking at the outstretched hand.

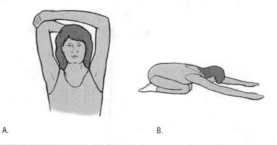

A.   B.

C.   D.

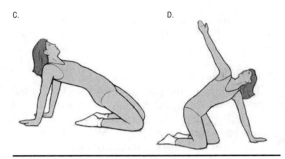

Figures 3.3 A-D (below) – A. Full spinal segmental extension stretch. Begin on the hands and knees. Initiate extension of the sacrum, arching the back (extend) segment by segment, completing full extension from the lumbar to the cervical spine. B. Full spinal segmental flexion stretch. Begin on hands and knees. Initiate flexion of sacrum, then lumbar, thoracic, and cervical spine. Protracting both scapulae increases flexion in the thoracic spine. C. Seated adductor stretch. Start in seated posture with an erect spine. Touch soles of feet together and bend knees, sliding the feet toward the midline. Allow knees to drop for increased hip abduction. With a straight back, lean forward to increase stretch in adductors. D. Combined spinal rotation, hip extension, and rotator stretch. Begin seated with an erect spine, both knees flexed. Cross left leg over right leg. Right arm reaches for left knee and uses the knee to assist the torso into left rotation. Inhale; on an exhalation, attempt further spinal rotation. Reverse the stretch for right rotation.

A.   B.

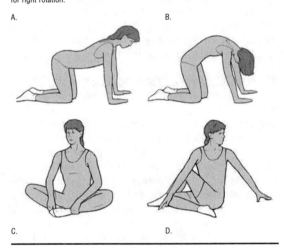

C.   D.

Figures 3.4 A-D (below) – A. Bilateral knee to chest stretch. Begin supine. Pull both thighs to chest, supporting the back of the thigh with the hands. B. Full spinal extension press-up stretch. Begin prone. Place hands on the mat just below the shoulder level and press up slowly. Maintain contact with the mat with front of thighs and pelvis. Evenly distribute extension throughout the entire spine. Precaution: Tightness in the thoracic spine restricts thoracic extension. This is a vulnerable area in the presence of osteoporosis. Propped on elbows is preferable for those with osteoporosis. C. Quadriceps stretch. Begin prone. To relieve stress on the low back, use a towel roll under the hips. Bend one knee toward the buttocks and hold the foot with one hand. A towel or rope can be used to assist reaching the lower leg. D. Hip rotator stretch. Begin supine. Cross one leg over, forming a figure 4, and flex both hips to or past 90°. The stretch is felt in the buttocks of the figure 4 leg.

A.   B.

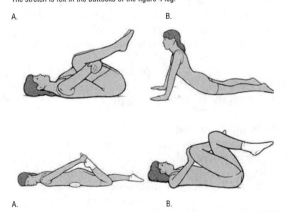

A.   B.

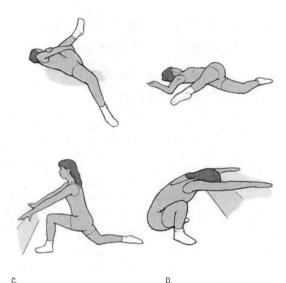

C.   D.

Figures 3.5 A-D (above) – A. Hip flexion stretch. Begin supine. With one leg over the side of the exercise bench, flex the opposite leg as close to the chest as possible. The stretch is felt anteriorly in the hip and thigh of the hanging leg. B. Hip internal rotation, adduction and knee extension stretch. Begin supine. The stretch is horizontal adduction and internal rotation of the hip with fully extended knees. Rotate head in the opposite direction to aid in keeping the shoulders flat against the mat. Allowing knee flexing is a simpler technique. C. Forward lunge stretch. Begin standing. Step forward with one leg, leaving the trailing leg in contact with the floor. The trailing leg stretches the anterior hip and thigh. The forward leg is flexed at 90° at the knee and the hip, causing a proximal hamstring stretch. D. Full squat stretch. Begin standing while holding a chair or table. Allow full adduction, external rotation, and flexion at the hips. Careful attention to hip, knee, and ankle alignment is important. Try to maintain both heels in contact with the floor.

A.   B.

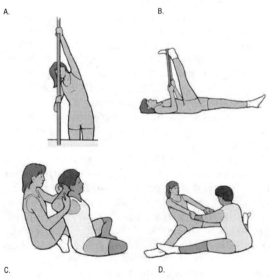

C.   D.

Figures 3.6 A-D (above) – A. Long dowel rod prop stretch, arm and torso stretch. Begin standing. Place the pole on an exercise bench and slide the arm up the pole, lengthening the shoulder girdle, spine, torso, and ribs. Use deep breathing to increase stretch between ribs. B. Assisted hamstring stretch (using a long piece of rope). Begin supine. Do a straight-leg raise with the rope hooked around the sole of the foot and pull the leg to increase hip flexion. Simpler technique requires the rope to be placed on the back of the calf. C. Partner-assisted pectoralis major stretch. Begin with one partner sitting behind the other. The partner receiving the stretch interlocks hands behind head. The assisting partner places the knees against the stretcher's back and pulls gently on the arms, creating an extension stretch for chest and upper back. Precaution: this may be contraindicated in patients with osteoporosis. D. Partner-assisted stretch of the hip adductors. Begin seated facing a partner in full knee extension, full hip abduction, bracing the feet against feet. One partner gently pulls forward to increase the inner thigh stretch. Alternate stretching between partners, asking for and giving feedback to ensure safety.

D. Specificity of Exercise Training and Testing

Energy Systems And Fiber Type

Most athletes use training techniques that mimic movements used in competition in an attempt to train the same muscle groups required for the competitive event. For example, a soccer player spends most of the time in lower body training, while a kayak competitor requires mainly upper body training. In addition, athletes work to enhance specific energy systems used in competition.

Although the concept of specificity remains a premise of exercise training, cross-training has become particularly popular. Cross-training is the use of more than one mode of exercise (*e.g.*, swimming and running) and/or training for more than one aspect of fitness (e.g., endurance, flexibility, and/or strength). Cross-training is often used to prevent injury, to maintain fitness while recovering from injury, or to supplement specific training. As described in this section, this type of training has both benefits and limitations.

Specificity also applies to exercise testing. Testing protocols that assess muscular strength do not accurately assess cardiorespiratory fitness. To test specific aspects of fitness, an activity-specific testing mode yields the most accurate results. Specificity is therefore an important consideration in testing or training for athletic competition, physical fitness, or rehabilitation after disease or injury. This section discusses specificity in terms of energy systems and movement and the applicability of combining different modes of exercise.

Activities requiring sudden, high-intensity work, such as throwing, primarily use stored ATP (i.e., ATP that is already in muscle cells). In short, high-speed events, such as the 100-m run, most of the ATP is derived from the phosphocreatine system. In sustained sprint events, such as the 400-m run, energy is derived mainly through anaerobic glycolysis. Finally, endurance activities (*e.g.*, cross-country skiing or a marathon) rely primarily on oxidative (aerobic) metabolism for energy. Specific training is required to enhance the energy system that is predominant in energy production for a given event or sport. Likewise, an accurate assessment of the physiological characteristics required for an event requires an exercise test protocol that is specific for that event.

Endurance Training

Endurance training is also accompanied by enhanced oxygen and substrate transport, and increased capillary density. An increase in capillary density decreases the diffusion distance for oxygen and metabolic substrates (*e.g.*, glucose and fatty acids) from blood to muscle. The concentration of myoglobin, which transports and stores oxygen within muscle, also increases during endurance training.

Strength Training

The primary change in skeletal muscle structure resulting from prolonged resistance training is increased muscle size (hypertrophy) due to an increased number of myofibrils (actin and myosin) and increased amounts of connective tissue. These changes occur in all major fiber types. During the first few weeks of training, however, these changes are disproportionate to the gain in strength (61). Neural adaptations, such as improved motor unit recruitment and efficiency rather than an increased amount of tissue seems to be responsible for initial gains in muscle strength (61).

Endurance and Strength Training

Endurance athletes often supplement training with resistance exercise. Athletes participating in events requiring strength often add endurance exercise to their training regimen.

Effects of Endurance Training on Strength

Endurance athletes have a lower than normal vertical jump. In fact, vertical jump decreases with endurance training, yet increases with cessation of endurance training (62). Conversely, previously inactive subjects undergoing simultaneous endurance and resistance training of the legs demonstrate improvement in leg strength and maximal oxygen consumption ($\dot{V}O_{2max}$) (63, 64). However, these training protocols have failed to elicit strength improvements similar to improvements identified when identical resistance training programs were administered without endurance training.

These investigations used intensive interval training (3–5 repetitions of 5 min each near $\dot{V}O_{2max}$) to improve $\dot{V}O_{2max}$. In research conditions, less intensive interval and continuous endurance training protocols have demonstrated that combined endurance and resistance training elicits improvement in strength comparable with that seen with strength training alone (64, 66). In addition, continuous endurance training was accompanied by an increase in $\dot{V}O_{2max}$ of approximately 18%, similar to that seen with intensive interval training (64).

Specificity Of Muscle Group

Endurance Training

Athletes often use a variety of activities to improve performance. Performance may improve through cardiovascular, muscular, and neural changes. This section discusses how training these systems may cross over to different activities.

Cross-training benefits are probably derived through central adaptations. This is suggested by comparisons between arm and leg performances in which transfer of biochemical and neural factors is unlikely.

Although cardiovascular changes are primarily responsible for increasing $\dot{V}O_{2max}$, endurance may be enhanced more through changes in oxidative enzymes and glycogen storage. Finally, while transfer of training between different activities has been demonstrated, most studies of training transfer were conducted on previously inactive subjects. Therefore, whether cross-training (*i.e.*, the supplementation of training with an alternative activity) enhances performance is unresolved.

Resistance Training

Since resistance training does not produce cardiovascular improvement, it is logical to expect resistance training to be specific, with little or no transfer among motor units. However, neural adaptations occurring early during strength training are not entirely specific.

Single-limb resistance training is accompanied by strength gains in contralateral inactive muscle groups. Moritani and deVries (67) found increased strength (35%) in trained and untrained (24%) elbow flexors. Ploutz et al. (68) demonstrated increased strength in trained (14%) and untrained (7%) knee extensors, along with limited hypertrophy in trained muscle groups and no hypertrophy in untrained muscle groups. Integrated electromyography and magnetic resonance imaging indicate that fewer motor units are recruited per unit of force applied in both trained and untrained muscle groups (67, 68). These results suggest that the transfer of strength to contralateral untrained muscle groups is due to neural adaptation. No evidence suggests that strength gain transfers to additional untrained muscle groups (*e.g.*, legs to arms or quadriceps to gastrocnemius).

Specificity Of Movement Pattern

Specificity applies not only to energy systems and muscle groups but also to movement patterns. Motor units used during training demonstrate the most physiological alterations; therefore, movement patterns are also specifically trained. The following factors affect motor unit recruitment:
- Body position and movement pattern
- Static or dynamic contraction
- Concentric or eccentric contraction
- Intensity, frequency, and duration of contraction

Body Position and Movement Pattern

Strength gain is specific to the angle of the joint at which training occurs. Thorstensson et al. (69) trained subjects for 8 wk, with free weights (squat training) and with the vertical jump and standing long jump. Following training, a significant increase in squat strength was demonstrated, while leg press strength improved only about half as much. Leg extension strength (measured statically) did not improve.

Body position may also affect the response to endurance exercise. In the supine position, stroke volume (SV) is near maximum. Therefore, at a given submaximal work rate in this position, the passive increase in SV results in a lower heart rate and lower myocardial oxygen demand. These changes may permit some cardiac clients to exercise safely in a recumbent position at higher workloads, perhaps facilitating enhanced improvement of functional capacity.

Static versus Dynamic Contractions

Static (isometric) tension/force development is applied against an immovable object, and no joint movement occurs, whereas movement accompanies a dynamic contraction because the force overcomes the resistance or vice versa. Overload training using either type of contraction increases strength. However, the manner in which strength increases may be different. Static training increases strength at joint angles similar to those used in training. Therefore, static training has little use for activities requiring dynamic movement. Duchateau and Hainaut (70) demonstrated greater increase in static strength of the adductor pollicis following static training than following dynamic resistance training. However, a greater increase in the speed of contraction was seen following dynamic training than following static training.

In addition, static exercise accompanied by a Valsalva maneuver is contraindicated for most high-risk populations because it can produce a marked increased in blood pressure. The prolonged contraction increases total peripheral resistance and inhibits blood flow through muscle, and the Valsalva maneuver increases intrathoracic pressure, which can reduce venous return and SV. These changes increase myocardial oxygen demand when cardiac output is reduced.

Concentric versus Eccentric Contractions

There are two types of dynamic contraction, concentric (force is greater than the resistance, and the muscle shortens) and eccentric (force is less than the resistance, and the muscle lengthens). Lowering of a weight during a biceps curl is one example of eccentric contraction.

Although neither concentric nor eccentric contractions appear better suited for improving strength, eccentric contractions may enhance other types of adaptation. For example, both bodybuilders and ultramarathoners have large amounts of connective tissue within skeletal muscle, which may be a protective adaptation to cope with the high levels of force that must be exerted in these events (71). One disadvantage of having excess connective tissue may be that it inhibits motion in the antagonistic muscle. Excessive eccentric exercise also predisposes the athlete to overuse syndromes and muscle soreness (71).

Intensity, Frequency, and Duration of Contractions

In resistance training, resistance moved and the number of repetitions and sets performed affect physiological adaptation. Competitive body builders, who typically use less resistance and more repetitions and sets than competitive weight lifters, often have greater gains in muscle girth. This may in part be due to an increased amount of connective tissue (71). Furthermore, although elite weight lifters may not have continuous hypertrophy, strength may increase substantially, perhaps because of an ability to recruit more motor units (61).

Fox et al. (72) studied 8-wk interval training programs of high power (19 repetitions of 30 s each) and low power (7 repetitions of 120 s each). Figure 3.7 illustrates that both groups had similar increases in $\dot{V}O_{2max}$, and although both groups had lower blood lactate concentrations after a 2-min posttraining run near $\dot{V}O_{2max}$, the lactate concentration in the low-power group was significantly lower than in the high-power group. Subsequently, long-duration training at a low intensity was accompanied by decreased anaerobic enzyme activity in both slow-twitch and fast-twitch muscle fibers, and increased aerobic enzyme activity in type I and type IIA muscle fibers (73). Training at a higher intensity for a shorter duration increases anaerobic capacity in type IIA muscle and type IIB muscle, and aerobic metabolism in type IIB muscle. These data indicate that intensive interval training is more beneficial for middle-distance events that rely on a blend of aerobic and anaerobic metabolism than for endurance performers, who benefit more from longer, less intensive training intervals and long-distance training. In fact, serious competitors generally apply both types of training, but the ratio depends on the event.

Specificity and Other Components of Fitness

There are five major categories of health-related physical fitness:
1. Cardiorespiratory endurance
2. Muscular strength
3. Muscular endurance
4. Flexibility
5. Body composition

This section discusses application of specificity to each component in terms of both exercise testing and training.

Cardiorespiratory Endurance

Specificity and endurance training were discussed previously. Cross-over of training effects between one mode of endurance activity and another is limited. The most effective way to train for a particular activity is to practice that activity regularly. In addition, resistance training of the same muscle group may increase endurance, but no evidence suggests that endurance training increases strength.

Muscular Endurance

Muscular endurance is the ability of a muscle or muscle group to repeat dynamic movements or to sustain static force over time. There is no clear distinction between cardiorespiratory and muscular endurance activities; both require contraction of skeletal muscle over extended time. However, cardiovascular endurance activities (*e.g.,* distance running) are affected by cardiorespiratory limitations, and muscular endurance activities may be less affected. Muscular endurance activities (*e.g.,* push-ups) generally require the athlete to overcome greater resistance and usually cannot be maintained as long as cardiorespiratory endurance activities. Muscular endurance activities also generally require greater anaerobic metabolic activity (anaerobic glycolysis) than aerobic metabolic activity for energy.

Training for muscular endurance can improve the efficiency of movement and acid–base buffering capacity. Trained athletes therefore often tolerate higher blood lactate concentrations than untrained persons.

Literature concerning the specificity of muscular endurance is scarce. Although some transfer from strength training is likely, optimal improvement in muscular endurance probably requires specific training. Therefore, training and testing should be activity specific. Position, movement

Figure 3.7 – Effects of high-power (19 repetitions of 30 seconds each) and low-power (7 repetitions of 120 seconds each) treadmill interval training on VO2max and net blood lactate accumulation (increased lactate concentration following a single exercise session). Similar increases occurred in VO2max, but net lactate accumulation decreased more as a result of low-power training than as a result of high-power training (P < .05). (Adapted with permission from Fox EL, Bartels RL, Klinzing J, et al. Metabolic responses to interval training programs of high and low power output. Med Sci Sports 9:191-196, 1977.)

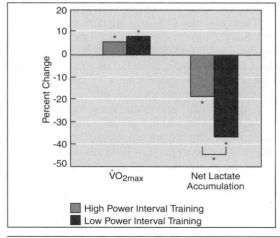

pattern, type of contraction (i.e., static versus dynamic, concentric versus eccentric), and rate and resistance of contractions should be replicated during training.

Muscular Strength

Muscular strength is the amount of static or dynamic force that can be produced. Specificity of muscular strength was discussed earlier in this chapter. Strong evidence supports the importance of specific strength testing with respect to body position, movement pattern (including number of repetitions), and type of contraction. Single-repetition maximum testing is an excellent way of measuring strength; however, a 10-repetition maximum test may be a better indicator of muscular endurance.

Flexibility

Flexibility is the range of motion about a given joint or group of joints. Range of motion is limited primarily by the amount of soft tissue (including muscle and the joint capsule) surrounding the joint (74). Therefore, strength training resulting in hypertrophy and increased connective tissue mass may reduce the flexibility of joints involved in training. Flexibility can be increased or maintained through a regular stretching program and strength training exercises that move a *specific* joint through its full range of motion.

Body Composition

The two basic components of the body (fat and lean mass) respond differently to exercise training. Following several weeks of exercise training, the body composition may change slightly. Changes most often seen are a decrease in fat with endurance exercise and an increase in lean mass with resistance training. Methods of assessing body composition (*e.g.,* skinfold measurements), may not be sensitive to certain components of body composition and hence may produce inaccurate estimates of exercise-related changes in body composition.

For a significant amount of fat loss to occur, more energy must be expended than consumed. This is best achieved by reducing caloric intake and increasing physical activity. Endurance activity can be performed longer than resistance activity and is generally more useful for increasing caloric expenditure and fat loss. However, resistance training is more likely to preserve fat-free mass during weight loss and may help reduce fat (75). Therefore, weight loss programs should include both endurance and resistance training as part of the exercise program. Exercise should be prescribed to maximize total energy expenditure without undue fatigue. The optimal exercise prescription for weight control using resistance exercise remains unclear.

E. Medical Complications of Exercise

The possible medical complications of exercise are numerous (76). Fortunately, serious complications are rare, and common complications are minor. Musculoskeletal and traumatic injuries, the most frequent hazards of exercise, are usually self-limited, with only 10–20% requiring medical attention (77, 78). However, serious and even fatal events do occur during increased levels of activity, particularly in individuals who are not habitually active. This chapter focuses on these complications.

Cardiovascular Complications Of Exercise

Cardiovascular complications are cause for the most concern. Almost all such complications occur in individuals with underlying acquired heart disease or congenital abnormalities; individuals without heart disease have a low risk of a cardiac event during exercise. These complications can be divided into two general groups based on

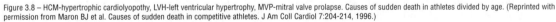

Figure 3.8 – HCM-hypertrophic cardiolyopothy, LVH-left ventricular hypertrophy, MVP-mitral valve prolapse. Causes of sudden death in athletes divided by age. (Reprinted with permission from Maron BJ et al. Causes of sudden death in competitive athletes. J Am Coll Cardiol 7:204-214, 1996.)

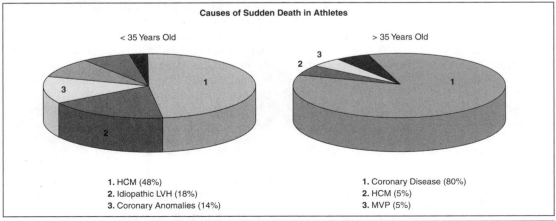

Causes of Sudden Death in Athletes

< 35 Years Old
> 35 Years Old

1. HCM (48%)
2. Idiopathic LVH (18%)
3. Coronary Anomalies (14%)

1. Coronary Disease (80%)
2. HCM (5%)
3. MVP (5%)

age. Cardiac problems in those older than 35 tend to be due to coronary heart disease (CHD), while those that occur in persons younger than 35 are usually secondary to cardiovascular structural abnormalities (4–6) (Fig. 3.8).

Complications in Those with Coronary Heart Disease

Coronary heart disease (CHD) is the leading cause of serious injury and death during high activity levels in those over 35 years of age. In a healthy population, a cardiac event during exercise is uncommon, but in those with underlying CHD, exercise may trigger an acute myocardial infarction (MI) and/or sudden cardiac death (79, 82–84).

Complications in Those with Cardiac Structural Defects

While CHD is the leading cause of death during exercise in the elderly, anatomical defects are the foremost cause of sudden death in young athletes. All of these congenital abnormalities are rare; the most common are hypertrophic cardiomyopathy, coronary artery anomalies, and Marfan syndrome. These three defects account for almost three-quarters of 158 deaths in young competitive athletes examined by Maron *et al.* (81) between 1985 and 1995.

Anomalous Coronary Artery

The second-largest group of structural defects in young athletes who die suddenly are abnormalities in coronary arteries. These arteries arise from and/or course through atypical locations, and occasionally, because of their anatomical position, an interruption of blood flow results in sudden death. The risk of occlusion (blockage) is particularly high during and immediately after exercise. All coronary artery anomalies are rare, but most common are the following:

1. Left coronary artery arising from the anterior sinus of Valsalva (right cusp of the aortic valve) and coursing between the aorta and pulmonary trunk (86).
2. Mural left anterior descending artery (artery tunneled into the ventricular wall) (87).

Less common coronary artery anomalies resulting in sudden death include the following:

1. Single artery
2. Hypoplasia (small size or short course)
3. Intussusception (inward convulsion)
4. Aneurysm
5. Acute-angled takeoff of the left main coronary artery (88, 89)

Coronary artery anomalies are difficult to identify prospectively. However, there may be prior episodes of syncope, exertional angina, or resting electrocardiographic (ECG) abnormalities (86). Some types of anomalous arteries may be excluded by echocardiography but may be clearly visualized with magnetic resonance imaging. Those who are identified, particularly with the left coronary artery arising from the right cusp of the aorta, should not participate in competitive sports unless they have undergone surgical correction (85).

Marfan Syndrome

Marfan syndrome is an inherited connective tissue disease that predisposes affected individuals to develop aortic aneurysm. It is suspected in tall, thin individuals, such as basketball and volleyball players, with physical characteristics consistent with Marfan's and a family history of sudden death. Possible physical findings include an outflow murmur and the presence of a pulsatile mass in the abdomen. If suspected, aneurysms can be screened with ultrasound. If undetected, these aneurysms may rupture during vigorous activity and cause death (90).

Complications of Exercise Testing

An exercise test is heavy physical exertion by an individual in a controlled setting. As such, the same complications seen in the general population during increased activity may occur. Most of these complications are, as in the general population, rare, and range from minor to serious.

In those without known heart disease, exercise testing is a very low risk procedure. For example, no complications occurred in 380,000 exercise tests done in young individuals presumed to be free of heart disease (92). In addition, in 71,914 exercise tests performed at a single institution as part of a preventive medicine program, only one cardiac complication occurred among persons without known CHD (93).

Arrhythmic Complications

Arrhythmias can be precipitated by exercise and so may be encountered during exercise testing and cardiac rehabilitation. Two of the most serious arrhythmias are ventricular fibrillation and ventricular tachycardia. Most cases of ventricular fibrillation during exercise in the general population are fatal because they are not identified and treated. During exercise testing and cardiac rehabilitation, however, participants are closely monitored, and ventricular fibrillation may be identified and its prevalence determined.

Ventricular tachycardia is a rapid arrhythmia of the ventricles that can degenerate to ventricular fibrillation which usually suggests myocardial scar rather than myocardial ischemia. It is slightly more common than ventricular fibrillation and was found to arise 29 times in 50,000 exercise tests (5.8/10,000 tests) (91). Both ventricular tachycardia and ventricular fibrillation require immediate treatment with direct current cardioversion with a defibrillator.

Other far less common arrhythmias that may occur during exercise testing are atrial tachycardia, sinus bradycardia, atrial fibrillation, atrioventricular nodal tachycardia, atrial flutter, second-degree atrioventricular block, and left bundle branch block (91). Arrhythmias are most likely to occur in those with a history of arrhythmia.

Contraindications to Exercise Testing

Because exercise testing can be dangerous, it is crucial to identify those who are at increased risk for complications and exclude them when necessary. All personnel involved in performing exercise testing should be familiar with contraindications and precautions. There are published guidelines for contraindications to exercise testing (Box 3.1) (94, 95).

In general, contraindications are conditions that may be aggravated by exercise or that may affect exercise performance. For example, exercise testing in an individual with unstable angina may precipitate MI or fatal arrhythmia. Severe aortic stenosis, dissecting aneurysm, and myocarditis increase the risk of a fatal complication. These contraindications are empirical rather than based on clinical studies.

The experience level of the personnel conducting the test, access to emergency medical equipment and services, and the benefit of testing should be considered in the decision as to whether a safe exercise test can be performed on persons whose health indicates precautions. In some cases, a decision to defer testing until the individual is treated and more stable is appropriate. Changes in the mode and protocol for exercise and/or end points for stopping the test can contribute to the safety of the test in some cases. The ability to monitor changes in the ECG and blood pressure is critical, and the presence of a health care professional with extensive experience in exercise testing and a low threshold for stopping the test is crucial for testing.

Indications to Stop an Exercise

Terminating an exercise test depends on the expertise and judgment of those supervising it (94, 96, 97). As with contraindications, the setting and indications for the test may influence termination. Increasing angina (chest pain), hypotension (very low blood pressure), signs and symptoms of myocardial ischemia (lack of oxygenated blood flow to the heart), and serious arrhythmias are serious problems that may precipitate test termination (Box 3.2). Other reasons, such as the technical inability to monitor the ECG and request by the client, are self-evident. The decision to continue with the test should be made by an experienced health care professional, preferably with a physician in attendance or accessible during the test. Clients should be treated cautiously, with a tendency to stop the test sooner rather than later.

Box 3.1 – Contraindications to Exercise Testing*

Absolute
- A recent significant change in the resting ECG suggesting significant ischemia, recent myocardial infarction (within 2 days) or other acute cardiac event
- Unstable angina
- Uncontrolled cardiac arrhythmias causing symptoms or hemodynamic compromise
- Severe symptomatic aortic stenosis
- Uncontrolled symptomatic heart failure
- Acute pulmonary embolus or pulmonary infarction
- Acute myocarditis or pericarditis
- Suspected or known dissecting aneurysm
- Acute infections

Relative†
- Left main coronary stenosis
- Moderate stenotic valvular heart disease
- Electrolyte abnormalities (e.g., hypokalemia, hypomagnesemia)
- Severe arterial hypertension (i.e., systolic BP of >200 mm Hg and/or a diastolic BP of >110 mm Hg) at rest
- Tachyarrhythmias or bradyarrhythmias
- Hypertrophic cardiomyopathy and other forms of outflow tract obstruction
- Neuromuscular, musculoskeletal, or rheumatoid disorders that are exacerbated by exercise
- High-degree atrioventricular block
- Ventricular aneurysm
- Uncontrolled metabolic disease (e.g., diabetes, thyrotoxicosis, or myxedema)
- Chronic infectious disease (e.g., mononucleosis, hepatitis, AIDS)

*Modified from Gibbons RA, Balady GJ, Beasely JW, et al. ACC/AHA guidelines for exercise testing. J Am Coll Cardiol 1997;30:260–315.

†Relative contraindications can be superseded if benefits outweigh risks of exercise. In some instances, these individuals can be exercised with caution and/or using low-level end points, especially if they are asymptomatic at rest.

Box 3.2 – General Indications for Stopping an Exercise Test in Low-Risk Adults*

- Onset of angina or angina-like symptoms.
- Significant drop (20 mm Hg) in systolic blood pressure or a failure of the systolic blood pressure to rise with an increase in exercise intensity.
- Excessive rise in blood pressure: systolic pressure > 260 mm Hg or diastolic pressure > 115 mm Hg.
- Signs of poor perfusion: light-headedness, confusion, ataxia, pallor, cyanosis, nausea, or cold and clammy skin.
- Failure of heart rate to increase with increased exercise intensity.
- Noticeable change in heart rhythm.
- Subject requests to stop.
- Physical or verbal manifestations of severe fatigue.
- Failure of the testing equipment.

*Assumes that testing is nondiagnostic and is being performed without direct physician involvement or electrocardiographic monitoring. For clinical testing, Box 5-3 provides more definitive and specific termination criteria.

Follow-up after Terminating an Exercise Test

If an exercise test is terminated, the health care personnel supervising the test must carry out the appropriate course of action. Appropriate follow-up may include any or all of the following:

1. Notification of and attendance by a physician if one was not present during the exercise test
2. Careful observation of ECG, blood pressure, and other signs and symptoms until the condition subsides or stabilizes
3. Treatment (*i.e.*, of arrhythmias or angina) when qualified medical personnel are in attendance
4. Phone contact with primary and/or referring physicians

5. Transport to an emergency department or physician's office
6. Access to the emergency medical system

Regardless of the course of action, documentation, including ECG tracings, blood pressure recordings, and all test results, should be provided to the physician.

Noncardiovascular Complications of Exercise

Heat Complications

Overheating is a leading cause of noncardiovascular deaths in young athletes (80). Heat injury is a function of environment, degree of exposure, intensity of exercise, prior conditioning, and preexisting physical illness. Athletes are most prone to develop heat illness when they are not acclimated to hot weather, are wearing heavy clothing (such as full football gear), are dehydrated, have sickle cell trait, and/or are in a hot and humid climate (98).

Under these conditions complications range from minor to fatal. The illnesses that may be precipitated by exercise in warm climates are heat rash, heat cramps, heat syncope, heat exhaustion, and exertional heat stroke. Most of these problems are benign and self-limited, but heat exhaustion and exertional heat stroke may be fatal if not properly treated.

Heat exhaustion is characterized by intense thirst, goose bumps, dizziness, fatigue, rapid pulse, muscle cramps, nausea, vomiting, syncope, and, in advanced stages, circulatory failure. Heavy sweating usually persists throughout the course of illness. Core temperature remains below 40°C (104°F) and there is no tissue injury. Heat exhaustion may progress to heat stroke.

Heat stroke is different from heat exhaustion in that core temperature rises above 41°C (105.8°F), resulting in significant tissue injury. The skin may feel cool and the athlete often shivers, making it important to measure core temperature for the diagnosis. Sweating may cease in heat stroke, in contrast to heat exhaustion. When this occurs, body temperature regulation is lost and a true medical emergency arises. There may be mental status changes; victims sometime progress to convulsions and/or coma. Rhabdomyolysis, acute renal failure, hemolysis, myocardial infarction, hyperkalemia, and hepatic necrosis can also develop, and, if untreated, death often follows (99).

To treat heat exhaustion and exertional heat stroke, the victim should be moved to a cooler environment and the body cooled with fans, ice, and wet cloths. Excessive clothing must be removed and the feet elevated. Intake of oral fluids should be encouraged. Heat stroke requires additional more intensive treatment (chilled intravenous saline and possibly hospitalization), but these actions may be performed until trained medical personnel are present.

Heat illness may be prevented by avoiding the extremes of weather or by gradual adaptation to activity in hot climates. It is recommended that athletes curtail activities when the wet bulb–globe temperature, an index of temperature, humidity, and radiation, is greater than 28°C (82°F) (100). In addition, maintaining adequate hydration is an important aspect of prevention.

Hydration-Related Complications

To maintain body temperature in a physiological range during exercise, sweating is necessary to promote heat loss. Water and electrolytes, mainly sodium and chloride, are lost in sweat. During prolonged exercise, this loss leads to dehydration (a loss of more water than sodium with a resulting rise in serum sodium), which impairs exercise performance. The amount lost is determined by the rate of sweating (which depends on the intensity of exertion), ambient temperature, humidity, amount of clothing, and acclimation level of the athlete, as well as individual variation. Depending on these factors, sweat rates can range from 0.5 to 3.7 $L \cdot h^{-1}$. Children have lower sweat rates than adults.

Fluid ingestion during prolonged exercise is recommended to prevent significant dehydration (100). The ideal fluid is an isotonic carbohydrate–electrolyte solution that fulfills dual purposes of replacing sweat loss and providing carbohydrate fuel, such as glucose, to supplement tissue stores. Fluid replacement is generally not necessary for exercise lasting less than 30 min, but it becomes more important with prolonged activity (101).

Table 3.9 – Suggested Guidelines for Fluid Replacement During Prolonged Exercise

1. Immediately prior to exercise or during warm-up, ingest up to 300 mL of cool (about 10°C) flavored water.
2. For the initial 60–75 min of exercise, ingest 100–150 mL of a cool, dilute (5 g/100 mL) glucose polymer solution at regular (10–15 minute) intervals. It seems unwarranted to consume CHO in amounts much greater than 30 g during this period, since only 20 g of ingested CHO are oxidized in the first hour of moderate-intensity exercise, irrespective of the type of CHO consumed or the drinking regimen.
3. After 75–90 min of exercise, increase concentration of ingested glucose polymer solution to 10–12 g/100 mL plus 20 mEq/L sodium. Higher sodium concentrations, although possibly may promote rapid intestinal fluid absorption, are not palatable to most athletes. Small amounts of potassium (2–4 mEq/L), which may facilitate rehydration of the intracellular fluid compartment, may be included. For the remainder of the exercise, consume 100–150 mL of this solution at 10–15-min intervals. Such a regimen ensures optimal rates of fluid and energy delivery, limiting any dehydration-induced decreases in plasma volume and maintaining the rate on ingested CHO oxidation at about 1 g/min late in exercise.

CHO, carbohydrate.

Reprinted with permission from Nokes TD et al. Fluid and energy replacement during prolonged exercise. Curr Ther Sport Med 517–520, 1995.

The exact amount of fluid that should be ingested during exercise is not established. The American College of Sports Medicine "Position Paper on the Prevention of Thermal Injuries during Distance Running" (100) recommends that participants in foot races be encouraged to drink 100–200 mL of water every 2–3 km of the race. This is only a guideline; it may be too much or too little, depending on the environment and the pace and sweat rate of the athlete. Overconsumption of water can lead to hyponatremia (low serum sodium), a rare condition that may cause medical problems (102). Thus, correct fluid intake, neither too much nor too little, is key to optimal performance and avoidance of medical complications. Guidelines to help achieve this balance are presented in Table 3.9.

Complications in Special Populations

Exercise considerations for some special populations are beyond the scope of practice of the certified Personal Trainer. Further information is available *in ACSM's Guidelines For Exercise Testing and Prescription*, 6th Edition, Lippincott Williams & Wilkins Publishers, 2000 and *ACSM's Resource Manual for Guidelines For Exercise Testing And Presciption*, 4th Edition, Lippincott Williams & Wilkins Publishers, 2001.

SECTION III References

1. Casperson CJ, Powell KE, Christenson GM. Physical activity, exercise and physical fitness: Definitions and distinctions for health-related research. Public Health Rep 100:126, 1985.
2. Pate RR, Pratt M, Blair SN, et al. Physical activity and public health: A recommendation from the Centers for Disease Control and Prevention and the American College of Sports Medicine. JAMA 273:402, 1995.
3. American College of Sports Medicine. ACSM Guidelines for Exercise Testing and Prescription. Philadelphia: Lippincott Williams & Wilkins, 2000.
4. Fletcher GF, Balady G, Blair SN, et al. Statement on exercise: Benefits and recommendations for physical activity programs for all Americans. Circulation 94:857, 1996.
5. American College of Sports Medicine. The recommended quantity and quality of exercise for developing and maintaining CR, muscular fitness and flexibility in healthy adults. Med Sci Sports Exerc 30:975, 1998.
6. Harris SS, Caspersen CJ, DeFriese GH, et al. Physical activity counseling for healthy adults as a primary preventive intervention in the clinical setting: Report for the US Preventive Services Task Force. JAMA 261:3590, 1989.
7. NIH Consensus Development Panel. Physical activity and cardiovascular health. JAMA 276:241, 1996.
8. U.S. Surgeon General. Physical activity and health: A report of the Surgeon General. Washington: U.S. Government Printing Office, 1996.
9. McArdle WD, Katch FI, Katch VL. Exercise Physiology. Baltimore: Williams & Wilkins, 1996.
10. MacAlpin RH, Kattus AA. Adaptation to exercise in angina pectoris: The electrocardiogram during treadmill walking and coronary angiographic findings. Circulation 33:183, 1966.
11. Powell KE, Thompson PD, Caspersen CJ, et al. Physical activity and the incidence of coronary heart disease. Ann Rev Public Health 8:253, 1987.
12. Blair SN, Kohl HW, Paffenbarger RS, et al. Physical fitness and all-cause mortality: A prospective study of healthy men and women. JAMA 262:2395, 1989.
13. Blair SN, Kohl HW, Barlow CE, et al. Changes in physical fitness and all-cause mortality: A prospective study of healthy and unhealthy men. JAMA 273:1093, 1995.
14. Lee IM, Hsieh CC, Paffenbarger, RS Jr. Exercise intensity and longevity in men: The Harvard alumni study. JAMA 273:1179, 1995.
15. Haskell WH. Dose-response issues from a biological perspective. In: Bouchard C, Shepard RJ, Stephens T, eds. Physical Activity, Fitness, and Health. Champaign, IL: Human Kinetics, 1994.
16. Cahill B, ed. Proceedings of the Conference on Strength Training and the Prepubescent. Chicago: American Orthopaedic Society for Sports Medicine, 1988.
17. Kraemer WJ, Fleck SJ. Strength Training for Young Athletes. Champaign, IL: Human Kinetics, 1993.
18. Tanner SM. Weighing the risks: Strength training for children and adolescents. Phys Sportsmed 21:105, 1993.
19. Peterson JA, Bryant CX. The StairMaster Fitness Handbook. Champaign, IL: Sagamore, 1995.
20. Munnings F. Strength training: Not only for the young. Phys Sportsmed 21:133, 1993.
21. Bryant CX, Peterson JA. Strength training for the heart? Fitness Manag 2:32, 1994.
22. Franklin BA, Bonzheim K, Gordon S, et al. Resistance training in cardiac rehabilitation. J Cardiopulm Rehab 11:99, 1991.
23. McKelvie RS, McCartney N. Weightlifting training in cardiac patients: considerations. Sports Med 10:355, 1990.
24. Fleck SJ, Kraemer WJ. Designing Resistance Training Programs. 2nd ed. Champaign, IL: Human Kinetics, 1997.
25. American College of Sports Medicine. ACSM's Guidelines for Exercise Testing and Prescription. 6th ed. Philadelphia: Lippincott Williams & Wilkins, 2000.
26. American Association of Cardiovascular and Pulmonary Rehabilitation. Guidelines for Cardiac Rehabilitation Programs. 3rd ed. Champaign, IL: Human Kinetics, 1999.
27. Hakkinen K. Factors influencing trainability of muscular strength during short term and prolonged training. Natl Strength Cond Assoc J 7:32, 1985.
28. Kraemer WJ, Deschenes MR, Fleck SJ. Physiological adaptations to resistance exercise: Implications for athletic conditioning. Sports Med 6:246, 1988.
29. DiNubile NA. Strength training. Clin Sports Med 10:33, 1991.
30. Peterson JA, Bryant CX, Peterson SL. Strength Training for Women. Champaign, IL: Human Kinetics, 1995.
31. National Strength and Conditioning Association. Position statement on prepubescent strength training. Natl Strength Condit Assoc J 7:27, 1985.
32. Ettinger WH, Burns R, Messier SP, et al. A randomized trial comparing aerobic exercise and resistance exercise with a health education program in older adults with knee osteoarthritis: The Fitness Arthritis and Seniors Trial (FAST). JAMA 277:25–31, 1997.
33. Webster's Ninth New Collegiate Dictionary. Merriam-Webster, 1991.
34. Morris HF. Sports Medicine Handbook. 1st ed. Dubuque, IA: William C. Brown 1984:45–51.
35. Per-Olof A, Rodahl K. Textbook of Work Physiology. 2nd ed. St Louis: McGraw Hill, 1977:72–79.
36. Garfin SR, Tipton CM, MuBarak SJ, et al. Role of fascia in maintenance of muscle tension and pressure. J Appl Physiol 51:317–319, 1981.
37. Mozam K, Lawrence J, Keagy R. Muscle relationships in functional fascia. Clin Orthop 150:403–409, 1978.
38. Anderson B. Stretching: 20th Anniversary, Bolinas, CA: Shelter Publications, 2000.
39. Altrig Z, Hoffman J, Martin J. Clinical Exercise Testing Prescription and Rehabilitation. 5th ed. Philadelphia: Lea & Febiger, 1992:123–126.
40. Chu D. Plyometrics. Livermore, CA: Bittersweet, 1989:8–15, 78–79.
41. Beaulieu JE. Stretching for All Sports. Pasadena, CA: Athletic, 1980:5–50.
42. Moffatt RJ. Strength and flexibility considerations for exercise prescription. In: Blair SN, Painter P, Pate R, et al., eds. Resource Manual for ACSM Guidelines for Exercise Testing and Prescription. Philadelphia: Lea & Febiger, 1988.
43. Bersin D, Bersin K, Reese M. Relaxercise Based on Feldenkrais Theory. New York: Harper & Row, 1990:3–97.
44. Satchidananda YS. Integral Yoga-Hatha. Holt, Rinehart & Winston, 1970 11–65.
45. Hittleman A. Hittleman's Yoga 28 Day Exercise Plan. New York: Workman, 1969.
46. American College of Sports Medicine. ACSM's Guidelines for Exercise Testing and Prescription. Philadelphia: Lippincott Williams & Wilkins, 2000.
47. deVries H. Evaluation of static stretching procedures for flexibility. Res Q Exerc Sport 33:222–229, 1962.

48. deVries H. Physiology of Exercise: Flexibility 1981. J Phys Ed Recreat Dance 52:41, 1980.

49. Anderson B. 8 Minute Stretch. Women Sports Fitness Nov–Dec:46–52, 1989.

50. Krusen's Handbook of Physical Medicine and Rehabilitation. 4th ed. By Frederic J. Kottke, MD, Professor Emeritus, Department of Physical Medicine and Rehabilitation, University of Minnesota Medical School, Minneapolis, MN; and Justus F. Lehmann, MD, Professor, Department of Rehabilitation Medicine, University of Washington School of Medicine, Seattle, WA.

51. Kuland D. The Injured Athlete. Philadelphia: Lippincott, 1982:165–176.

52. Karpovich PV, Hale C. Effects of warming up upon physical performance. JAMA 162:1117–1119, 1956.

53. Jensen C. Pertinent facts about warm up. Athlet J 56:72–75, 1975.

54. Martin BJ. Effects of warm up on metabolic responses to strenuous exercise. Med Sci Sports Exerc 7:146–149, 1975.

55. Kisner C, Colby LA. Therapeutic Exercise Foundations and Techniques. 2nd ed. Philadelphia: Davis, 1990.

56. Knott M, Voss D. Proprioceptive Neuromuscular Facilitation. 2nd ed. New York: Harper & Row, 1968.

57. Hutton A. Three Techniques Comparing Stretching of the Hamstrings. University of California, 1979. (Abstract reported).

58. Etnyre BR, Lee EJ. Chronic and acute flexibility of men and women using three different stretching techniques. Res Q Exerc Sport 59:222–228, 1988.

59. Agre JC. Static Stretching for Athletes. Arch Phys Med 59:561, 1978.

60. Logan H, Egstrom GH. The effects of slow and fast stretching on sacrofemoral angle. J Assoc Phys Mental Rehabil 15:85, 1988.

61. Kraemer WJ, Fleck SJ, Evans WJ. Strength and power training: Physiological mechanisms of adaptation. Exerc Sport Sci Rev 24:363–397, 1996.

62. Dudley GA, Fleck SJ. Strength and endurance training: Are they mutually exclusive? Sports Med 4:79–85, 1987.

63. Hickson RC. Interface of strength development by simultaneously training for strength and endurance. Eur J Appl Physiol 45:255–263, 1980.

64. Dudley GA, Djamil R. Incompatibility of endurance- and strength-training mode of exercise. J Appl Physiol 59:1446–1451, 1985.

65. Sale DG, MacDougall JD, Jacobs I, Garner S. Interaction between concurrent strength and endurance training. J Appl Physiol 68:260–270, 1990.

66. McCarthy JP, Agre JC, Graf BK, et al. Compatibility of adaptive responses with combining strength and endurance training. Med Sci Sports Exerc 27:429–436, 1995.

67. Moritani T, DeVries HA. Neural factors versus hypertrophy in the time course of muscle strength gain. Am J Phys Med 58:115–130, 1979.

68. Ploutz LL, Tesch PA, Biro RL, et al. Effect of resistance training on muscle use during exercise. J Appl Physiol 6:1675–1681, 1994.

69. Thorstensson A, Karlsson J, Viitasalo JH, et al. Effect of strength training on EMG of human skeletal muscle. Acta Physiol Scand 98:232–236, 1976.

70. Duchateau J, Hainaut K. Isometric or dynamic training: Differential effects on mechanical properties of a human muscle. J Appl Physiol 56:296–301, 1984.

71. Stauber WT. Eccentric action of muscles: Physiology, injury, and adaptation. Exerc Sport Sci Rev 17:157–185, 1989.

72. Fox EL, Bartels RL, Klinzing J, et al. Metabolic responses to interval training programs of high and low power output. Med Sci Sports Exerc 9:191–196, 1977.

73. Gillespie AC, Fox EL, Merola AJ. Enzyme adaptations in rat skeletal muscle after two intensities of treadmill training. Med Sci Sports Exerc 14:461–466, 1982.

74. Johns RJ, Wright V. Relative importance of various tissues in joint stiffness. J Appl Physiol 17:824–828, 1962.

75. Walberg JL. Aerobic exercise and resistance weight-training during weight reduction: Implications for obese persons and athletes. Sports Med 47:343–346, 1989.

76. Levine BD, Stray-Gundersen J. The medical care of competitive athletes: The role of the individual and the individual assumption of risk. Med Sci Sports Exerc 26:1190–1192, 1994.

77. Kraus JF, Conroy C. Mortality and morbidity from injuries in sports and recreation. Ann Rev Pub Health 5:163–192, 1984.

78. Koplan JP, Siscovick DS, Goldbaum GM. The risks of exercise: A public health view of injuries and hazards. Pub Health Rep 100:189–195, 1985.

79. Albert CM, Mittleman MA, Chae CU, Lee IM, Hennekens CH, Manson JE. Triggering of sudden death from cardiac causes by vigorous exertion. N Engl J Med 343:1355–1361, 2000.

80. Van Camp SP, Bloor CM, Mueller FU, et al. Nontraumatic sports deaths in high school and college athletes. Med Sci Sports Exerc 27:641–647, 1995.

81. Maron BJ, Shirani J, Poliac LC, et al. Sudden death in young competitive athletes. JAMA 276:199–204, 1996.

82. Opie LH. Sudden death and sport. Lancet 1:263–266, 1975.

83. Mittleman MA, MaClure M, Tofler GH, et al. Triggering of acute myocardial infarction by heavy physical exertion. N Engl J Med 329:1677–1683, 1993.

84. Willich SN, Lewis M, Lowel H, et al. Physical exertion as a trigger of acute myocardial infarction. N Engl J Med 329:1684–1690, 1993.

85. Maron BJ, Mitchell JH. 26th Bethesda Conference. Recommendations for determining eligibility for competition in athletes with cardiovascular abnormalities. Revised recommendations for competitive athletes with cardiovascular abnormalities. J Am Coll Cardiol 24:845–899, 1994.

86. Barth CW, Roberts WC. Left main coronary artery originating from the right sinus of Valsalva and coursing between the aorta and pulmonary trunk. J Am Coll Cardiol 7:366–373, 1986.

87. Morales AR, Romanelli R, Bovcek RJ. The mural left anterior descending coronary artery, strenuous exercise and sudden death. Circulation 62:230–237, 1980.

88. Roberts WC, Glick BN. Congenital hypoplasia of both right and left circumflex coronary arteries. Am J Cardiol 70:121–123, 1992.

89. Roberts WC, Silver MA, Sapala JC. Intussusception of a coronary artery associated with sudden death in a college football player. Am J Cardiol 57:179–180, 1986.

90. Tahernia AC. Cardiovascular anomalies in Marfan's syndrome: The role of echocardiography and beta-blockers. South Med J 86:305–310, 1993.

91. Atterhog JH, Bjorn J, Samuelsson R. Exercise testing: A prospective study of complication rates. Am Heart J 98:572–579, 1979.

92. Wendt TH, Scherer D, Kaltenbach M. Life-threatening complications in 1,741,106 ergometries. Dtsch Med Wochenschr 109:123–127, 1984.

93. Gibbons L, Blair SN, Kohl HW, et al. The safety of maximal exercise testing. Circulation 80:846–852, 1989.

94. Young DZ, Lampert S, Graboys TB, et al. Safety of maximal exercise testing in patients at high risk for ventricular arrhythmias. Circulation 70:184–191, 1984.

95. American College of Sports Medicine. ACSM's Guidelines for Exercise Testing and Prescription. 6th ed. Philadelphia: Lippincott Williams & Wilkins, 2000.

96. Dubach P, Froelicher VF, Klein J, et al. Exercise-induced hypotension in a male population. Circulation 78: 1380–1387, 1988.

97. Fletcher GF, Balady G, Froelicher VF, et al. Exercise standards: A statement for healthcare professionals from the American Heart Association. Circulation 91:580–615, 1995.

98. Kark JA, Posey DM, Schumacher HR, et al. Sickle-cell trait as a risk factor for sudden death in physical training. N Engl J Med 317:781–787, 1987.

99. Knochel JP. Pathophysiology of heat stroke. In: Hopkins, Ellis, eds. Hyperthermia and Hypermetabolic Disorders. Cambridge, UK: Cambridge University Press, 1996:42–62.

100. American College of Sports Medicine. Position statement on the prevention of thermal injuries during distance running. Med Sci Sports Exerc 19:529–533, 1987.

101. Noakes TD. Dehydration during exercise, what are the real dangers. J Clin Sport Med 5:123–128, 1995.

102. Frizell RT, Lang GH, Lowance DC, et al. Hyponatremia and ultramarathon running. JAMA 255:772–774, 1986.

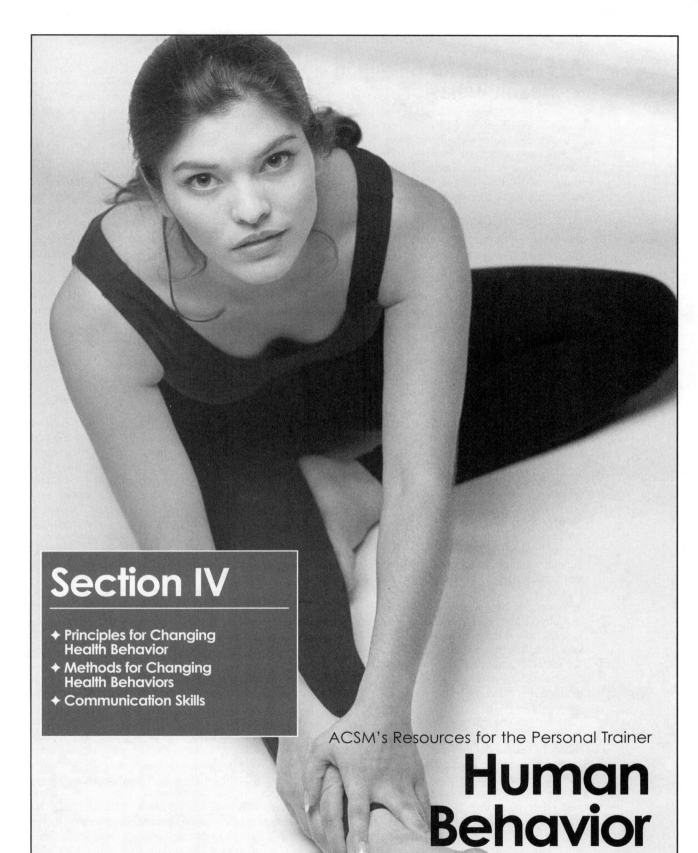

Section IV

- ✦ **Principles for Changing Health Behavior**
- ✦ **Methods for Changing Health Behaviors**
- ✦ **Communication Skills**

ACSM's Resources for the Personal Trainer

Human Behavior

A. Principles for Changing Health Behavior

Assisting clients to begin and maintain health behavior change is a challenge even for the most experienced certified Personal Trainer (cPT). Nevertheless, behavioral scientists have identified strategies that if systematically applied, are useful in helping an individual begin and sustain health behavior change (1). The transtheoretical model, developed by Prochaska and DiClimente, has had the greatest influence in recent years on designing exercise interventions and has been applied to a number of health behavior change areas (2–4). This model predicts a progression of behavior change through a series of stages: precontemplation (no intent and no exercise), contemplation (intent, but no exercise), preparation (intent and occasional exercise), action (regular exercise), and maintenance (exercising for six months or more). Progression through these stages is related to use of various behavior change strategies, the expected outcomes of exercise (both pros and cons), and self-confidence, or self-efficacy. Marcus *et al.* (5) showed that a work site exercise program designed to account for a level of motivation had a significantly stronger effect than one that did not.

The transtheoretical model is partly derived from social learning theory, a comprehensive analysis of human functioning in which human behavior is assumed to be developed and maintained on the basis of three interacting systems: behavioral, cognitive, and environmental (6). Social learning theory emphasizes the human capacity for self-directed behavior change. Willingness to change is related to self-confidence, which is influenced by four main factors: persuasion from an authority, observation of others, successful performance of the behavior, and physiological feedback. Social learning theory is a useful model to help in the understanding of why people change; behavioral therapy provides the methods and strategies for effecting and maintaining behavior change. Many excellent and detailed discussions of behavior change programs are available (7–10).

Other theoretical models have added useful ideas for conceptualizing behavior change. The theory of reasoned action and the theory of planned behavior describe the relations among health beliefs, attitudes, intentions, behavior, and perceived behavioral control as applied to exercise and other behaviors (11–13). The health belief model also emphasizes the role of beliefs in determining health care behavior (14). In this model, the important variables influencing behavior include the readiness to make a change, the perceived benefit of the change, cues to action, and modifying factors, such as knowledge and socioeconomic background. Also, the cognitive and behavioral processes used in changing health behaviors have been examined, particularly in relation to exercise (4). Finally, comprehensive models of behavior change, including systems and even community factors, may provide helpful ideas for designing more effective programs (15, 16).

Health Behavior Change Model

Health behavior change can be conceptualized as occurring in stages, arbitrarily divided into the antecedent, adoption, and maintenance phases. The antecedent stage includes the precontemplation, contemplation, and preparation components of the transtheoretical model (3). Antecedents refer to all conditions that can assist, initiate, hinder, or support change. For example, observing the benefits a friend receives from exercising may serve as an antecedent or stimulus for motivation to begin an exercise program. Adoption (or the action phase in the transtheoretical model) comprises the early phases of a behavior change program. Maintenance applies to later phases when the participant is undergoing behavior change.

Antecedents

People sometimes decide to change for reasons that they do not understand or that are beyond their control. A chance encounter with a friend who has made important changes and looks better, an illness, a caustic remark from a coworker, and loose clothes that become tight are all events that may initiate a health behavior change. Nevertheless, social learning theory and the transtheoretical model predict that certain antecedents to behavior change are useful in increasing intention to change. If you ask a person to rate intention on a scale from 0 to 10 in which 0 indicates no intention to change and 10 indicates certainty, people with little intention are not likely to change, whereas those persons with higher scores of intention are more likely to change (17). Intentions frequently change and can be influenced by many factors. For motivated individuals, environmental cues such as posters or notes on bulletin boards may stimulate a behavior change.

Information

Intention to change often begins with information, which should be presented in simple and clear ways using language that is understandable. About 30–40% of the public read at a seventh-grade level or lower. Information is most effective when combined with instructions about how to make the changes. Information about benefits to change rather than risks from no change may be emphasized for more impact. Although pamphlets, self-help books, and handouts are often used to communicate health information, most people read no more than 10–15% of such material unless they are extremely interested or are held accountable. Some audiences who would seem to benefit most from information may ignore it. For instance, smokers ignore messages about the risks of smoking, nonexercisers know less about the benefits of physical activity than exercisers, and poorly educated groups may not read long with complicated materials. Knowledge critical to behavior change should be tested prior to the program so myths and misperceptions can be corrected.

Instructions

Instructions to change a particular behavior (persuasion) from a person of authority are a powerful antecedent to behavior change. The public considers health care professionals the most credible source of information. Persuasion from an authoritative figure should occur in a kind, but firm manner. People reluctant to make health behavior change listen for ambivalence in the message. They are not, for example, likely to follow this message: "Smoking is bad for your health; you should think about stopping." They are more likely to be affected by this: "You must stop smoking." Instructions should be clear, achievable, and accompanied by necessary information about how to bring about change. In addition, reminders and feedback should reinforce instructions. Participants should be asked to repeat the critical information.

Models

Role models, whether family, friends, or other credible sources (*e.g.,* health professionals), can facilitate change by allowing the participant to see how other individuals make change, react to change, generalize change to different types of situations (*e.g.,* how people practice food changes at home, in restaurants, and in grocery stores), and cope with difficult situations to maintain healthy habits. People undergoing health behavior change can benefit from being asked to think of persons they know or admire who have made changes. Videotapes or films demonstrating how individuals have made changes and the effect of change can be effective in increasing intention to change.

Experience

Experience is a major factor in determining initiation of a new health behavior. People are more likely to repeat a behavior if it was helpful in the past. Experience may also lead to superstitious health traps. A cold that seemed to resolve more rapidly than usual may, for example, be associated with taking a vitamin whether or not the vitamin is helpful. The level of confidence to try a new behavior is largely determined by experience. Review of previous success or failure may assist with the change process. Examination of a previously unsuccessful attempt at exercise, for example, may reveal ways to encourage adoption of the behavior in a future attempt. People often need to develop new skills to be more effective before

change can occur. Developing new skills leads to increased confidence and intention to change.

Other Incentives and Disincentives

Other incentives and disincentives are important antecedents for health behavior change. Incentives should be built into a program and should outweigh the disincentives. Clients should be encouraged to answer the question, "How can I make sure that I benefit from this program?" Some of the benefits may be obvious, such as exercising to feel and look better, while other benefits may not be as obvious, such as exercising to prevent disease. Reducing disincentives when beginning an exercise program is equally important. Participants may begin exercise at an inconvenient time, in a place that does not appeal to them, or with an activity that is not enjoyable. Such disincentives almost ensure that a program will be short lived.

Careful attention to antecedents can influence intention to adopt behavior change. With sufficient information, compelling instructions, appropriate models to change, positive physiological feedback, increased confidence to change, and maximized incentives and minimized disincentives, a health behavior change is likely to be adopted. An examination of the antecedents for change answers these questions:

- What does the client need to know about the reasons for and methods of bringing about the desired change?
- What instructions (persuasion) have been given from significant people about the importance of making changes?
- What are existing and potential models for change?
- What is the past success with making this or comparable changes?
- How confident is the client that change can be accomplished this time?
- What can be done to increase confidence?
- What are the incentives and disincentives?

Adoption

When to intervene or encourage adoption of a new behavior should be guided by clinical experience and science and facilitated by carefully listening to the client's needs and interests. Continued gentle reminders may be useful, even for a chronic smoker who has refused to quit many times in the past. Simply asking a person to try a new behavior (e.g., increase activity or alter diet) may be sufficient to instigate change. Medical or personal crises may present an incentive and often an opportunity for change. However, at times it is important not to push the participant beyond willingness to change. Questions such as, "Are you ready to try to stop smoking?" or "Do you want to consider a healthier diet?" may tell the cPT whether to encourage further change.

Goal setting is an important part of the adoption phase. Asking clients to list goals and to identify areas where assistance is needed may be effective. A number of studies have demonstrated that flexible, individually tailored, achievable goals increase adherence to change. Goals should be specific, not global, and short-term, but linked to longer-term goals. A useful way to determine whether a goal is likely to be achieved is to determine level of confidence (using a scale from 0–100%, no confidence to entirely certain) for attaining the goal in a given time frame. Clients reporting 70% or more are likely to be able to do so. In setting goals it is important to ensure that needs, goals, and preferences are included in the goal-setting process.

Once a person intends to make a behavior change and is confident of success, the adoption of change is often precipitated by cues to action. For instance, many people begin a health care program on the basis of symptoms or general state of being. Such physiological and emotional feedback cues people to change and is critical in influencing maintenance. Smoking relapse often occurs in the first few days after quitting because withdrawal symptoms overwhelm intentions. Poorly conditioned people may stop exercising at the beginning of an exercise program because of unpleasant feelings, such as shortness of breath.

Certain environmental and physical prerequisites are often necessary for health behavior change and should be discussed with participants. Such prerequisites for exercising:

- Clothing and equipment
- Access to facilities
- Necessary written materials
- A release from a physician if appropriate

The early stages of change are often the most difficult. Replacing one activity, even a self-destructive one, with another involves many subtle and important shifts in life. Cigarette smokers who quit often say they feel as if they have lost a good friend. Support is particularly important at such times.

Maintenance

Once a behavior is adopted, other factors determine maintenance. Behavior that satisfies (reinforcing) or reduces discomfort is likely to be maintained. Four strategies may prove useful in enhancing maintenance:

1 Monitoring and feedback of change (monitoring)
2 Making the activity as satisfying as possible (reinforcement)
3 Anticipating relapse or interruptions (relapse prevention)
4 Making a formal commitment (a contract)

Monitoring

Self-report, diary, physiological, or other types of monitoring are useful for maintaining behavior change and assisting exercise professionals in determining progress. Monitoring forms may be used by cPTs for review and problem solving. In addition, monitoring through use of self-reports and diaries provides clients with important feedback that may increase the likelihood of maintenance. Goals vary, but cognitive-behavioral and physiological goals should be developed as appropriate. Monitoring forms should be simple and convenient.

Reinforcement

Positive reinforcement is a powerful factor for sustaining change. Many environmental stimuli, such as food, water, sexual activity, and warmth are natural reinforcers. Social and/or symbolic reinforcers include attention, praise, money, and awards. Recognition from peers or games and competition can help maintain a behavior. However, it is important to realize that reinforcers are idiosyncratic, that is, reinforcement to one participant may not be reinforcement to another person. Several excellent discussions of reinforcement are available (18–20).

Relapse Prevention

Various techniques assist participants with relapse or prepare for interruptions or other events that may cause discontinuation of a program. The relapse prevention model is derived from studies of alcoholics and smokers attempting to change. Marlatt and Gordon observed that even one cigarette might lead to total relapse and that preparation for the situations in which the cigarette urge is strongest (e.g., while drinking or under stress) could help to prevent this relapse (20). The model can be applied to other behaviors. For instance, the Stanford Cardiac Rehabilitation Program staff encourages people to monitor exercise to improve maintenance and identifies clear signals for relapse, such as an actual or anticipated reduction in exercise frequency, and to develop strategies to deal with possible relapse (4).

Upon initiation of an exercise program, clients are encouraged to write what they will do when illness, injury, or changes in schedule interrupt exercise. Some examples:

- Asking a jogging partner for a reminder after return from vacation
- Leaving a money deposit with a friend that is refundable when restarting exercise after an illness
- Asking an exercise professional to call periodically to inquire about exercise

Clients who stop exercising for an extended time may require additional effort to overcome the lapse, but the principles are similar. Note that relapse prevention focuses on decreasing rather than increasing behavior.

Contracts

Written contracts are also extremely useful to maintain change and to help with maintenance. Exercise professionals should not make contracts that are unrealistic or unlikely to be achieved. Behavior change is dynamic, and goals should be assessed, updated, and revised as necessary. Problem solving may be important for goals that are not achieved. In problem solving, a participant identifies a list of possible solutions, develops a plan for implementing these solutions, tries them, evaluates results, and repeats the process if the initial solutions are unsuccessful.

Developing a Program

A program consists of the antecedent, adoption, and maintenance phases of behavioral change, how the interventions associated with this phase are sequenced and integrated, and the interaction between the exercise professional and the client.

Organization

Implementing behavior change takes time. Programs should ensure that such time is available for both the exercise professional and the participant. A session immediately prior to exercise class devoted to education and behavior change may be helpful. This session can be used to present new information, review progress toward goals, share solutions for problems, and so on. It is also important to allow exercise professionals time with peers and administrators for formal review of behavioral aspects of the program. Such sessions can be spent evaluating educational material, reviewing progress of clients, solving problems, and designing new aspects of intervention.

The initial step is asking a participant to consider change. Often people intend to adopt one behavior, but recommending additional health behavior changes may be important, such as recommending that an exerciser also stop smoking. Suggesting such changes can be difficult, but few people resent a thoughtful attempt to assist in improving health.

The second and perhaps most important step is to provide information, instructions, and models for change. This includes reviewing the past, building confidence for change, reducing disincentives, and increasing incentives to change.

The third step is to request a commitment that is specific in time and place for when the new behavior will occur. The final step is to develop, with the participant, a way to monitor progress of the new behavior and to determine when and how progress will be reviewed. Early in the adoption phase, the client should be trained in relapse prevention. Problem solving should be used as necessary to help overcome difficulties. Such problem solving can occur in the whole group, at the beginning or the end of a session, via telephone, or in a face-to-face counseling session.

Exercise Professional Qualities

Different exercise professionals achieve different outcomes, even within the same program. Exercise professionals seem to be most effective when participants feel that the exercise professional is competent, likes them, understands them, and is interested. This relationship translates into a bond between exercise professional and participant that helps to make the program effective. Role playing of typical participant situations with peers and receiving feedback is a particularly good way for exercise professionals to develop interpersonal skills.

Overpersistence with an unwilling participant is a problem for some exercise professionals. Exercise professionals who assume too much responsibility for the actions of another person are particularly likely to be overpersistent. Unfortunately, overpersistent exercise professionals often begin to resent inaction, feel chronic frustration, or devote too much time to that participant. To avoid these problems, exercise professionals should have guidelines about when a program or request for change may be discontinued.

B. Methods for Changing Health Behaviors

Fitness and rehabilitation professionals face the challenge of working with clients and their families, as well as the community, to develop methods of changing negative health-related behaviors. To achieve positive changes in health-related behaviors, a clear understanding of adult learning processes and the psychological influences on learning and behavior change are important. This chapter addresses the challenge of exercise compliance, concepts of adult learning, and psychological components of successful behavior change, and suggests practical strategies to improve behavioral change outcomes.

Exercise Compliance

To understand why people sometimes lack the motivation for regular physical activity, one must first acknowledge a simple yet important fact: exercise is voluntary and time-consuming. Therefore, it may extend the day or compete with other valued interests and responsibilities of daily life. The traditional approach to the exercise compliance problem has involved attempting to persuade dropouts to become reinvolved. An alternative approach, however, involves the identification and subsequent monitoring of "dropout prone" individuals, with an aim toward preventing relapse.

Figure 4.1 – Self-motivation assessment scale to determine likelihood of exercise compliance.

A	B	C	D	E	
5	4	3	2	1	1. I get discouraged easily.
5	4	3	2	1	2. I don't work any harder than I have to.
1	2	3	4	5	3. I seldom if ever let myself down.
5	4	3	2	1	4. I'm just not the goal-setting type.
1	2	3	4	5	5. I'm good at keeping promises, especially the ones I make myself.
5	4	3	2	1	6. I don't impose much structure on my activities.
1	2	3	4	5	7. I have a very hard-driving, aggressive personality.

Directions: Circle the number beneath the letter corresponding to the alternative that best describes how characteristic the statement is when applied to you. The alternatives are:

    A. *extremely* uncharacteristic of me.
    B. *somewhat* uncharacteristic of me.
    C. neither characteristic nor uncharacteristic of me.
    D. *somewhat* characteristic of me.
    E. *extremely* characteristic of me.

Scoring: Add together the seven numbers you circled. A score ≤24 suggests dropout-prone behavior. The lower the self-motivation score, the greater the likelihood toward exercise noncompliance. If the score suggests dropout proneness, it should be viewed as an incentive to remain active, rather than a self-fulfilling prophecy to quit exercising.

(Copyright © 1978 by Dishman RK, Ickes W, Morgan WP. Self-motivation and adherence to habitual physical activity. J Appl Social Psychol 1980;10:115-132. From Falls HB, Baylor AM, Dishman RK. Essentials of Fitness. Appendix A-13, Philadelphia: Saunders College, 1980. Reproduced by permission of the copyright holders.)

Box 4.1 – Variables Predicting the Exercise Dropout*

Personal Factors
  Smoker
  Inactive leisure time
  Inactive occupation
  Blue collar worker
  Type A personality
  Increased physical strength
  Extroverted
  Poor credit rating
  Overweight and/or low ponderal index
  Poor self-motivation
  Depressed
  Hypochondriacal
  Anxious
  Introverted
  Low ego strength
Program Factors
  Inconvenient time and/or location
  Excessive cost
  High-intensity exercise
  Lack of exercise variety, e.g., running only
  Exercising alone
  Lack of positive feedback or reinforcement
  Inflexible exercise goals
  Low enjoyment ratings for running programs
  Poor exercise leadership
Other Factors
  Lack of spouse support
  Inclement weather
  Excessive job travel
  Injury
  Job change and/or move

*Adapted from Franklin BA. Program factors that influence exercise adherence: practical adherence skills for clinical staff. In: Dishman R, ed. Exercise Adherence: Its Impact on Public Health. Champaign, IL: Human Kinetics, 1988:237–258.

Principal factors related to long-term exercise noncompliance include cigarette smoking, blue collar employment, inactive leisure time, and inactive occupation. A brief questionnaire designed to assess "self-motivation" can be used, along with measures of intention and self-efficacy, to predict male and female dropout-prone behavior (21, 22) (Fig. 4.1 and Box 4.1).

The Learning Process

Stages of Learning

To design movement experiences for clients that result in positive learning and ultimately behavior change, cPTs must understand the nature of learning and the factors that influence its outcomes. Because each client will present themselves with unique characteristics and varied stages of readiness, their ability to learn in a new environment may also differ. When learning a new skill, individuals typically progress through three stages before they can reproduce a skilled movement consistently on request. These phases are the cognitive phase, the associative phase, and the automatic phase. The cognitive phase is where the general concepts of the skill and its proper sequencing are being learned. The cognitive phase usually requires significant concentration by the individual and it is also when many performance errors are made. The associative phase allows the individual to begin focusing on specific subcomponents of the skill and timing and flow of the entire movement become more consistent and natural. Feedback is highly effective for individuals in the associative phase. Finally, the automatic phase is where the skill has developed to the point where it is performed consistently, and under a wide variety of conditions and circumstances. Having an understanding of these three stages and their function serves as foundational information for cPTs who deliver skill instruction to their clients.

Types of Learners

Individuals can perceive, organize, and process information in one or more of the following ways: Visual, tactile (kinesthetic), and auditory. Visual learners obtain information primarily through the written word (they tend to be readers) and benefit from handouts. Tactile (kinesthetic) learners obtain information by practicing a skill or behavior and benefit from demonstrations. Auditory learners obtain information best by listening and benefit from discussions and question/answer opportunities.

Adult Learning

Learning and changing behavior involves a clear understanding of many factors that influence learning potential. Adults learn largely based on their beliefs, culture, prior experiences, and knowledge. Generally accepted principles of learning indicate that adults:

- Are self-directed
- Participate in decision-making
- Base learning on past experiences
- Use problem solving as a basis for learning
- Learn only when they are "ready" to learn, for example, when they are physically and emotionally stable and are aware that there is a need to learn (23, 24)

Psychological Components of Successful Behavior Change

Successful behavior change is based upon an understanding of certain psychological theories. Behavior modification, social cognitive theory, and stages of motivational readiness (also known as the transtheoretical model) are fundamental to guiding our behavioral interventions. Behavior modification theory has added greatly to our ability to effect long-term behavior change. This theory actively involves the client in the change process. This is achieved by clients doing the following:

- Setting short- and long-term, realistic, and measurable goals
- Determining their "confidence" to achieve each goal
- Signing a contract with a clear description of the desirable goal and means to achieve the goal
- Receiving feedback on their success and revising the plan as appropriate
- Receiving lifestyle physical activity counseling, including specific cognitive and behavioral counseling strategies (*e.g.*, diaries, prompts) to increase the adoption and maintenance of physical activity in daily living (25–27)
- Developing social support systems to provide encouragement and help during difficult times (28–30)

Readiness for change theory has received wide acceptance and use by health care practitioners. This theory addresses the individual's ability to make permanent change based upon his or her emotional and intellectual "readiness to change" (31). Clients or patients can be evaluated as to the stage of readiness they express before being given the challenge to change a behavior. The stages, as modified for physical activity interventions, are defined as precontemplation, contemplation, preparation, action, and maintenance. Box 4.2 describes each of these stages (25, 26, 30, 32, 33). Individuals should also be counseled to deal with hypokinetic lapses or relapses, and to recognize that these behaviors are not necessarily tantamount to failure.

Strategies to Improve Behavioral Change Outcomes

Using self-efficacy measures and integrating the stages of change into educational strategies can greatly influence behavioral and lifestyle outcomes. In addition, providing written and visual materials as well as experimental educational tools (*e.g.*, yoga classes for relaxation) can influence and support behavioral change. Written plans and documentation of progress should be integrated into the client record.

Use of behavior modification strategies, such as setting goals, making agreements or contracts,

Box 4.2 – Stages of "Readiness to Change" Model*

1. Precontemplation—patients express lack of interest in making change. Moving patients through this stage involves utilization of multiple resources to stress the importance of the desired change. This can be achieved through written materials, educational classes, physician and family persuasion and other means.
2. Contemplation—patients are "thinking" about making a desired change. This stage can be influenced by helping patients define the risks and benefits of making or not making the desired change (e.g., starting an exercise program).
3. Preparation—patients are doing some physical activity but not meeting the recommended criteria, i.e., 30 minutes of moderate-intensity physical activity for ≥5 days/week or 3 to 5 days/week of vigorous-intensity activity for ≥20 minutes.
4. Action—patients are meeting the above-referenced (preparation) criteria on a consistent basis but they have not maintained the behavior for 6 months.
5. Maintenance—patients have been in action for 6 months or more.

*Modified for physical activity interventions (see references 12,13).

Box 4.3 – Behavioral Management Strategies for Initiating and Maintaining Exercise Adherence*

Techniques	Practical Applications/Recommendations
Initiation of Exercise	
Preparation	The exercise professional should establish realistic expectations among new participants. Overly pessimistic or optimistic expectations should be corrected.
Shaping	This strategy is analogous to the physiologic principle of progression. Begin the exercise program at a dosage (intensity, frequency, duration) that is comfortable for the participant, and increase the volume slowly until the optimal level is attained.
Goal-setting	Goals should be individualized and based upon the participant's physiologic and psychosocial status. Goals can be set for both supervised and unsupervised exercise. Short-term goals that are specific, yet flexible, are more effective than longer-term goals.
Reinforcement	Participants should be queried as to what reinforcers (rewards) would work for them. One of the most effective rewards may be praise from program staff that is specific to each individual. Certificates, patches, and attendance charts can also be used as reinforcers.
Stimulus control	Environmental cues or stimuli (e.g., written notes, watch alarms) may be used to remind participants to maintain their exercise commitment. Having a routine time and place for exercise establishes powerful stimulus control.
Contracting	A behavioral contract has been shown to enhance the commitment to exercise. Signing the contract formalizes the agreement and makes it more significant.
Cognitive strategies	Participants should be oriented to the advantages and disadvantages of exercise. Individuals who select their own flexible goals generally demonstrate better adherence as compared with those whose goals are rigidly set by exercise professionals.
Maintenance of Exercise	
Generalization training	Specific steps should be taken to "generalize" the exercise habit from the gymnasium or home setting to other environments (e.g., walk breaks at work, using stairs, gardening, parking the car away from stores).
Social support	The support of family, friends, and coworkers should be sought from the beginning. Finding a compatible exercise partner often serves to enhance exercise adherence.

Box 4.3 (continued) – Behavioral Management Strategies for Initiating and Maintaining Exercise Adherence*

Self-management	Participants should be encouraged to be their own behavior therapists. They should practice self-reinforcement by focusing on increased self-esteem, enjoyment of the exercise itself, and the anticipated health and fitness benefits.
Relapse prevention training	Exercise professionals should prepare participants for situations that may produce a relapse and ways of coping with them so that a complete relapse is avoided. Relapses should be viewed as inevitable challenges, rather than failures.

*Adapted from Martin JE, Dubbert PM. Behavioral management strategies for improving health and fitness. J Cardiac Rehabil 1984;4:200–208.

providing frequent feedback, scheduling appropriate rewards, assessing and integrating social support, and providing prompts are critical in modulating health behavior change (28). Box 4.3 further defines these strategies with specific reference to techniques to initiate and maintain exercise behaviors (34).

We must be careful not to define our beliefs and practices as the "gold standard" of behavior. Labeling clients as "noncompliant" because they do not participate in behaviors that we believe are beneficial to their health is not necessarily the optimal approach to understanding and facilitating healthy behavior change. A more successful approach is to assess an individual's educational level, resources to facilitate change, readiness to learn, and personal beliefs. Such individually tailored education and counseling are more likely to result in long-term change. In addition, health care professionals should live the life they prescribe. In doing this, their actions as "role models" can positively influence the behaviors of those they counsel and educate.

Methods of behavior change are often effective in altering many health-related behaviors, but their use does not guarantee success. The techniques presented here should be integrated into the exercise program in a way that is appropriate to the population, the setting, and the expertise of the staff. An effective program would selectively incorporate several of these techniques into a focused multifactorial program; however, it is not necessary to use all of them (25, 26). The techniques are only introduced in this chapter; additional readings, relevant training, or consultation from an expert in behavior change should be used to complement this information.

Practical Recommendations to Enhance Exercise Adherence

In addition to educating people about exercise, it is necessary to motivate them to act and maintain a personal fitness program (35). Unfortunately, exercise testing and exercise prescription are often overemphasized in relation to the behavioral components of the program. As a result, negative forces often outweigh the positive forces contributing to sustained participant interest and adherence. Such imbalance (Fig. 4.2) leads to a decline in adherence while program effectiveness diminishes. Research and empiric experience suggest that the following program modifications and motivational strategies may enhance participant interest, enthusiasm, and long-term adherence.

Recruit Physician Support of the Exercise Program

According to a recent clinical study, the single most important factor determining client's participation in exercise was receiving a strong recommendation from their primary care physician (36). Simple physician counseling has also been shown to be highly effective in motivating clients to make other significant lifestyle changes (*e.g.,* smoking cessation).

Figure 4.2 – Variables affecting adherence to a physical conditioning program. Negative variables often outweigh positive variables, resulting in poor adherence.

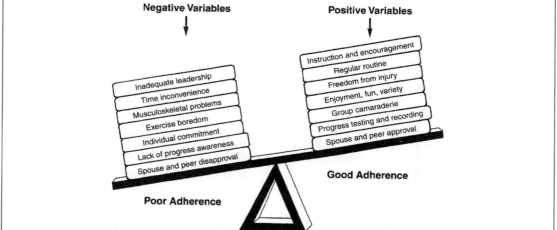

Minimize Injuries and/or Complications with a Moderate Exercise Prescription

Oftentimes, novice exercisers become discouraged due to muscular soreness or injury from increasing the activity dosage too abruptly. Excessive intensity (+ 85% $\dot{V}O_{2max}$), frequency (+5 $d \cdot wk^{-1}$), or duration of training (+45 min per session) offer the participant little additional gain in aerobic fitness, yet the incidence of orthopedic injury increases substantially. Attention to warm-up, proper walking or running shoes, and training on appropriate terrain (i.e., avoiding hard and uneven surfaces) should aid in decreasing attrition due to injury. Participants should be counseled to discontinue exercise and seek medical advice if they experience excessive muscle soreness, orthopedic injury, or premonitory signs or symptoms, including abnormal heart rhythms (palpitations), chest pain or pressure, or dizziness.

Advocate Exercising with Others

Poorer long-term adherence has been reported in programs in which an individual exercises alone compared with those that incorporated group dynamics (37). Commitments made as part of a group tend to be stronger than those made independently (38). The social support provided by others may offer the incentive to continue even during periods of sagging interest.

Emphasize Variety and Enjoyment in the Exercise Program

The type of physical activity program has also been shown to influence long-term exercise adherence. Calisthenics, when relied on too heavily in an exercise program, readily becomes monotonous and boring, leading to poor exercise adherence. The most successful physical conditioning regimens are those that are pleasurable and offer the greatest diversification.

Provide Positive Reinforcement through Periodic Testing

Exercise testing, body fatness assessment, and serum lipid profiling may be done at the start of the exercise program and at regular intervals thereafter to assess the individual's response to the conditioning stimulus. Favorable changes in these measures can serve as powerful motivators that produce renewed interest and dedication.

Recruit Support of the Program Among Family and Friends

Lack of social support is frequently found to be a precursor to exercise noncompliance. Accordingly, attention should be focused not only on the participant, but also on family and friends. Spouse support and approval appears to play a key role in this regard. The importance of this influence became evident in one study that showed that the husband's adherence to the exercise program was directly related to the wife's attitude toward it (38). Of those men whose spouses had a positive attitude toward the exercise program, 80% demonstrated good-to-excellent adherence, and only 20% exhibited fair-to-poor adherence. In contrast, when the spouse was neutral or negative, 40% showed good-to-excellent adherence and 60% demonstrated fair-to-poor adherence.

Include an Optional Recreational Game to the Conditioning Program Format

The standard warm-up, endurance phase, and cool-down used in most exercise programs offer little in terms of fun or variety. A recreational game may be included as an option to this format. Game modifications that serve to minimize skill and competition and maximize participant success are particularly important in preventive and rehabilitative exercise programs. Through such modifications the leader is better able to emphasize the primary goal of the activity: enjoyment of the game for its own sake (39).

Establish Regularity of Workouts

If individuals start their workouts at the same time each day, they will accept them as part of their routine schedule and exercise will become habitual. Availability of morning and evening sessions should serve to further increase the compatibility of an exercise commitment with the varied schedules of participants.

Use Progress Charts to Record Exercise Achievements

The importance of immediate, positive feedback on reinforcement of health-related behaviors is well documented. A progress chart that allows participants to document daily and cumulative exercise achievements (e.g., mileage) can facilitate this objective.

Recognize Participant Accomplishments through a System of Rewards

Peer recognition is another powerful motivator. Recognition of lifestyle, health, or exercise achievements can be made in the form of inexpensive trophies, plaques, ribbons, certificates, or "iron-on" insignias. To this end, an annual awards ceremony or banquet is recommended.

Provide Qualified, Enthusiastic Exercise Professionals

Although numerous variables affect exercise adherence, perhaps the single most important is the exercise leader (40, 41). Exercise staff should be well-trained, compassionate, sensitive, empathetic, tactful, innovative, and enthusiastic. Box 4.4 lists recommended behavioral strategies of the good exercise professional.

Box 4.4 – Behavioral Strategies of the Good Exercise Professional

1. Show a sincere interest in the participant. Learn why participants have gotten involved in your program and what they hope to achieve.
2. Be enthusiastic in your instruction and guidance.
3. Develop a personal association and relationship with each participant: learn clients' names and greet them by shaking hands.
4. Consider the various reasons why adults exercise (i.e., health, recreation, weight loss, social, personal appearance) and allow for individual differences.
5. Remove or reduce as many initial barriers to participation as possible. If cost, distance, child care, or other factors make it difficult for clients to attend, assist them to overcome these obstacles whenever possible.
6. Initiate participant follow-up (e.g., postcards or telephone calls) when several unexplained absences occur in succession. Novice exercisers should be advised that an inevitable slip in attendance does not imply failure.
7. Practice what you preach. Participate in the exercise sessions yourself.
8. Honor special days (e.g., birthdays) or exercise accomplishments with extrinsic rewards such as T-shirts, ribbons, or certificates.
9. Attend personally to orthopedic and musculoskeletal problems. Provide alternatives to floor exercise.
10. Counsel participants on proper foot apparel and exercise clothing.
11. Avoid constant references to complicated medical or physiologic terminology. Concentrate on a few selected terms to provide a little education at a time.
12. Arrange for occasional visits by personal physicians.
13. Provide a constant flow of newspaper or magazine articles to the participants on topics related to physical activity and other relevant information.
14. Encourage an occasional visitor or participant to lead activity.
15. Have a designated area for participant counseling with an appropriate decor.
16. Give clear and concise information. Listen, summarize, and clarify to ensure that your communications have been correctly understood.
17. Introduce "first-time" exercisers on the gymnasium floor or in the locker room. This orientation will encourage a sense of belonging to the group.
18. Reinforce participants by complimenting them on their appearance as they are exercising. Your conversation during exercise may also serve as a distracter from any unpleasant sensations that they may be experiencing.
19. Use goal setting as a motivational tool. Build on areas of participant perceived interest, "How would he or she like to be different?"
20. Show your optimism. This creates a positive self-fulfilling prophesy where the participant succeeds largely because of your belief that he or she can persevere.

Population-Specific Barriers to Physical Activity

Women, older adults, and obese individuals are faced with several unique barriers to exercise participation, which may account for their lower initial enrollment, poorer attendance, and higher drop-out rates. The role of caregiver is typically the woman maintaining the home and caring for children, an older spouse, or a family member. Women are also less likely to drive to an exercise facility. Some women may be uncomfortable participating in a male-dominated physical conditioning program. Several factors may restrict physical activity with clients of increasing age: poor health, fear of injury, and inaccessibility to fitness facilities. Among obese individuals, unique barriers include previous negative experiences with exercise (feelings of inadequacy, limited physical skills) and the physiologic and psychosocial bur-

den of their excess weight. Nevertheless, these obstacles can oftentimes be overcome with careful program design (42). The role of the cPT is to facilitate the decision to participate in regular exercise and other health-related habits, to support these lifestyle changes over time, and to provide training to prevent relapse to the former undesirable behavior.

C. Communication Skills

Communication skills pertinent to the cPT serve three significant functions. The first is to develop rapport and convey a sense of empathy for the challenges clients confront in making and maintaining lifestyle changes. The second function is to assess health-related behaviors with respect to the effect on optimal functioning and risk of disease, which includes understanding the perspective of the client on how these behaviors contribute to health and quality of life. This second function also includes assessing the state of readiness for change. The third function is to facilitate change through discussion of potential benefits and problems associated with implementing a lifestyle change. This function allows the client to make informed decisions consistent with personal values.

Function 1: Developing Rapport and Conveying Empathy

Acceptance

The cPT should set a tone of openness and acceptance during initial conversations with the client. It is particularly important to refrain from appearing to make judgments about lifestyle or health history. Such a perception on the part of the client may affect the type of information the client is willing to disclose and/or the accuracy of the information. To behave neutrally is not easy, particularly if values conflict, as is often the case in the area of health behaviors. Therefore, it is important for the cPT to separate personal values and beliefs from those of the client. Only then can the cPT respond in an objective and empathic manner, both verbally and nonverbally.

Expressing Empathy through Active Listening

Empathy has been defined as the ability to understand people from their frame of reference rather than your own (43). Failure to acknowledge the importance of personal events in the life of a client can diminish understanding of the emotional state and its effect on health-related behaviors.

There are a number of barriers to discussing such sensitive issues for both clients and cPTs (44). These may include cultural expectations that the interview focus on medical issues only, logistical concerns about wasting time, and personal preferences not to address emotional issues. To be an effective cPT, however, the practitioner must make an effort to understand what the person feels and convey to the client that desire to comprehend.

Empathy can be conveyed through the use of active listening responses. This entails having participants describe experiences, after which the cPT responds by rephrasing what has been said. Such paraphrasing ensures that the cPT has made an accurate interpretation and also conveys that the cPT is attempting to listen and understand what is being said. For example, a cPT might respond to complaints by saying, "You seem frustrated with not being able to jog as fast as you would like." This response is particularly effective, as it identifies and reflects the emotional component of the experience. Such statements facilitate the development of rapport and self-disclosure.

In contrast, expressing sympathy conveys an attempt to share another's feelings (*e.g.*, "I've had the same thing happen to me") or to imply pity for the experience (*e.g.*, "I'm sorry you are having a problem"). Although such responses are useful in some limited situations, in general cPTs should be careful not to convey that their personal experiences are exactly the same as the client's or that an expression of sympathy is only given because it is socially appropriate. Active listening can also be conveyed through the use of questions designed to clarify a statement or probe for additional information. For example, a client may say, "I've tried to stop smoking, but every time I do I gain a ton of weight and go right back to smoking again anyway. The only thing I change is my weight, and that's not a good change."

Nonverbal Communication

Communication between cPT and client includes both verbal and nonverbal components. Although the verbal portion of a message is often easiest to describe, the nonverbal component is also extremely important (43). Nonverbal communication, such as maintaining good eye contact, is essential to the development of rapport and expression of empathy. Humans respond to nonverbal communication, even if they are not specifically aware of what they are sensing and responding to. Experienced cPTs, however, are particularly alert to seeing and hearing nonverbal communication. For example, when asked about his diet, a client may report, "I kept up with it fairly well." The verbal report may suggest that the participant is doing well. However, poor eye contact, inflections in the tone of voice, and hesitant, low-energy speech may suggest that compliance with the prescribed diet was less than fairly good. These types of inconsistencies between verbal and nonverbal components should prompt the cPT to con-

sider a gentle, inquisitive confrontation regarding the issue (*e.g.*, "You say you are keeping up with your diet, but you seem hesitant when talking about it. I'm wondering if you could share with me any problems you might be having.").

Nonverbal communication can be divided into three main categories. Kinesics refers to body movements that convey information, such as eye contact, hand gestures, winking, body position, and facial expressions. Poor eye contact, extremely low levels of body movement, or a flat or sad facial expression are particularly important cues. Characteristics of speech, such as voice inflections and changes in volume, are collectively referred to as paralinguistics. These characteristics often modify the meaning of the verbal content. Finally, characteristics of interpersonal space, such as seating arrangements and interpersonal distance, are included in the nonverbal component of proxemics. Awareness of proxemics is vital to creating a comfortable environment for your client.

Function 2: Assessing Readiness to Change

Behavioral Assessment

The importance of obtaining a comprehensive history of health-related behaviors cannot be overemphasized. In addition to self-report, a particularly useful strategy for gathering data during the assessment phase is to have the client track or self-monitor health behaviors over a prescribed period. It may also be helpful to involve family members and significant others in the interview process. Frequently, people close to the client have valuable insight into health behaviors and can provide information that the client may not be aware of or is not able, willing, or ready to disclose. Thus, these supplementary sources often fill in holes in what a cPT has been able to glean. Such input can also provide the cPT with a better understanding of the social environment in which the client will attempt to make lifestyle changes.

Motivational Assessment

Health-related behaviors must be understood in the context of the values and overall lifestyle of the client. Whereas one cannot motivate individuals directly, one can appeal to what motivates them. Motivations for health-related behavior change may not be the same for the client and the cPT. The challenge is to find common ground where health-enhancing recommendations also meet a client's goal. For instance, the cPT may suggest a regimen of regular aerobic exercise to increase cardiopulmonary endurance. The initial response may be a lack of perception of a significant need to engage in such activity, since the client can perform most daily activities. Careful questioning, however, may reveal that the client discontinued hunting several years ago because of lack of strength and endurance. In this case, the task would be to connect the need for cardiopulmonary endurance with the desire to participate once again in a valued recreational activity. Once this match is realized and appreciated, the task is to help the client develop clear goals and a well-designed program to achieve them within a specific time.

Function 3: Facilitating Change

The certified Personal Trainer's Role

The task of the cPT is to facilitate change rather than simply to prescribe it. Thus, the cPT and client should work together to discuss, develop, and agree on a plan for change. In doing so, the cPT should be wary of the tendency to overwhelm the client with a barrage of verbal instructions and written materials designed to promote compliance. Simplicity is often a key to success.

During this partnership, the cPT should always keep in mind that the ultimate goal for the client is to accept and maintain responsibility for personal behavior. Dependency on the cPT is a real threat to long-term maintenance, one that is not readily apparent to those new to the cPT role. Therefore, it is critical that the cPT encourage independence. For example, the cPT may facilitate social support and link rewards for success to family and friends rather than solely to the cPT. In addition, the client must be encouraged to accept personal responsibility for making the change and solving related problems that arise on a day-to-day basis.

In preparing for behavior change, it is often helpful to assist the client in identifying all of the benefits as well as the costs of the behavior change. Consider having the client list the benefits on one side and costs on the other side of a piece of paper. Next, ask them to compare and to determine whether the benefits truly outweigh the costs. The role of the cPT during this process is to help the client explore all of the possibilities in terms of costs and benefits, including those that have not been considered. Once they are identified, discussion can be focused on methods to decrease the costs and improve the benefits. Unfortunately, although this exercise puts the behavior change into perspective and provides a frame of reference that can be used to advantage during difficult times in the process, it is often bypassed in the haste to get on with the behavior change. For instance, the written list can be saved for use during relapse, when the participant may have lost perspective, to bring back the original frame of reference in terms of the cost–benefit ratio.

Clients often have mixed feelings regarding the adoption of a new behavior (*e.g.,* exercise) or cessation of a valued behavior (*e.g.,* smoking, high-fat diet). It is therefore fairly common to hear a client say, "I want to lose weight," only later to admit that he or she doesn't want to change eating habits. When the cPT suspects a conflict, gentle confrontation may be a very useful technique. This entails restating the two conflicting points and probing for clarification. For example, "Mary, I need you to help me. You've said that you really want to exercise more often and that 5:30 P.M. is the best time for you. Still, you rarely are able to make it. What are you saying to yourself when you are making the decision not to exercise?" Although an extremely useful technique, confrontation, if not carefully worded, can be uncomfortable for both client and cPT. Hence, gentle confrontation is generally employed once rapport has been established.

Using Feedback Appropriately

Feedback, when used correctly, can be a compelling component to effective learning and skill performance. Feedback is any information, both verbal and nonverbal that the learner receives about the performance. The input received may contain information about the execution of the movement and/or the learner's effort throughout the movement. A cPT's response to a client's behavior may significantly influence future behaviors. Clients tend to modify their behaviors based on what they interpret from the cPT's feedback. Thus, it is important that your feedback (both verbal and nonverbal) is in context with the movement performed. Effective feedback is specific, relevant to the behavior or activity, and provides useful information for the client in modifying subsequent attempts at the activity.

Accurate and appropriate use of cues becomes an invaluable tool for the cPT when giving feedback. Typical verbal cues are "good job," "nice work," "great," "excellent," "much better," etc. Nonverbal feedback takes the form of facial expressions and gestures and in some cases, can be more effective than verbal feedback. Examples of positive nonverbal feedback cues include smiles, thumbs-up sign, clapping of hands, nodding in approval, *etc.* Nonverbal negative feedback may include frowning, looking away, thumbs down, tapping fingers, rolling eyes. Cues should always be used in a relevant and appropriate fashion. Giving mixed messages can create frustration and be very confusing for the client.

SECTION IV References

1. Elder JP, Ayala GX, Harris S. Theories and intervention approaches to health-behavior change in primary care. Am J Prev Med 17:275–284, 1999.
2. Prochaska JO, DiClimente CC. Stage process of self-change of smoking: Toward an integrative model of change. J Consul Clin Psych 51:390, 1983.
3. Prochaska JO, Velicer WF, Rossi JS, et al. Stages of change and decisional balance for 12 problem behaviors. Health Psychol 13:39, 1994.
4. Marcus BH, Simkin LR. The transtheoretical model: Applications to exercise behavior. Med Sci Sports Exerc 26:1400, 1994.
5. Marcus BH, Emmons KM, Simkin-Silverman LR, et al. Evaluation of motivationally tailored vs. standard self-help physical activity interventions at the workplace. Am J Health Promot 12:246, 1998.
6. Bandura A. Self-Efficacy: The Exercise of Control. San Francisco: WH Freeman, 1997.
7. Agras WS, Kazdin AE, Wilson CT. Behavior Therapy: Toward an Applied Clinical Science. San Francisco: WH Freeman, 1979.
8. Miller NH, Taylor CB. Lifestyle Management in Patients with Coronary Heart Disease. Champaign, IL: Human Kinetics, 1995.
9. Watson DL, Tharp RC. Self-Directed Behavior Change. Monterey, CA: Brooks/Cole, 1981.
10. Blumenthal JA, McKee DC. Applications in Behavioral Medicine and Health Psychology: A Clinician's Source Book. Sarasota, FL: Professional Resource Exchange, 1987.
11. Fishbein M, Ajzen I. Belief, Attitudes, Intention and Behavior. Reading, MA: Addison-Wesley, 1975.
12. Ajzen I. From intentions to actions: a theory of planned behavior (pp. 11–40). In: Kuhl J, Beckmann J, eds. Actional Control: From Cognition to Behavior. New York: Springer-Verlag, 1985.
13. Courneya KS. Understanding readiness for regular physical activity in older adults: An application of the theory of planned behavior. Health Psychol 14:80, 1995.
14. Becker MH, Maiman LA. Sociobehavioral determinants of compliance with health and medical care recommendations. Med Care 13:10, 1975.
15. Winett RA, King AC, Altman D. Psychology and Public Health: An Integrative Approach. New York: Pergamon, 1989.
16. Green LW, Kreuter MW. Health Promotion and Planning: An Education and Environmental Approach. Mountain View, CA: Mayfield, 1991.
17. Taylor CB, Houston-Miller N, Killen JD, DeBusk RF. Smoking cessation after acute myocardial infarction: Effects of a nurse-managed intervention. Ann Intern Med 113:118, 1990.
18. Goldfried M, Davison CC. Clinical Behavior Therapy. New York: Holt, Rinehart & Winston, 1976.
19. Cautela JR, Kastenbaum RA. Reinforcement survey schedule for use in therapy, training, and research. Psychol Rep 29:115, 1967.
20. Marlatt GA, Gordon JR, eds. Relapse Prevention: Maintenance Strategies in the Treatment of Addiction. New York: Guilford, 1985.
21. Dishman RK, Ickes W, Morgan WP. Self-motivation and adherence to habitual physical activity. J Appl Social Psychol 1980;10:115–132.
22. Falls HB, Baylor AM, Dishman RK. Essentials of fitness. Appendix A–13. Philadelphia: Saunders College, 1980.
23. Comoss PM. Education of the coronary patient and family: Principles and practice. In: Wenger NK, Hellerstein HK, eds. Rehabilitation of the Coronary Patient. 3rd ed. New York: Churchill Livingston, 1992:439–460.
24. Cupples SA. Inpatient cardiac rehabilitation: patient education implementation and documentation. J Cardiopulm Rehabil 1995;15:412–417.
25. Dunn AL, Marcus BH, Kampert JB, et al. Reduction in cardiovascular disease risk factors: 6-month results from Project Active. Prev Med 1997;26:883–892.
26. Dunn AL, Marcus BH, Kampert JB, et al. Comparison of lifestyle and structured interventions to increase physical activity and cardiorespiratory fitness. JAMA 1999;281:327–334.
27. Andersen RE, Wadden TA, Bartlett SJ, et al. Effects of lifestyle activity vs structured aerobic exercise in obese women. JAMA 1999;281:335–340.
28. Taylor CB, Miller NH. Principles of health behavior change. In: Roitman J, Southard D, eds. ACSM's Resource Manual for Guidelines for Exercise Testing and Prescription. 3rd ed. Baltimore: William & Wilkins, 1998:542–547.
29. Miller NH, Taylor CB. Lifestyle Management for Patients with Coronary Heart Disease. Champaign, IL: Human Kinetics, 1995.
30. Miller NH, Hill M, Kottke T, et al. The multilevel compliance challenge: recommendations for a call to action. A statement for healthcare professionals. Circulation 1997;95:1085– 1090.
31. Prochaska J, DiClemente C. Transtheoretical therapy, toward a more integrative model of change. Psych Theory Res Prac 1982;19:276–288.
32. Prochaska JO, DiClemente CC. Common processes of change in smoking, weight control and psychological distress. In: Schiffman S, Wills TA, eds. Coping and Substance Use. San Diego: Academic Press, 1985:345–363.
33. Marlatt GA, Gordon JR, eds. Relapse Prevention: Maintenance Strategies in the Treatment of Addictive Behaviors. New York: Guilford Press, 1985.
34. Martin JE, Dubbert PM. Behavioral management strategies for improving health and fitness. J Cardiac Rehabil 1984;4:200–208.
35. Wilmore JH. Individual exercise prescription. Am J Cardiol 1974;33:757–759.
36. Ades PA, Waldmann ML, McCann WJ, et al. Predictors of cardiac rehabilitation participation in older coronary patients. Arch Intern Med 1992;152:1033–1035.
37. Massie JF, Shephard RJ. Physiological and psychological effects of training a comparison of individual and gymnasium programs, with a characterization of the exercise `drop-out.' Med Sci Sports 1971;3:110–117.
38. Heinzelman F, Bagley RW. Response to physical activity programs and their effects on health behavior. Public Health Rep 1970;85:905–911.
39. Franklin BA, Stoedefalke KG. Games-as-aerobics: activities for cardiac rehabilitation programs. In: Fardy PS, Franklin BA, Porcari JP, et al., eds. Training Techniques in Cardiac Rehabilitation. Champaign, IL: Human Kinetics, 1998:106–136.
40. Oldridge NB. What to look for in an exercise class leader. Phys Sportsmed 1977;5:85–88.
41. Oldridge NB. Qualities of an exercise leader. In: Blair SN, Painter P, Pate RR, et al., eds. ACSM's Resource Manual for Guidelines for Graded Exercise Testing and Exercise Prescription. Philadelphia: Lea and Febiger, 1988:239–243.
42. Blair SN, Horton E, Leon AS, et al. Physical activity, nutrition, and chronic disease. Med Sci Sports Exerc 1996;28:335–349.
43. Cormier WH, Cormier LS. Interviewing Strategies for Helpers: Fundamental Skills and Cognitive Behavioral Interventions. Pacific Grove, CA: Brooks/Cole, 1993.
44. Egener B. Empathy. In: Feldman MD, Christensen JF, eds. Behavioral Medicine in Primary Care: A Practical Guide. Stamford, CT: Appleton & Lange, 1997:8–14.

Section V

- ◆ Preparticipation Health Appraisal in the Nonmedical Setting
- ◆ Cardiorespiratory Assessment of Apparently Healthy Populations
- ◆ Assessment of Muscular Strength and Endurance
- ◆ Flexibility and Range of Motion
- ◆ Body Composition

ACSM's Resources for the Personal Trainer

HEALTH APPRAISAL, FITNESS EXERCISE TESTING

A. Preparticipation Health Appraisal in the Nonmedical Setting

It is clear that a physically active lifestyle provides partial protection against several major chronic diseases. Regular exercise is beneficial in the primary prevention of coronary artery disease (CAD) and the reduction of mortality after myocardial infarction. CAD remains the leading cause of death in Western industrialized countries and there is little doubt that regular exercise can decrease your chances of dying prematurely. Therefore, inactive (sedentary) individuals can greatly benefit from becoming more active.

The many health-related benefits of a physically active lifestyle are well documented. However, it is essential to realize that to be most effective, regular exercise must be combined with other positive lifestyle interventions. Furthermore, although exercise is extremely safe for most individuals, it is prudent to take certain precautions to optimize the benefit-to-risk ratio.

To ensure an optimal benefit-to-risk ratio, the exercise professional should incorporate some form of health appraisal before performing fitness testing or initiating an exercise program. The purpose of such an appraisal is to provide information relevant to the safety of fitness testing before beginning exercise training, to identify known diseases and risk factors for CAD and other preventable chronic diseases so that appropriate lifestyle interventions can be initiated, and to identify additional factors that require special consideration when developing an appropriate exercise prescription and programming that optimize adherence, minimize risks, and maximize benefits.

It is essential that the preparticipation health appraisal be both cost-effective and time-efficient so that unnecessary barriers to exercise can be avoided. The precise nature and extent of the appraisal should be determined by the age, sex, and perceived health status characteristics of the partic-

Table 5.1 – Physical Activity Readiness Questionnaire: Matching Questions of Original and Revised Versions

Original	Revised
1. Has your doctor ever said you have heart trouble?	1. Has your doctor ever said that you have a heart condition and that you should only do physical activity recommended by a doctor?
2. Do you frequently have pains in your heart and chest?	2. Do you feel pain in your chest when you do physical activity?
3. Do you often feel faint or have spells of severe dizziness?	4. Do you lose your balance because of dizziness or do you ever lose consciousness?
4. Has a doctor ever said your blood pressure was too high?	6. Is your doctor currently prescribing drugs (for example, water pills) for your blood pressure or heart condition?
5. Has your doctor ever told you that you have a bone or joint problem such as arthritis that has been aggravated by exercise or might be made worse with exercise?	5. Do you have a bone or joint problem that could be made worse by a change in your physical activity?
6. Is there a good physical reason not mentioned here why you should not follow an activity program even if you wanted to?	7. Do you know of any other reason you should not do physical activity?
7. Are you over 65 and not accustomed to vigorous exercise?	(No matching question. Introductory comments state: If you are over 69 years of age, and you are not used to being very active, check with your doctor.)
(No matching question)	3. In the past month, have you had chest pain when you were not doing physical activity?

Table 5.2 – Physical Activity Readiness Questionnaire (PAR-Q)

For most people, physical activity should not pose any problem or hazard. PAR-Q has been designed to identify the small number of adults for whom physical activity might be inappropriate and those who should have medical advice concerning the type of activity most suitable.

1. Has a doctor ever said that you have a heart condition and that you should only do physical activity recommended by a doctor?
   (**Significance/clarification:** Persons with known heart disease are at increased risk for cardiac complications during exercise. They should consult a physician and undergo exercise testing before starting an exercise program. The exercise prescription should be formulated in accordance with standard guidelines for cardiac patients. Medical supervision may be required during exercise training.)

2. Do you feel pain in your chest when you do physical activity?

3. In the past month, have you had chest pain when you were not doing physical activity?
   (**Significance/clarification:** A physician should be consulted to identify the cause of the chest pain, whether it occurs at rest or with exertion. If ischemic in origin, the condition should be stabilized before starting an exercise program. Exercise testing should be performed with the patient on his or her usual medication and the exercise prescription formulated in accordance with standard guidelines for cardiac patients. Medical supervision may be required during exercise training.)

4. Do you lose your balance because of dizziness or do you ever lose consciousness?
   (**Significance/clarification:** A physician should be consulted to establish the cause of these symptoms, which may be related to potentially life-threatening medical conditions. Exercise training should not be undertaken until serious cardiac disorders have been excluded.)

5. Do you have a bone or joint problem that could be made worse by a change in your physical activity?
   (**Significance/clarification:** Existing musculoskeletal disorders may be exacerbated by inappropriate exercise training. Persons with forms of arthritis known to be associated with a systemic component (for example, rheumatoid arthritis) may be at an increased risk for exercise-related medical complications. A physician should be consulted to determine whether any special precautions are required during exercise training.)

6. Is your doctor currently prescribing drugs (for example, water pills) for your blood pressure or heart condition?
   (**Significance/clarification:** See question 1. Medication effects should be considered when formulating the exercise prescription. The exercise prescription should be formulated in accordance with guidelines for the specific cardiovascular disease for which medications are being used. A physician should be consulted to determine whether the condition or factor requires special precautions during exercise training or contraindicates exercise training.)

7. Do you know of any other reason you should not do physical activity?
   (**Significance/clarification:** The exercise prescription may have to be modified in accordance with the specific reason provided. Depending on the specific reason, a physician may have to be consulted.)

If a person answers yes to any question, vigorous exercise or exercise testing may have to be postponed. Medical clearance may be necessary.

ipants, as well as the available economic, personnel, and equipment resources. Health appraisals can range from a short questionnaire to interviews and sophisticated computerized evaluations.

Safety of Exercise

Most prospective participants in exercise programs conducted in nonmedical settings are apparently healthy individuals whose goals are to enhance fitness and well-being, reduce weight, and reduce risk of chronic disease. For such individuals, the primary safety goal of a preparticipation health appraisal is to identify individuals who should receive further medical evaluation to determine whether there are contraindications to exercise testing or training, or whether referral to a medically supervised exercise program is necessary.

According to ACSM guidelines, asymptomatic, apparently healthy men under age 45 and women under age 55 with fewer than two CAD risk factors do not require medical clearance before beginning a vigorous exercise program. It is also considered unnecessary for asymptomatic apparently healthy men and women, irrespective of age or CAD risk factors, to have a medical evaluation by a physician before embarking on a program of moderate exercise training (i.e., exercise intensity 40–60% $\dot{V}O_{2max}$) (1). For such individuals, preparticipation screening can be accomplished using validated self-administered questionnaires, such as the Physical Activity Readiness Questionnaire (PAR-Q).

Although many preexercise questionnaires are available, the PAR-Q is well developed and most widely used. Modifications to any preexercise screening tool should be determined primarily by the population served.

Some limitations to consider when using the PAR-Q should include:

1. Inability to screen out persons with two or more major CAD risk factors (who require a medical examination before participation in vigorous exercise)
2. Automatic referral for medical evaluation by a physician of asymptomatic, apparently healthy individuals over age 65, even if participation in moderate exercise is the goal
3. Inability to identify medications that may affect exercise safety
4. Inability to identify pregnant women, for whom special safety precautions may be required
5. From an overall health perspective, the absence of questions aimed at the identification of adverse health behaviors other than a sedentary lifestyle

The original and newest revisions of the PAR-Q are shown in Table 5.1. The significance/clarification of each of the question in the new version of

the PAR-Q is outlined in Table 5.2. Customized questionnaires can be developed to address the limited capability of the PAR-Q; to obtain information about risk factors, personal history, and health behaviors; and to obtain other information that may warrant special considerations.

ACSM Risk Stratification

It is recommended that persons interested in participating in organized exercise programs be evaluated for selected risk factors associated with the development of coronary artery disease (CAD) (3.7) and for signs or symptoms suggestive of cardiovascular, pulmonary, or metabolic disease (Box 5.1) (8). The risk factor list presented in Table 5.3 should not be viewed as an all-inclusive list of risk factors for CAD, but rather as a list of risk factors with clinically relevant thresholds which should be considered collectively when making decisions about the level of medical clearance, the need for exercise testing prior to program entry, and the level of supervision for both exercise testing and exercise program participation. Other variables (e.g., major depression) have also been suggested as positive risk factors in the primary and secondary prevention of CAD (2).

Once symptom and risk factor screening has occurred, it is recommended that individuals being considered for exercise testing or who plan to increase their physical activity be stratified based on the likelihood of untoward events. This stratification becomes increasingly important as disease prevalence increases in the population under consideration. Using age, health status, symptom, and risk factor information, participants and clients can be initially classified into one of three risk strata (Box 5.2) for triage and preliminary decision making.

No set of guidelines for exercise testing and participation can cover all situations. Local circumstances and policies vary, and specific program procedures are also properly diverse. To provide some general guidance on the need for a medical examination and exercise testing prior to participation in a moderate-to-vigorous exercise program, ACSM suggests the recommendations presented in Table 5.4 for determining when a diag-

Box 5.1 – Major Signs or Symptoms Suggestive of Cardiovascular and pulmonary Disease*

- Pain, discomfort (or other anginal equivalent) in the chest, neck, jaw, arms, or other areas that may be due to ischemia
- Shortness of breath at rest or with mild exertion
- Dizziness or syncope
- Orthopnea or paroxysmal nocturnal dyspnea
- Ankle edema
- Palpitations or tachycardia
- Intermittent claudication
- Known heart murmur
- Unusual fatigue or shortness of breath with usual activities

*These symptoms must be interpreted in the clinical context in which they appear because they are not all specific for cardiovascular, pulmonary, or metabolic disease. For clarification and discussion of the clinical significance of the signs or symptoms, see reference 11.

Table 5.3 – Coronary Artery Disease Risk Factor Thresholds for Use With ACSM Risk Stratification*

Risk Factors	Defining Criteria
Positive	
Family history	Myocardial infarction, coronary revascularization, or sudden death before 55 years of age in father or other male first-degree relative (i.e., brother or son), or before 65 years of age in mother or other female first-degree relative (i.e., sister or daughter)
Cigarette smoking	Current cigarette smoker or those who quit within the previous 6 months
Hypertension	Systolic blood pressure of $\geq$140 mm Hg or diastolic $\geq$90 mm Hg, confirmed by measurements on at least 2 separate occasions, or on antihypertensive medication
Hypercholesterolemia	Total serum cholesterol of >200 mg/dL (5.2 mmol/L) or high-density lipoprotein cholesterol of <35 mg/dL (0.9 mmol/L), or on lipid-lowering medication. If low-density lipoprotein cholesterol is available, use >130 mg/dL (3.4 mmol/L) rather than total cholesterol of >200 mg/dL
Impaired fasting glucose	Fasting blood glucose of $\geq$110 mg/dL (6.1 mmol/L) confirmed by measurements on at least 2 separate occasions (7)
Obesity†	Body Mass Index of $\geq$30 kg/m² (8), or waist girth of >100 cm (9)
Sedentary lifestyle	Persons not participating in a regular exercise program or meeting the minimal physical activity recommendations‡ from the U.S. Surgeon General's report (10)
Negative	
High serum HDL cholesterol§	>60 mg/dL (1.6 mmol/L)

*Adapted from Expert Panel on Detection, Evaluation, and Treatment of High Blood Cholesterol in Adults. Summary of the second report of the National Cholesterol Education Program (NCEP) expert panel on detection, evaluation, and treatment of high blood cholesterol in adults (Adult Treatment Panel II). JAMA 1993;269:3015–3023.

†Professional opinions vary regarding the most appropriate markers and thresholds for obesity; therefore, exercise professionals should use clinical judgment when evaluating this risk factor.

‡Accumulating 30 minutes or more of moderate physical activity on most days of the week.

§It is common to sum risk factors in making clinical judgments. If high-density lipoprotein (HDL) cholesterol is high, subtract one risk factor from the sum of positive risk factors because high HDL decreases CAD risk.

Box 5.2 – Initial ACSM Risk Stratification

Low risk
Younger individuals* who are asymptomatic and meet no more than one risk factor threshold from Table 2-1
Moderate risk
Older individuals (men $\geq$ 45 years of age; women $\geq$ 55 years of age) or those who meet the threshold for two or more risk factors from Table 2-1
High risk
Individuals with one or more signs/symptoms listed in Box 2-1 or known cardiovascular,† pulmonary,‡ or metabolic§ disease

*Men < 45 years of age; women < 55 years of age.

†Cardiac, peripheral vascular, or cerebrovascular disease.

‡Chronic obstructive pulmonary disease, asthma, interstitial lung disease, or cystic fibrosis (see reference 12).

§Diabetes mellitus (types 1 and 2), thyroid disorders, renal or liver disease.

nostic medical examination and exercise test are appropriate and when physician supervision is recommended. Although the testing guidelines are less rigorous for those individuals considered to be low risk, the information gathered from an exercise test may be useful in establishing a safe and effective exercise prescription for these individuals. The exercise testing recommendations reflect the notion that the risk of untoward events increases as a function of exercise intensity (*e.g.,* moderate versus vigorous). Although several descriptions of "moderate" and "vigorous" exercise are listed in Table 5.4, exercise professionals should choose the most applicable definition for their setting when making decisions about the level of screening prior to exercise training and physician supervision during exercise testing. The degree of medical supervision of exercise tests varies appropriately from physician-supervised tests to situations in which there may be no physician present. The degree of physician supervision may vary with local policies and circumstances, the health status of the client, and the experience of the laboratory staff. The appropriate protocol should be based on the age, health status, and physical activity level of the person to be tested.

In all situations where exercise testing is performed, site personnel should be trained and certified in cardiopulmonary resuscitation. Whenever possible, testing should be performed by ACSM-certified personnel because these certifications evaluate knowledge, skills, and abilities directly related to exercise testing.

B. Cardiorespiratory Assessment of Apparently Healthy Populations

Several physiological responses to exercise are used to evaluate cardiorespiratory (CR) fitness, including oxygen consumption ($\dot{V}O_{2max}$), heart rate, and blood pressure. Measuring these variables during exercise, particularly maximum exercise, increases the chance of detecting any coronary artery disease or pulmonary disease. Unfortunately, maximum exercise tests are impractical and very expensive. Therefore, maximal testing is reserved for clinical assessments, athletic evaluation, and research. Submaximal exercise tests cost less and carry a lower risk for the individual. Although less sensitive and specific for detecting disease or estimating maximal oxygen consumption ($\dot{V}O_{2max}$), when correctly performed, submaximal tests can provide a valid estimate of cardiorespiratory fitness.

Pretest Screening

Pretest health screening is essential for risk stratification and for determining the type of test that should be performed and the need for an exercise test prior to exercise training (9). A thorough pretest health screening includes the following:

- Complete medical history
- Medical contraindications to exercise
- Symptoms suggesting cardiac or pulmonary disease
- Angina or other forms of discomfort at rest or during exercise
- Unusual shortness of breath at rest or during exercise
- Dizziness or light-headedness
- Orthopaedic complications that may prevent adequate effort or compromise the validity of test results
- Other unusual signs or symptoms that may preclude testing
- Risk factors for coronary heart disease
- History of major cardiorespiratory events
- Current medications
- Activity patterns
- Nutritional habits
- Reading and signing an informed consent form

Along with the appropriate informed consent, the PAR-Q has been recommended as a minimum standard for entry into a moderate-intensity exercise program (9). In addition, the ACSM and the American Heart Association have published a preparticipation screening questionnaire for health and fitness facilities (10). If any concerns are raised by the health screen appraisal or readiness questionnaire, a medical referral should be obtained before proceeding with the test.

Submaximal Exercise Testing

During submaximal exercise testing, predetermined workloads are used to elicit a steady state of exertion (plateau of heart rate and $\dot{V}O_2$). The steady-state heart rate at each work level is displayed graphically and extrapolated to the $\dot{V}O_2$ at the age-predicted maximal heart rate (max HR = 220 − age). A variety of protocols for different exercise modalities (*i.e.*, treadmill, stationary cycle, and step increments) can be used as long as the $\dot{V}O_2$ requirements of each selected workload can be estimated with accuracy.

The objectives of cardiovascular fitness assessments in the apparently healthy population are as follows:

- Determine the level of cardiovascular fitness and establish fitness program goals and objectives.
- Develop a safe, effective exercise prescription for the improvement of cardiovascular fitness.

Table 5.4 – ACSM Recommendations for (A) Current Medical Examination* and Exercise Testing Prior to Participation and (B) Physician Supervision of Exercise Tests

	Low Risk	Moderate Risk	High Risk
A.			
Moderate exercise[†]	Not necessary[‡]	Not necessary	Recommended
Vigorous exercise[§]	Not necessary	Recommended	Recommended
B.			
Submaximal test	Not necessary	Not necessary	Recommended
Maximal test	Not necessary	Recommended[∥]	Recommended

*Within the past year (see reference 2).

†Absolute moderate exercise is defined as activities that are approximately 3–6 METs or the equivalent of brisk walking at 3 to 4 mph for most healthy adults (13). Nevertheless, a pace of 3 to 4 mph might be considered to be "hard" to "very hard" by some sedentary, older persons. Moderate exercise may alternatively be defined as an intensity well within the individual's capacity, one which can be comfortably sustained for a prolonged period of time (~45 min), which has a gradual initiation and progression, and is generally noncompetitive. If an individual's exercise capacity is known, relative moderate exercise may be defined by the range 40–60% maximal oxygen uptake.

‡The designation of "Not necessary" reflects the notion that a medical examination, exercise test, and physician supervision of exercise testing would not be essential in the preparticipation screening; however, they should not be viewed as inappropriate.

§Vigorous exercise is defined as activities of >6 METs. Vigorous exercise may alternatively be defined as exercise intense enough to represent a substantial cardiorespiratory challenge. If an individual's exercise capacity is known, vigorous exercise may be defined as an intensity of >60% maximal oxygen uptake.

∥When physician supervision of exercise testing is "Recommended," the physician should be in close proximity and readily available should there be an emergent need.

- Document improvements in CR fitness as a result of exercise training or other interventions.
- Motivate individuals to initiate an exercise program or comply with an established program.
- Provide information concerning health status.

Although if done correctly, submaximal exercise tests provide valuable information concerning cardiovascular fitness, they have extremely limited diagnostic capabilities and should not be used as a replacement for clinical exercise tests or other clinical treatment or management modalities. Health care professionals should avoid detailed interpretation beyond the scope of the information obtained.

Considerations with Submaximal Exercise Testing

Considerations for selection of protocol and equipment include any physical or clinical limitations that may preclude certain types of exercise (*i.e.*, age, weight, arthritis, orthopaedic complications, individual comfort, level of fitness, type of exercise training that will be performed, and individual preference) (11–13). For example, some individuals may perform better on a non–weight-bearing modality (cycle versus treadmill), while others may not have the required range of motion in the hip or knee to pedal and may perform better walking. Deconditioned, weak, or elderly persons may have to start the test at a low work level and increase the workload in small increments.

Table 5.5 – Cost Comparison of Submaximal Testing Modalities

Costs	Treadmill	Cycle	Step	Field
Equipment	+++	++	+	+
Staff needs	+++	+++	+	+
Interpretation	++	++	++	++
Space	+++	++	++	+
Paper, forms	++	++	++	++
Other indirect costs	+++	+++	++	+

+++, Greater expense; +, lesser expense

Regardless of the type of exercise and protocol selected, the same type of exercise and protocol should be used for repeat testing if between-test comparisons are important.

Staffing

The staff administering the tests should be ACSM certified and academically trained in exercise science or at least have a basic knowledge of exercise physiology and exercise testing. Staff members should be able to do the following:

1. Establish rapport with the subject and make him or her feel comfortable.
2. Recognize normal acute and chronic responses to exercise.
3. Recognize abnormal signs and symptoms during exercise.
4. Provide basic life support measures competently.
5. Adhere to established procedures and protocols.
6. Clearly explain test results to the individual.

Table 5.5 provides a relative comparison of the costs of the various modalities used for submaximal exercise testing.

Test Type

Procedural guidelines for several submaximal-testing protocols are provided in the *ACSM Guidelines for Exercise Testing and Prescription* (9).

Cycle Ergometer Tests

For the following reasons, cycle ergometers are the most commonly used modality for submaximal exercise testing:

- Low expense
- Portability
- Small space requirements
- Ease of use by both clients and providers
- Heart rate and $\dot{V}O_2$ responses highly reproducible at standardized workloads
- A low rate of prediction errors (coefficient of variation of less than 10%) (14, 15)

Frequently used cycle protocols include the YMCA protocol and the Astrand–Rhyming protocol. Both tests have norms and reliably predict $\dot{V}O_{2max}$ (14, 16). For well-trained cyclists, commonly used protocols may prove inadequate.

Cycles with a high power output capacity and protocols employing faster pedaling rates may be necessary to elicit the desired range of physiological responses to ensure accuracy (17).

Stepping Protocols

Step testing is an excellent modality for predicting cardiorespiratory fitness by measuring the heart rate response to one or more step rates (or step heights), or by measuring postexercise recovery heart rates. Step tests require little or no equipment; steps are easily transportable; stepping skill requires no practice; the test is usually of short duration; and stepping is excellent for mass testing (21, 22). Postexercise (recovery) heart rates decrease with improved cardiorespiratory fitness and test results are easy to explain to participants (22). Special precautions might be needed for those who have balance problems or are extremely deconditioned.

With respect to equipment and staffing needs, stepping protocols are inexpensive because they allow testing of several subjects concurrently. Upon completion of the step test, the heart rate is counted for a fixed time. The use of a standard 8-inch step eliminates the need for different step heights and allows the test to be performed in any stairway.

The primary physiological assumption of the step test is that the rate of recovery indicates the level of cardiovascular endurance (18). The mean prediction error for step testing is 12%, and a 95% confidence interval of 16% has been demonstrated (19). Step tests are easily administered according to guidelines similar to those traditionally used by the YMCA (16).

Individual Monitoring and Abnormal Responses

Submaximal exercise tests allow the exercise professional to obtain data about individuals at varying levels of fitness. For those at high risk and who require much supervision, individual testing in a laboratory may be more appropriate than field testing. During treadmill or cycle ergometer tests, heart rate, electrocardiogram, blood pressure, rate of perceived exertion, signs, and symptoms can be easily recorded. Vital signs should be assessed prior to the test, at each workload, and during recovery for a total of at least four to eight minutes. Once the criterion heart rate or work rate has been obtained, the individuals should be given an adequate cool-down period. This may consist of slowing the pace of the treadmill, decreasing the resistance on an ergometer, or allowing subjects to walk freely. An adequate cool-down should last until the individual feels rested, ventilation and heart rate have slowed to near resting levels, and all symptoms resolve.

Field or group testing may be appropriate for

Table 5.6 – Original and Revised Scales for Ratings of Perceived Exertion

ORIGINAL SCALE		CATEGORY–RATIO SCALE	
6	0.0	Nothing at all	No intensity
7 Very, very light	0.3		
8	0.5	Extremely weak	Just noticeable
9 Very light	0.7		
10	1.0	Very weak	
11 Fairly light	1.5		
12	2.0	Weak	Light
13 Somewhat hard	2.5		
14	3.0	Moderate	
15 Hard	4.0		
16	5.0	Strong	Heavy
17 Very hard	6.0		
18	7.0	Very strong	
19 Very, very hard	8.0		
20	9.0		
	10.0	Extremely strong	Strongest intensity
	11.0		
		Absolute maximum	Highest possible

low-risk individuals. During field testing, it may be possible to record only time or distance during the test and heart rate at test completion. Furthermore, it may be possible to monitor for signs of distress only visually. However, close supervision and monitoring are crucial, and participants should be carefully assessed prior to the test. Throughout the testing and recovery periods, supervisors should position themselves so that they can maintain visual contact with each participant.

Although individuals may be thoroughly screened prior to testing, evidence of occult disease may arise at any time during testing and recovery. For this reason, the following variables should be monitored throughout the test and recovery periods:

- Rating of perceived exertion (Table 5.6)
- Signs or symptoms of cardiac or pulmonary distress or signs of overexertion, including chest pain or other discomfort, shortness of breath, dizziness or light-headedness, or profuse sweating and nausea
- Heart rate and rhythm
- Blood pressure

Test Termination

In the event of an abnormal response, the test should be terminated, the medical director of the facility and the individual's primary care physician notified, and all specified follow-up procedures performed. In the event of mechanical or electrical failure that may compromise the accuracy of the test results or monitoring capabilities, the test should be terminated until the problem is corrected.

Procedures and protocols for the most common emergencies that occur during exercise (e.g., angina, myocardial infarction, dysrhythmia, hypoglycemia, dizziness, and cardiac arrest) should be part of the institution's operations manual and clearly posted in the testing area, known by every staff member, and reviewed and practiced frequently. Make sure that all entrances are clear, staff members know their specific roles, and all telephone numbers and contact information are current and clearly posted. All professional exercise staff members should have the appropriate level of ACSM certification and a minimum of basic life support certification.

Psychological factors, such as pretest anxiety, may influence the heart rate, especially at rates below 120 bpm and at low workloads. It is not unusual for the heart rate and/or blood pressure to be higher at rest than during the initial stages of exercise in these cases. Having the subject repeat the first test may improve reliability, particularly if the subject has never previously performed such a test (20).

Factors that can cause variation in the heart rate response to testing:

- Dehydration
- Prolonged heavy exercise prior to testing
- Environmental conditions (e.g., heat, humidity, ventilation)
- Fever
- Use of alcohol, tobacco, or caffeine 2–3 h prior to testing

Because of these inherent inconsistencies, standard procedures for each test must be strictly followed to ensure the greatest accuracy and reproducibility possible:

- Standard testing protocol
- The same testing modality and protocol for repeat testing
- A constant pedal speed throughout cycle ergometry testing
- Cycle seat height properly adjusted, recorded, and standard for each test
- The time of day for repeat testing consistent
- All data collection procedures standardized and consistent
- Test conditions standard
- Subjects free of infection and in normal sinus rhythm
- Prior to the test, no intense or prolonged exercise for 24 h, smoking for 2–3 h, caffeine for 3 h, or heavy meal for 3 h
- Room temperature 18–20°C (64–68°F) with air movement provided

C. Assessment of Muscular Strength and Endurance

Muscular fitness is one of the primary components of physical health. It includes two basic physiological components: muscular strength and muscular endurance. Muscular strength refers to the ability to generate force at a given speed (velocity) of movement (23). Muscular endurance refers to the ability to persist in physical activity or to resist muscular fatigue (24). Muscular strength and endurance are developed by placing an overload on the targeted muscle or muscle groups. Through adaptation, the muscle groups become stronger or better able to sustain muscular activity.

Specificity of Training

The increase in strength resulting from resistance training is specific to the following:
- The type of contraction used in training
- The range of motion (ROM) through which training occurs
- The velocity of contraction during training
- Whether exercises are performed unilaterally or bilaterally

These examples of specificity of training are at least partially attributed to neural adaptation; however, for specificity of contraction, and type and velocity of contraction, evidence suggests that resistance training also has specific effects on the contractile properties of the muscle. There are two basic types of muscle activity: static and dynamic. In static muscular activity, the muscle attempts to shorten against a fixed or immovable resistance. There is no skeletal movement, and the muscle neither shortens nor lengthens forcibly. Dynamic muscle action involves movement, which may be concentric (*i.e.,* the force produced by the muscle is sufficient to overcome resistance and muscle shortening occurs) or eccentric (*i.e.,* the muscle exerts force, lengthens, and is overcome by the resistance).

Training a muscle group with dynamic actions (*e.g.,* lifting weights) produces a relatively large increase in dynamic muscle strength but only small increases in isometric strength. Isometric training, on the other hand, improves isometric strength more than dynamic strength (27).

Strength training at slow speeds results in relatively large increases in the ability of the muscle to generate force at slow speeds but relatively small increases during contractions at faster speeds. The carryover of strength from high-speed training to slow-speed testing is also reduced (28). An intermediate training velocity is best for increasing strength at all velocities of movement. Thus, for individuals interested in general fitness, an intermediate training velocity is recommended (25).

Measurement Devices

The dynamometer is used to measure static strength by recording the amount of force exerted. The most common type is the hand or grip dynamometer. Grip strength is measured as kilograms of force exerted by squeezing the hand dynamometer as hard as possible.

Dynamometers are popular for testing large numbers of people because they are easy to use and portable. Cumbersome setup procedures that often accompany other types of muscle performance measurements are not required. However, dynamometers can be used to measure only a few muscle groups, and their reliability is not well established. In addition, isolation of specific muscle groups is not accomplished, which makes standardization difficult.

One repetition maximum (1 RM) tests measure the greatest amount of weight that can be lifted one time for a specific weight-lifting exercise. The tests are usually limited to the amount of weight that can be lifted at the weakest position in the ROM and therefore do not assess muscle performance through a full ROM. Generally the test begins with an amount of weight that can be easily lifted. After a successful trial, a 2–3 min rest period is allowed. The weight is increased by 5–10 lb (or more, depending on the difficulty of the previous lift) and another trial is attempted. The 1 RM, the amount of weight for the last trial that can be successfully completed with good form, can usually be obtained in 4–6 trials. The 1 RM provides a measure of dynamic strength that can be applied to almost any weight lifting exercise. One-RM tests are commonly used because they are easy to administer and can often be performed with the same equipment used for training. They are highly reliable, although they do involve a skill factor, and subsequent tests may yield greater results due to practice. Thus, 1-RM tests may not be specific for muscle force production.

The application of computer technology and advancements in machine design has improved the accuracy and standardization of muscular strength testing. Some electromechanical instruments have been designed to measure dynamic muscular strength at a preset movement speed. In theory, these constant-velocity (isokinetic) dynamometers are thought to measure the maximum force that can be applied throughout the constant-velocity movement. Because a period of acceleration is required to reach the preselected velocity of movement and a period of deceleration is required at the end of the movement, isokinetic dynamometers cannot measure force production through a full ROM. In addition, oscillation in observed forces, called torque overshoot, can limit the accuracy of these devices. Torque overshoot represents impact forces between the moving body part and the measurement device.

Measurement of Muscular Strength

The primary function of skeletal muscle is to generate force. In most instances, forces generated by skeletal muscles are used to produce movement or for anatomical stabilization. The measurement of muscle force production is used for the following purposes:
- Assess muscular fitness

- Identify weakness
- Monitor progress in rehabilitation programs
- Measure the effectiveness of resistance training

The maximum amount of force that a muscle or group of muscles generates can be measured by a variety of methods, including a dynamometer, strain gauge device, 1-RM test, or computer-assisted force and work output determination. Each of these methods has been briefly described.

Regardless of the method chosen to assess muscular strength, certain conditions are required for accurate and reliable measurement of muscle force output. Body position must be stabilized to allow only the desired movement. In the case of measuring muscle force generation during an isometric contraction, the involved joint or joints at which movement would occur must be isolated.

Muscle force production varies throughout the ROM. The most descriptive measures of muscle function account for this. The term *strength curve* describes a plot of the resultant force exerted versus an appropriate measure of the joint configuration. Because of acceleration at the initiation and deceleration at the termination of all movements, and because dynamic strength is influenced by the speed of movement, dynamic strength tests are not appropriate for the quantification of muscle function through a ROM. In addition, if dynamic muscle actions are performed rapidly, kinetic forces that give an inaccurate measure of true force production may be recorded. Depending on the specific movement, these kinetic forces may be dangerous, especially for populations with orthopaedic problems, because of the impact that occurs upon rapid deceleration. Isometric tests can safely and accurately quantify muscle force production throughout the ROM if multiple joint angles are measured.

A final consideration required for the accurate assessment of muscle force production is whether the mass of the involved body part influences the measurement. For example, if the force generated by the quadriceps muscles during knee extension does not equal or exceed the mass of the lower leg, no measurable force is observed. Thus, the mass of the lower leg detracts from observed force production of the quadriceps muscles during knee extension testing. This mass must be accounted for to accurately quantify force. Although there is some controversy concerning the need for correction of the influence of gravitational forces during testing because most bodily actions are not corrected for gravity, the actual force generated by specific muscles in certain positions may be significantly influenced by body mass (29). Thus, although one cannot neglect the fact that in normal daily activities muscles are influenced by body mass, standardization of testing position and correction for gravitational forces are required for accurate quantification of muscle force production. The need for stabilization, positional standardization, compensation for gravitational influences, and measurement through a ROM have been recently discussed by Pollock et al. (26).

Measurement of Muscular Endurance

Almost all of the devices for measuring strength can also be used for assessing muscular endurance. Tests of muscular endurance should be designed to evaluate the ability of muscle groups to produce submaximal force for repeated contractions. More specifically, the length of time a muscle contraction can be held or the number of repeated submaximal contractions a muscle group can make should be determined. Accordingly, similar to strength, muscular endurance can be assessed either statically or dynamically.

Measuring Muscle Endurance Statically

Two basic methods can be used to assess static muscular endurance. One method involves performing a maximal static contraction and sustaining that level of contraction for 60 s. The force being exerted by the muscle should be recorded at 10-s intervals. Accordingly, individuals who have a slower rate of decline in force production are exhibiting a greater level of muscle endurance for that specific muscle group than those whose level of recorded force falls faster. A second method for assessing static muscular endurance is to determine the length of time a given percentage of a maximum voluntary contraction can be sustained.

Measuring Muscle Endurance Dynamically

Several ways to determine dynamic muscular endurance exist. One way dynamic muscle endurance is assessed is to perform the maximum number of repetitions possible using a set weight, a given percentage of maximum strength (*e.g.*, of 1 RM), or some set percentage of body weight. The endurance of a muscle group can be determined isokinetically through the performance of successive maximal repetitions. Isokinetic muscular endurance is measured as the number of repetitions completed before the torque production drops below 50% of the maximal torque value. Perhaps the most commonly used method for evaluating muscular endurance is calisthenics (*e.g.*, situps, push-ups, pull-ups). During such tests, the maximum number of times one can lift the body weight is used as the measure of endurance. For persons of below average muscular fitness or above average body weight, however, calisthenics exercises often involve more of a measure of muscular strength than muscular endurance.

D. Flexibility and Range of Motion

Joint flexibility is an important component of movement. The range of motion (ROM) of various joints is measured as a part of any evaluation of fitness or work capacity or clinical assessment of joint function

Flexibility Evaluation

There are many methods for evaluating joint ROM. Visual estimates and/or measurements are made, often with a special instrument. Movement may be produced actively or passively. Differences in technique vary from the use of warm-up exercises prior to measurement to changing the starting position. Measurement technique may vary, depending upon the joint and motion. Differences in methodology suggest that accuracy and consistency can be achieved by following procedural principles. Furthermore, precision in assessment techniques enhances both accuracy and reliability.

Visual Estimate versus Measured ROM

Visual estimates of ROM have been shown to be inaccurate for both extremity and spinal movements (30, 31). Gross or visual estimates of movement may, however, be useful for fitness screenings, group evaluations, and field testing, which are discussed later.

Active versus Passive Movement

Although ROM measurements are commonly taken for both passive and active movements, it is more difficult to obtain an accurate measurement during passive ROM (31). Passive joint movement can exert variable forces that may alter the ROM. When the individual is unable to move an extremity actively, for example because of paralysis or primary muscle disease, passive ROM can be measured reliably.

Technique can have significant effect on accuracy. Improper identification of anatomical landmarks is a source of error in the trunk and extremities (30, 31). Use of surface markings and standardized bony landmarks increases reliability, as does the correct positioning of the individual and the proximal joint segment (30, 32). Using a standard position that stabilizes the proximal segment and allows full range of movement in the distal segment improves reliability (30, 31, 33). It is not clear whether a single measure or multiple measures of a single movement improves reliability. Measurement of a simple hinge joint movement (*e.g.,* elbow flexion) is more accurate than the measurement of a complex movement (*e.g.,* ankle inversion). Repeated trials of passive straight leg–raising can increase the ROM as a result of moving the limb to the extremes of the ROM (34). When possible, measurements should be taken starting with the limb in an anatomically neutral position to increase reliability; this is particularly important when edema or contracture is present. Placement and stabilization of the measuring device can affect measurement reliability (30).

Measurement Devices

ROM is most often measured by goniometers, inclinometers, tape measures, and flexible rules. The selection of the device may depend upon the joint being measured.

Goniometers

Goniometers are the most commonly used measuring device for ROM because they are inexpensive and portable. The *universal goniometer* consists of two arms: a stationary arm that is stabilized on the proximal portion of the joint and a moving arm aligned with the distal portion of the joint, which is moved through the arc of motion during measurement. There are also dorsal and pendular goniometers (flexometers).

The reliability of goniometers is high if standard techniques are used. Goniometry may be inaccurate in spinal and complex movements (30).

Tape Measures

Tape measures can be used to measure spinal and finger movements. The skin distraction technique can be used to measure trunk flexion and lateral trunk flexion by comparing differences in position of two marks placed appropriately on the skin prior to and after movement (35). Variation for this was 10%. Tape measure techniques may be more reliable for lumbar flexion and lateral trunk flexion than inclinometry. Measurement of fingertip-to-floor distance using tape measure is unreliable (35).

Tape measures can also assess loss of ROM in the carpometacarpal and interphalangeal joints. These techniques are useful only if the individual cannot make a fist.

Flexible Rule

The flexible rule can be used to measure spinal movements. The tangent of an arc described by applying the rule to the contours of back during movement is the measure. Although the flexible rule is reliable, it is not widely used (30).

Group and Field Flexibility Screening

Group or field assessment of flexibility is most appropriate when highly accurate measures of ROM are not required. Field testing is commonly used to observe postural alignment (malalignment may make an individual prone to injury). The most common field tests are shown in Figures 5.1–5.4.

Tests that isolate trunk flexibility (Fig. 5.1C) from hamstring flexibility (Fig. 5.2C) are recommended because of the relationship to back injury. Figure 5.5 illustrates postural assessment.

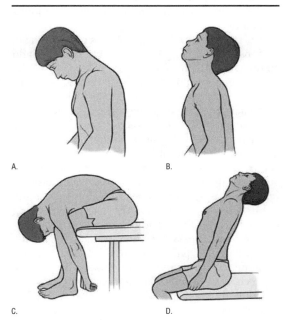

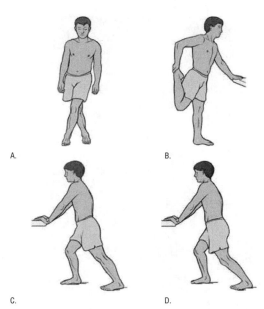

Figures 5.3 A-D (above) – Lower extremity flexibility. A. Illotibial band tightness. While standing, cross the lower extremity in from of the other limb and rotate hip internally. B. Rectus femoris length. With full hip extension, the leg should almost touch the buttocks. C. Gastrocnemius ROM. With knee straight and limb placed as far posteriorly as possible, the heel remains flat on the floor. D. Soleus ROM. Same position as gastrocnemius except with bent knee. Heel remains on floor.

Figures 5.1 A-D (above) – Neck and trunk flexion screening. A. Cervical flexion. The chin should touch the chest. B. Cervical extension. The head should bend as far as possible posteriorly. C. Vertebral flexion. With the hips and knees bent, the trunk should touch the anterior thighs. D. Vertebral extension. Backward movement of the trunk as far as possible without hip extension.

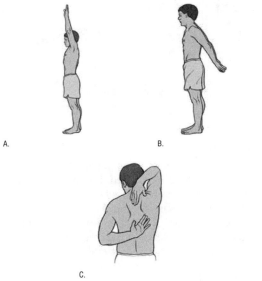

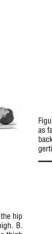

Figures 5.4 A-C (above) – Shoulder flexibility. A. Flexion. Reach forward and upwards as far as possible; the humerous with be parallel to the ear. B. Extension. Reach as far backward as possible. C. Combined bilateral rotation and elbow flexion. Normally fingertips should almost touch.

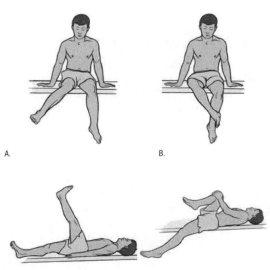

Figures 5.2 A-D (above) – Hip flexibility screening. A. Internal rotation. WHith the hip and knee flexed, move the leg as far to the side as possible by rolling the thigh. B. External rotation. Move the lef as far as possible past the midline by rolling the thigh outward. C. Straight leg raising. Keep the contralateral lower extremity in full extension while lifting the other extremity without bending the knee. Note limited hamstring flexibility. D. Combined test of hip flexion on the right. Bring the bent hip and knee as close to the chest as possible with a Thomas test for hip extension on the left by allowing the limb to drop over the edge of the table into extension.

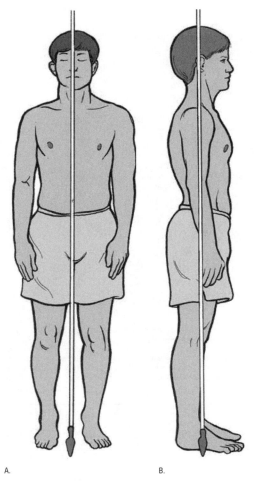

A.   B.

Figures 5.5 A-B (above) – Postural assessment with a plumb line. A. Anterior. Observe for symmetry and knee position. B. Lateral. Observe alignment of head, shoulders, hips, knees, and ankles.

Flexibility and Fitness

The relationship between level of fitness and flexibility is still being studied. It may be especially important in older adults, who usually exhibit a decline in movement capability. There is limited evidence to support the assumption that flexibility is related to fitness level in older adults.

The relationship between flexibility and injury is another pertinent issue. Decreased ROM is not always associated with injury.

Mobility is an important element in performing physical activities, but the ROM required may be specific to the activity. For example, a baseball player requires more dynamic shoulder flexibility than a soccer player. Flexibility assessment is often included in preseason evaluation as a means of preventing injuries, but the relationship between flexibility and injury remains unclear (36).

Identifying Risk Factors for Activity

Exercise professionals should be able to identify clients' conditions that require additional consultation before they begin an exercise program. An accurate and complete health history can elicit significant information. Persistent or recurrent joint pain may identify possibly arthritic joints. Medical consultation is advisable if pain, swelling, and /or heat in a joint or multiple joints is reported.

An individual who reports either recent acute back pain or a history of chronic back pain should be referred to a physician. Back pain is one of the most common and costly musculoskeletal problems in middle-aged adults. Although individuals with back pain are commonly able to participate in exercise programs, they should be referred to a physician and/or a physical therapist for an evaluation. Early intervention may reduce pain and decrease the likelihood that an acute problem will become chronic. This is consistent with the guide lines for management of acute back pain recently published by the Health Care Financing Administration (37). The chronicity of the problem impairs fitness by reducing activity during exacerbation of pain. An individualized exercise program for persons with chronic back pain, supervised by a physical therapist, may improve function, decrease disability, and reduce pain (38).

Complaints of musculoskeletal pain persisting and/or increasing with exercise is a primary reason for seeking a medical consultation. Understanding the underlying cause of pain and the effect exercise are important considerations for the exercise professional in planning exercise programs.

E. Body Composition

Body composition refers to the absolute and relative amounts of lean tissue, body fat, and water. There are many reasons to assess body composition. Most importantly, the strong associations between obesity, especially excessive intra-abdominal (visceral) fat, and increased risk of coronary artery disease, non–insulin-dependent diabetes, hypertension, and certain types of cancer, have received considerable attention in recent years. An excessively low level of fat is also detrimental, as evidenced by the physiological dysfunction of the chronically undernourished. In addition, assessment of body composition is useful to establish optimal weight for health and performance in athletes, to formulate dietary guidelines and exercise prescriptions for modifying body composition and evaluating efficacy, and to monitor changes in composition with growth, maturation, and aging to distinguish normal changes from disease states.

Although body fat is often the focus of assessment, lean tissue mass and its components (fluid, muscle, and bone) are at least as important. Low levels of lean mass and loss of lean tissue contribute to metabolic complications both directly

Table 5.7 – Ratings of the Validity and Objectivity of Body Composition Methods

METHOD	PRECISION	OBJECTIVITY	ACCURACY	VALID EQUATIONS	OVERALL
Body mass index	1	1	4, 5	4, 5	4
Near-infrared interactance	1	1, 2	4	4	3.5
Skinfolds	2	2, 3	2, 3	2, 3	2.5
Bioelectric impedance	2	2	2, 3	2, 3	2.5
Circumferences	2	2	2, 3	2, 4	3.0

1, excellent; 2, very good; 3, good; 4, fair; 5, unacceptable.
Precision is reliability within investigators; objectivity is reliability between investigators; accuracy refers to comparison with a criterion method; valid equations are cross-validated.

and indirectly, through impaired functional capacity and reduced physical activity and energy expenditure, hence a greater risk of fat gain. Low bone mass and density are primary predictors of the risk of osteoporotic fracture. The muscle wasting (sarcopenia) that occurs with certain diseases and with aging not only decreases muscle strength and the capacity for even routine activities but is also a strong correlate of mortality. Recently there has been increased emphasis on the development of interventions to increase lean tissue mass in healthy aging and clinical populations and in athletes. Assessment of lean mass is a crucial aspect of evaluating progress toward that goal.

There are both field and lab techniques to assess body composition. Lab techniques with relatively high accuracy include underwater weighing (also referred to as hydrostatic weighing or hydrodensitometry and considered the "gold standard" of estimating body composition for many years), air-displacement plethysmography (most often performed using an egg-shaped device called the Bod Pod), and Dual X-Ray Absorptiometry (DXA, pronounced "dex-a"). While DXA is used primarily in the lab and clinical setting, new versions of the Bod Pod device are user-friendly enough to be making their way into local health clubs. Exercise professionals generally use field techniques to assess body composition. Field techniques generally require less complex and more portable equipment, are less costly, and can be applied outside of controlled laboratory conditions. Anthropometric assessment using skinfolds and circumferences continues to be the most common approach, although newer techniques, such as bioelectric impedance analysis (BIA), are useful. There are numerous anthropometric and BIA equations for estimating body composition in various populations. As a result, one of the most difficult problems practitioners face is the selection of the most suitable method and equation.

To evaluate and choose the appropriate methods and equations for clients, exercise professionals must be familiar with the development of those methods.

Method Selection

Selection of an appropriate method is based on the relative precision, reliability, and accuracy of available methods, the availability of appropriate equations, and affordability (Table 5.7). Percent body fat and FFM can be estimated with field techniques with errors of more than 3% and more than 2.5–3 kg, respectively. Generally, they are adequate for screening and for following moderate changes in composition over time. When greater precision and accuracy are needed, laboratory techniques must be used.

Anthropometry

Weight-for-height indices and measurements of skinfold thicknesses, limb and trunk circumferences, and skeletal dimensions all have been used to estimate body composition. Circumferences are affected by both fat and muscle and do not provide accurate estimates of fatness in the general population. However, in obese persons, whose skinfold measurements can be difficult to obtain, circumferences can give useful estimates of fatness. Circumferences may also work well in athletic populations to estimate FFM, since athletes tend to vary more in muscularity than body fat.

Skinfolds and circumferences are also useful for assessing fat pattern and indirectly, distribution. The ratio of subscapular to triceps skinfolds, for example, has been used to reflect a central versus peripheral fat pattern, and the ratio of waist to hip circumferences (WHR) is a common index of upper versus lower body fat distribution. Epidemiological studies identify WHR as a predictor of chronic disease risk, and standards are available (Table 5.8). The assessment of fat pattern and distribution in combination with an estimate of total body fat is an

Table 5.8 – Waist-to-Hip Circumference Ratio (WHR) Standard for Men and Women

	AGE	RISK Low	RISK Moderate	RISK High	RISK Very High
Men	20–29	<0.83	0.83–0.88	0.89–0.94	>0.94
	30–39	<0.84	0.84–0.91	0.92–0.96	>0.96
	40–49	<0.88	0.88–0.95	0.96–1.00	>1.00
	50–59	<0.90	0.90–0.96	0.97–1.02	>1.02
	60–69	<0.91	0.91–0.98	0.99–1.03	>1.03
Women	20–29	<0.71	0.71–0.77	0.78–0.82	>0.82
	30–39	<0.72	0.72–0.78	0.79–0.84	>0.84
	40–49	<0.73	0.73–0.79	0.80–0.87	>0.87
	50–59	<0.74	0.74–0.81	0.82–0.88	>0.88
	60–69	<0.76	0.76–0.83	0.84–0.90	>0.90

(Reprinted with permission from Heyward VH, Stolarczyk LM. Applied Body Composition Assessment. Champaign, IL: Human Kinetics, 1996:82).

important aspect of the assessment of disease risk.

The body mass index (BMI), a weight-for-height ratio widely used in epidemiological studies, is calculated as weight in kilograms divided by height in meters squared. Obesity standards (Table 5.9) based on BMI have been developed, and high BMI is associated with increased risk of chronic disease. Ironically, BMI is a poor predictor of percent body fat and often misclassifies individuals as obese if they have above average muscularity and skeletal mass rather than excess fat. In children and the elderly, for whom the ratio of muscle and bone to height is changing, BMI is especially misleading. Although the BMI may be useful when no other method is available, the results must be interpreted cautiously, and a follow-up examination with a more accurate method should be sought for persons for whom interventions are considered.

Excess fat in the abdomen, out of proportion to total body fat, is an independent predictor of risk factors and morbidity. Waist circumference is positively correlated with abdominal fat and is an acceptable measurement for indirectly assessing abdominal fat before and during weight loss. The sex-specific cut points given in Table 5.9 can be used in combination with BMI to identify increased relative risk of the development of obesity-related risk factors in most adults with a BMI of 25–34.9 $kg \cdot m^{-2}$. These waist circumference cut points lose their incremental predictive power in people with a BMI above 35 $kg \cdot m^{-2}$ because these people exceed those cut points.

The reliability and validity of skinfolds and anthropometric methods are affected by the following:
- Skill of the measurer
- Type of caliper (due to pressure differences) or tape measure (if calibration is lost)
- Subject factors related to skinfold compressibility, tissue swelling (edema), and variability in fat pattern and distribution
- The prediction equation used to estimate fatness

Failure to locate and measure the site properly is a major source of technical error in the skinfold method. To avoid these errors, technicians must be trained and certified by an expert, and all measurements should be made according to standard techniques (41). Equipment error can be controlled by regular calibration with Vernier calipers or a meter stick.

The skinfold method assumes that the distribution of subcutaneous and internal fat is the same for everyone to whom a particular equation is applied. Moreover, it is assumed that the sites in a particular equation adequately represent the subcutaneous fat pattern of the individual to whom it is applied. For example, an equation that includes only limb sites underestimates fatness in a person with predominantly truncal fat. Similarly, fatness is underestimated if an equation that includes only upper body sites is applied to a person with a predominantly lower body fat pattern. Equation error can be reduced by basing the selection of prediction equations on the age, sex, race, and level of physical activity in the population being assessed.

Bioelectrical Impedance Analysis

Bioelectrical impedance analysis (BIA) is a rapid, noninvasive, and relatively inexpensive method of estimating fat and FFM. Although the relative prediction accuracy is similar to that of the skinfold method, BIA may be preferable in some settings because it does not require a high degree of technical skill and is generally more comfortable, requires minimal cooperation, and intrudes less on privacy. Baumgartner (42) and Kushner (43) have published excellent overviews of BIA.

Given that the FFM contains large amounts of water (about 73%) and electrolytes, it is a good conductor, unlike fat, which is anhydrous and a poor conductor of electrical current. Thus, total body impedance primarily reflects the volumes of water (intracellular and extracellular fluid) and muscle compartments constituting the FFM.

As with anthropometry, the accuracy and precision of BIA are affected by the instruments used, subject factors, technical skill, and the prediction equation used to estimate FFM (43). Factors such

Table 5.9 – Body Mass Index Standards and Risk of Disease

| WEIGHT | BMI[b] | CLASS | DISEASE RISK[a] | |
			MEN ≤ 102 CM (40 IN) WOMEN ≤ 88 CM (35 IN)	MEN >102 CM (40 IN) WOMEN >88 CM (35 IN)
Underweight	<18.5		—	—
Normal	18.5–24.9		—	—
Overweight	25.0–29.9		↑	↑↑
Obese	30.0–34.9	I	↑↑	↑↑↑
	35.0–39.9	II	↑↑↑	↑↑↑
Extremely obese	≥40.00	III	↑↑↑↑	↑↑↑↑

[a] Disease risk for NIDDM, hypertension, and CVD relative to normal weight and waist circumference.
[b] BMI is expressed in kilograms per square meter.
Adapted with permission from Expert Panel. Clinical Guidelines on the Identification, Evaluation, and Treatment of Overweight and Obesity in Adults. Bethesda, MD: National Institutes of Health, National Heart, Lung, and Blood Institute. U.S. Department of Health and Human Services, Public Health Service, 1998(22).

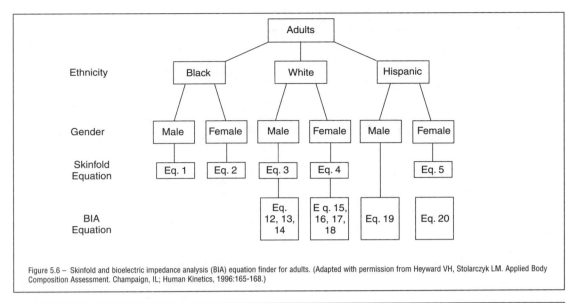

Figure 5.6 – Skinfold and bioelectric impedance analysis (BIA) equation finder for adults. (Adapted with permission from Heyward VH, Stolarczyk LM. Applied Body Composition Assessment. Champaign, IL; Human Kinetics, 1996:165-168.)

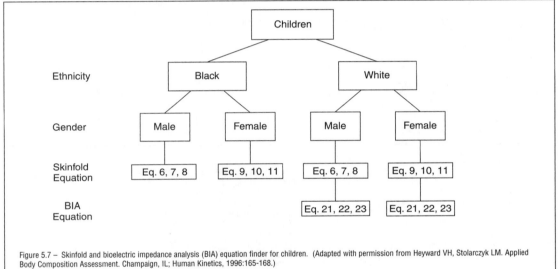

Figure 5.7 – Skinfold and bioelectric impedance analysis (BIA) equation finder for children. (Adapted with permission from Heyward VH, Stolarczyk LM. Applied Body Composition Assessment. Champaign, IL; Human Kinetics, 1996:165-168.)

as eating, drinking, and exercising must be controlled, since hydration status, fluid distribution, and temperature are sources of error in resistance measurements. Technician error is minor if standard procedures for electrode positioning and subject positioning are followed. Finally, as with skinfolds, equation error can be reduced by selecting prediction equations according to age, sex, race, and level of physical activity.

Equation Selection

Prediction equations are either population specific or general. Population-specific equations are derived for use in a specific homogeneous population (*e.g.*, prepubescent white boys or elderly African American women). Thus, they usually systematically underestimate or overestimate body composition if applied to individuals from other populations. In contrast, general equations can be applied to individuals who differ greatly in physical characteristics. General equations are developed from diverse, heterogeneous samples, and they account for differences in age, sex, race, ethnicity, and other characteristics by including these variables as predictors in the equation.

Recommended Equations

Heyward and Stolarczyk (39) recently made easier the task of equation selection. They reviewed the available equations and developed decision trees for selecting the most useful equations (Figs. 5.6 and 5.7). Decision trees can be used to find appropriate equations for African Americans, Whites, and Hispanics of both genders. The mathematical formulas for each equation are given in Tables 5.10 and 5.11. Equations for other minority groups (*e.g.*, Asians and Native Americans) and athletes are also available (39).

Table 5.10 – Skinfold Prediction Equations

	ETHNICITY	GENDER	AGE	EQUATION	REFERENCE
1	Black	Men	18–61	$Db (g/cc) = 1.1120 - 0.00043499$ (Σ 7SKF chest, abdomen, thigh, triceps, subscapular, suprailiac, madaxillary) $+ 0.00000055$ (Σ 7SKF)^2 $- 0.00028826$ (age).	19
2	Black	Women	18–55	$Db (g/cc) = 1.0970 - 0.00046971$ (Σ 7SKF chest, abdomen, thigh, triceps, subscapular, suprailiac, midaxillary) $+ 0.00000056$ (Σ 7SKF)^2 $- 0.00012828$ (age).	20
3	White	Men	18–61	$Db (g/cc) = 1.109380 - 0.0008267$ (Σ 3SKF chest, abdomen, thigh) $+ 0.0000016$ (Σ 3SKF)^2 $- 0.0002574$ (age).	19
4	White	Women	18–55	$Db (g/cc) = 1.0994921 - 0.0009929$ (Σ 3SKF triceps, suprailiac, thigh) $+ 0.0000023$ (Σ 3SKF)^2 $- 0.0001392$ (age).	20
5	Hispanic	Women	20–40	$Db (g/cc) = 1.0970 - 0.00046971$ (Σ 3SKF chest, abdomen, thigh, triceps, subscapular, suprailiac, midaxillary) $+ 0.00000056$ (Σ 7SKF)^2 $- 0.00012828$ (age).	20
6	Black & white	Boys	≤18	% BF $= 0.735$ (Σ 2SKF triceps, calf) $+ 1.0$	23
7	Black & white	Boys (SKF > 35 mm)	≤18	%BF $= 0.735$ (Σ 2SKF triceps, subscapular) $+ 1.6$	23
8	Black & white	Boys (SKF > 35 mm)	≤18	%BF $= 0.783$ (Σ 2SKF triceps, subscapular) $- 0.008$ (Σ 2SKF)^2 $+ 1^*$.	23
9	Black & White	Girls	≤18	% BF $= 0.610$ (2SKF triceps, calf) $+ 5.1$	23
10	Black & white	Girls (SKF > 35 mm)	≤18	%BF $= 0.546$ (Σ 2SKF triceps, subscapular) $+ 9.7$	23
11	Black & white	Girls (SKF > 35 mm)	≤18	%BF $= 1.33$ (Σ 2SKF triceps, subscapular) $- 0.013$ (Σ 2SKF)^2 $- 2.5$.	23

Db, body density; SKF, skinfolds; %BF, percent body fat.
* Intercept substitutions based on maturation and ethnicity for boys:

Age	Black	White
Prepubescent	-3.2	-1.7
Pubescent	-5.2	-3.4
Postpubescent	-6.8	-5.5

Adapted with permission from Heyward VH, Stolarczyk LM. Applied Bondy Composition Assessment. Champaign IL: Human Kinetics, 1996:173-185.

Table 5.11 – Bioelectric Impedance Analysis Prediction Equations

	ETHNICITY	GENDER	AGE	EQUATION	REFERENCE
12	White	Men	18–29	FFM (kg) $= 0.485$ (HT^2/r) $+ 0.338$ (BW) $+ 5.32$	13
13	White	Men (<20% BF)	17–62	FFM (kg) $= 0.00066360$ (HT^2) $- 0.02117$ (R) $+ 0.62854$ (BW) $- 0.12380$ (age $+ 9.33285$)	24
14	White	Men (≥20% BF)	17–62	FFM (kg) $= 0.00088580$ (HT^2) 0.02999 $+ 0.42688$ (BW) 0.07002 (age) $+ 14.52435$	24
15	White	Women	18–29	FFM (kg) $= 0.476$ (HT^2/r) $+ 0.295$ (BW) $+ 5.49$	13
16	White	Women	30–49	FFM (kg) $= 0.493$ (HT^2/r) $+ 0.141$ (BW) $+ 11.59$	13
17	White	Women	50-70	FFM (kg) $- 0.474$ (HT^2/r) $+ 0.180$ (BW) $+ 7.3$	13
18	White	Women	22–74	FFM (kg) $= 0.00151$ (HT^2) $- 0.0344$ (R) $+ 0.140$ (BW) $- 0.158$ (age) $+ 20.387$	25
19	Hispanic	Men	19-59	FFM (kg) $= 13.74 + 0.34$ (HT^2/r) $+ 0.33$ (BW) $- 0.14 +$ (age) $+ 6.18$	26
20	Hispanic	Women	20–40	FFM (kg) $= 0.00151$ (HT^2) $- 0.0344$ (R) $+ 0.140$ (BW) $- 0.158$ (age) $+ 20.387$	25
21	White	Both	6–10	TBW (L) $= 0.593$ (HT^2/r) $+ 0.65$ (BW) $+ 0.04$	17
22	White	Both	10–19	FFM (kg) $= 0.61$ (HT^2/r) $+ 0.25$ (BW) $+ 1.31$	27
23	White	Both	8–15	FFM (kg) $= 0.62$ (HT^2/r) $+ 0.21$ (BW) $+ 0.10$ (Σc) $+ 4.2$	13

HT, height (cm); BW, body weight (kg); R, resistance (Ω); Σc, reactance (Ω); TBW, total body water (L).
To convert TBW to FFM, use the following hydration constants:

Boys   5–6 yr FFM (kg) = TBW/0.77   Girls   5–6 yr FFM (kg) TBW/0.78
      7–8 yr FFM (kg) = TBW/0.768   7–8 yr FFM (kg) = TBW/0.776
      9–10 yr FFM (kg) = TBW/0.762   9–10 yr FFM (kg) = TBW/0.77

Adapted with permission from Heyward VH, Stolarczyk LM. Applied Body Composition Assessment. Champaign IL: Human Kinetics, 1996:173-185.

Body Fat Standards

There are no accepted percent body fat standards for all ages. Most body composition studies use small groups, usually young adults. These studies demonstrate that body fat typically ranges from 10 to 20% for men and 20 to 30% for women. Based on these studies, recommendations of 15% for men and 25% for women have been made. These "standards" essentially are the average percent fat for young adults. Their usefulness in other groups has not been established.

National data for describing percent fat for the U.S. population are not available. However, there are skinfold data from the National Health and Nutrition Examination Survey (NHANES II) on a large (20,000) representative sample of U.S. men and women. Using this approach, new percent fat health standards have been recently proposed (Fig. 5.8) (41). Some increase in percent fat with age was allowed. This was done in consideration of

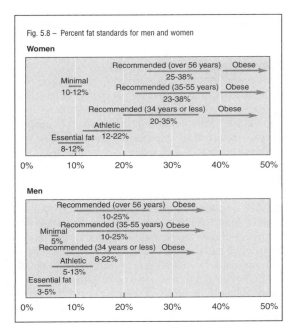

Fig. 5.8 – Percent fat standards for men and women

Women

Recommended (over 56 years)   Obese
25-38%
Minimal
10-12%   Recommended (35-55 years)   Obese
23-38%
Recommended (34 years or less)   Obese
20-35%
Athletic   12-22%
Essential fat
8-12%

0%   10%   20%   30%   40%   50%

Men

Recommended (over 56 years)   Obese
10-25%
Minimal   Recommended (35-55 years)   Obese
5%   10-25%
Recommended (34 years or less)   Obese
Athletic   8-22%
5-13%
Essential fat
3-5%

0%   10%   20%   30%   40%   50%

Table 5.12 – Percent Fat Standards for Active Men and Women

	NOT RECOMMENDED	RECOMMENDED BODY FAT LEVELS (%)		
		LOW	MID	UPPER
Men				
young adult	< 5	5	10	15
middle adult	< 7	7	11	18
elderly	< 9	9	12	18
Women				
young adult	< 16	16	23	28
middle adult	< 20	20	27	33
elderly	< 20	20	27	33

Adapted with permission from Lohman TG, Houtkooper LB, Going SB. Body composition assessment: Body fat standards and methods in the field of exercise and sports medicine. ACSM Health Fitness J 1:30–35, 1997.

recent studies showing that lower body fat or reduced body fat in middle-aged women is associated with a lower bone mineral content, putting those women at risk for osteoporosis and bone fractures. Thus, the emphasis on lower percent fat to prevent heart disease, especially in women, must be balanced against the increased risk of bone fractures, especially if bone mineral content is already low.

Standards for active men and women have also been developed (Table 5.12). These standards are not necessarily associated with better health but may be associated with improved physical performance.

Recently, a unique approach to derive percent fat standards for children and adolescents has been reported (44). In this study, the authors sought to develop criterion-referenced standards by assessing risk of high levels of blood pressure, total cholesterol, and low-density lipoprotein and low levels of high-density lipoprotein in girls and boys aged 6–18 years at different levels of body fatness. No excess risk was found until percent fat exceeded 25% in boys and 30% in girls. Age and race were not significant predictors of risk in this age group. Thus, 25% fat in boys and 30% fat in girls have been proposed as useful health standards for African Americans and Whites aged 6–18 years. A similar criterion-referenced approach would be useful in adults to determine whether risk varies with age and percent fat, or one standard is valid for all ages.

Resources for Body Composition Assessment

A number of excellent resources offer additional information on both laboratory and field methods for assessing body composition For informa-

tion on field techniques, the monograph by Heyward and Stolarcyzk (39) is particularly helpful, as is the *Anthropometric Standardization Reference Manual* (40) from the Arlie conference, which describes recommended standard techniques for anthropometry. Videotapes, manuals, and software packages for training and standardizing procedures, and for simplifying calculations and reporting results are available from Human Kinetics Publishers, Champaign, Illinois. The recent evidence report, *Clinical Guidelines on the Identification, Evaluation, and Treatment of Overweight and Obesity in Adults* (45), is an important resource for practitioners involved in obesity prevention and treatment.

Details Regarding Anthropometric Data

Anthropometric data are based on measurements of the following:

- Height
- Weight
- Body mass index (BMI)
- Body composition
- Waist-to-hip ratio

These measurements are compared to norms that consider age, gender, body frame, and ethnicity. Anthropometry has many advantages. These measurements are usually less expensive and easier to obtain than clinical data. They are also safer for the patient because they can be obtained non-invasively. Anthropometric measurements may be obtained in the field as well as in clinical settings and can be taken by individuals with minimal training. However, field work presents a few disadvantages: 1) The measurements may be less accurate when taken by untrained or poorly trained individuals, and 2) measurements may be affected by the testing environment (46). The equipment used for assessment must be properly maintained and calibrated regularly for accurate results. To ensure the most accurate measures possible, the same person should assess the patient on each visit.

Height

It is usually more important to measure height in children than in adults. However, periodic measurements in adults (every 3 years) are recommended. Unfortunately, height is often self-reported by adults and thus may be inaccurate. An inaccurate measurement may make it difficult to assess body weight.

Weight

Weight is most commonly measured using a platform balance scale. Weight without shoes, without objects in pockets, and while wearing light clothing is standard. If a change in weight is crucial for a diagnosis or for selecting a treatment, it should be measured at least 2 h after food or liquid intake and while wearing light clothing (46).

A weight history may help the health care professional determine patterns of nutrition and exercise behavior. Typical questions regarding weight history include highest and lowest adult weight, preferred weight, usual weight, and weight change during the past 6–12 months (46).

The Metropolitan Life Insurance Company introduced normative tables for weight in 1959. Different norms have been introduced because of the increased weight in the general population, and the 1959 tables are no longer used (47, 48).

An alternative method for determining ideal body weight is presented in the following (49):

Women: ideal body weight
100 lb for the first 5 ft + 5 lb for each inch over 5 ft

Men: ideal body weight
106 lb for the first 5 ft + 6 lb for each inch over 5 ft

Body Mass Index

Body mass index (BMI) is a ratio of weight to height in adults that indicates body composition (50). BMI can be used to define the degree of adiposity without accounting for body frame size. It is calculated by the Quetelet equation (51):

$$BMI = \frac{weight\,(kg)}{[height\,(m)]^2}$$

The BMI correlates the least with body height and the most with independent measures of body fatness in adults, including the elderly. A BMI score of 20–25 is associated with the lowest risk of excessive or deficient adipose tissue. Obesity is divided into three grades:

- Grade I = 25.0–29.9
- Grade II = 30–40
- Grade III = 40+

A BMI of at least 27 indicates obesity and increased health risk. Body mass index increases with age; therefore, age-specific guidelines for interpreting the BMI in the elderly have been recommended.

Body Composition

Percent body fat can be used to stratify the risk of cardiovascular disease in patients. The amount of body fat can be estimated by underwater weighing, skin-fold thickness measurements, circumferences, bioelectric impedance, and dual x-ray absorptiometry.

Waist-to-Hip Ratio

The waist-to-hip (W:H) ratio is used to estimate the risk of coronary artery disease (CAD). Values greater than 0.8 for women and greater than 0.9 for men indicate an increased risk for cardiovascular disease and diabetes. A W:H value greater than 1.0 indicates a significantly increased risk of CAD. For lean and normal-weight individuals, the most accurate method of estimating the risk of CAD may be to combine the W:H ratio and BMI (52).

Assessment throughout the Life Cycle

Pediatric Population

One of the best indicators of nutritional status in children may be physical growth. Length or stature and weight are commonly used to assess growth. Anthropometric measures commonly used in children include the weight-for-height index, height-for-age index, weight-for-age index, head circumference, mid-upper-arm circumference, and triceps skinfold thickness. These indexes can be plotted on standardized forms. The mid-upper-arm circumference and triceps skinfold thickness can help identify wasting, since these measures correlate with lean body mass (54, 55). The triceps skinfold can help determine whether excessive weight is due to excessive fat or excessive lean tissue (*e.g.,* muscle hypertrophy in athletes); however, this measurement is not the most reliable measure of body composition (46). Assessments of children should also consider activity level.

Adolescent Population

The patient is considered an adolescent on reaching puberty. Up to 20% of adult height and 50% of weight may be gained during this period. Both body fat and lean muscle mass increase. Girls generally gain more body fat than boys, and boys usually gain more lean tissue (56). It is important to use age-specific norms in assessing adolescents (53). Nutrient needs increase significantly during adolescence to accommodate rapid growth. The development of body image concerns during adolescence may lead to a desire to change the growth rate or body proportions with further dietary manipulation and often has a negative consequence.

Adult Population

Weight is particularly useful in assessing the nutritional status of adults. Height and weight should both be measured, as adults commonly overestimate height and underestimate weight. Weight loss reflects an acute inability to meet nutritional requirements and may indicate a nutritional risk factor or illness (56). The use of the Metropolitan Life Insurance table and/or the BMI can help determine appropriate body weight (48, 50). The previously mentioned methods of assessing body composition may also be used to determine nutritional status. Assessments for adults should consider activity and exercise levels.

Elderly Population

Aging is marked by a progressive loss of lean body mass and increased body fat, and is accompanied by changes in most physiological systems (56). Lean body mass in the healthy elderly is 30–40% less than in young adults. This represents the loss of both muscular and visceral protein and leads to functional and metabolic changes. Basal metabolic rate and therefore energy requirements decrease by 20% between ages 30 and 90, mainly because of decreased lean body mass (56). The Harris-Benedict equation can be used to estimate caloric requirements in this population. Physical activity helps maintain bone and muscle mass and functional capacity in this population, and also helps maintain a normal metabolic rate.

SECTION V References

1. American College of Sports Medicine. Guidelines for Exercise Testing and Prescription, 6th ed. Baltimore: Lippincott Williams & Williams, 2000.
2. Miller M, Vogel RA. The practice of coronary artery disease prevention. 1st ed. Baltimore: Williams & Wilkins, 1996:2.
3. Gastelli WB, Anderson K, Wilson PW, Levy D. Lipids and risk of coronary heart disease: The Framingham Study. Ann Epidemiol 2:23–28, 1992.
4. Stamler J, Stamler R, Neaton JD. Blood pressure systolic and diastolic, and cardiovascular risk: years population data. Arch Intern Med 153:598–615, 1993.
5. Grundy SM. Primary prevention of coronary heart disease. Circulation 100:988–998, 1990.
6. McGinnis JM, Foege WH. Actual causes of death in the United States. JAMA 270:2207–2212, 1993.
7. McGill HC Jr. The cardiovascular pathology of smoking. Am Heart J 115:250–257, 1988.
8. Willett WC, Green A, Stampfe MJ, et al. Relative and absolute excess risk of coronary heart disease among women who smoke cigarettes. N Engl J Med 317:1303–1309, 1987.
9. Franklin BA, ed. ACSM's Guidelines for Exercise Testing and Prescription. 6th ed. Philadelphia: Williams & Wilkins, 2000:22–29.
10. Balady GJ, Chaitman B, Driscoll D, et al. American College of Sports Medicine and American Heart Association Joint Position Statement: Recommendations for cardiovascular screening, staffing, and emergency policies at health/fitness facilities. Med Sci Sports Exerc 30:1009–1018, 1998.
11. O'Brien CP. Are current exercise test protocols appropriate for older patients? Coron Artery Dis 10:43–46, 1999.
12. McInnis KJ, Bader DS, Pierce GL, Balady GJ. Comparison of cardiopulmonary responses in obese women using ramp versus step treadmill protocols. Am J Cardiol 83:289–291, 1999.
13. Bader DS, Maguire TE, Balady GJ. Comparison of ramp versus step protocols for exercise testing in patients > or = 60 years of age. Am J Cardiol 83:11–14, 1999.
14. Astrand PO, Rhyming I. A nomogram for calculation of aerobic capacity (physical fitness) from pulse rate during submaximal work. J Appl Physiol 7:218–221, 1954.
15. deVries H, Klafs C. Predicting maximal oxygen intake from submaximal tests. J Sports Med 4:207, 1965.
16. Golding LA, Myers CR, Sinning WE, eds. The Y's Way to Physical Fitness. Rosemont, IL: YMCA of the USA, 1982:88–101.
17. Baron R, Bachl N, Petschnig R, et al. Measurement of maximal power output in isokinetic and non-isokinetic cycling. Int J Sports Med 20:532–537, 1999.
18. Blomqvist CG. Cardiovascular adaptations to physical training. Ann Rev Physiol 45:169–189, 1983.
19. Brouha L. The step test: A simple method of measuring physical fitness for muscular work in young men. Res Q Exerc Sport 14:31–35, 1943.
20. Capriotti PV, Sherman WM, Lamb DR. Reliability of power output during intermittent high-intensity cycling. Med Sci Sports Exerc 31:913–915, 1999.
21. Shephard RJ, Allen C, Benade AJS, et al. Standardization of submaximal exercise tests. Bull World Health Organ 1968;38:765–775.
22. Jette M, Campbell J, Mongeon J, et al. The Canadian home fitness test as a predictor of aerobic capacity. Can Med Assoc J 1976;114:680–682.
23. Knuttgen HG, Kraemer WJ. Terminology and measurement in exercise performance. J Appl Sport Sci Res 1:1–10, 1987.
24. Baumgartner TA. Jackson AS. Measurement for Evaluation in Physical Education and Exercise Science. Dubuque, IA: William C. Brown, 1987.
25. Fleck SJ, Kraemer WJ. Designing Resistance Training Programs. 2nd ed. Champaign, IL: Human Kinetics, 1997.
26. Pollock ML, Graves JE, Carpenter DM, et al. Muscle, In: Hockshuler SH, Colter HB, Colter RD, et al, eds. Rehabilitation of the Spine: Science and Practice. St. Louis: Mosby, 1993:263–284.
27. Amusa LO, Obajuluwa VA. Static versus dynamic training programs for muscular strength using the knee-extensors in healthy young men. J Ortho Sports Phys Ther 8:243–247, 1986.
28. Kanehisa H, Miyashita M. Specificity of velocity in strength training. Eur J Appl Physiol 52:104–106, 1983.
29. Ford WJ, Bailey SD, Babich K, et al. Effect of hip position on gravity effect torque. Med Sci Sports Exerc 26:230–234, 1994.
30. Lea RD. Current concepts review: range of motion measurements. J Bone Joint Surg 77A:78A, 1995.
31. Gajdosik RL, Bohannon, RW. Clinical measurement of range of motion: Review of goniometry emphasizing reliability and validity. Phys Ther 67:1867, 1987.
32. Keeley I, Mayer TG, Cox R, et al. Quantification of lumbar function: 5. Reliability of range-of-motion measures in the sagittal plane and an in vivo torso rotation measurement technique. Spine 11:31, 1986.
33. Watkins MA, Riddle DL, Lamb RI, et al. Reliability of goniometric measurements and visual estimates of knee range of motion obtained in a clinical setting. Phys Ther 71:90, 1991.
34. Atha J, Wheatley DW. The mobilising effects of repeated measurement of hip flexion . Br J Sports Med 10:22, 1976.
35. Merritt JL, McLean TJ, Erickson RP. Measurement of trunk flexibility in normal subjects: Reproducibility of three clinical methods. Mayo Clin Proc 61:192, 1986.
36. Knapik JI, Bauman CL, Jones. BH, et al. Preseason strength and flexibility imbalances associated with athletic injuries in female collegiate athletes. Am J Sports Med 19:76, 1991.
37. Agency of Health Care Policy and Research. Clinical practice guidelines: Acute low back problems in adults. Washington: US Department of Health and Human Services, Public Health Service #14, 1995.
38. Beekman CE, Axtell L. Ambulation, activity level, and pain: Outcomes of a program for spinal pain. Phys Ther 65:1649, 1985.
39. Heyward VH, Stolarczyk LM. Applied Body Composition Assessment. Champaign, IL: Human Kinetics, 1996.
40. Lohman TG, Roche AF, Martorell R, eds. Anthropometric Standardization Reference Manual. Champaign, IL: Human Kinetics, 1988.
41. Lohman TG, Houtkooper LB, Going SB. Body composition assessment: Body fat standards and methods in the field of exercise and sports medicine. ACSM Health Fitness J 1:30–35, 1997.
42. Baumgartner RN. Electrical impedance and total body electrical conductivity. In: Roche AF, Heymsfield SB, Lohman TG, eds. Human Body Composition. Champaign, IL: Human Kinetics, 1996:79–107.
43. Kushner RF. Bioelectrical impedance analysis: A review of principles and applications. J Am Coll Nutr 11:199–209, 1992.

44. Williams DP, Going SB, Lohman TG, et al. Body fatness and risk for elevated blood pressure, total cholesterol, and serum lipoprotein ratios in children and adolescents. Am J Public Health 82:358–363, 1992.

45. National Heart, Lung, and Blood Institute. Clinical Guidelines on the Identification, Evaluation, and Treatment of Overweight and Obesity in Adults: The Evidence Report. Bethesda, MD: National Institutes of Health, National Heart, Lung, and Blood Institute. U.S. Department of Health and Human Services, Public Health Service, 1998.

46. Simko MD, Cowell C, Gilbride JA. Nutrition Assessment: A Comprehensive Guide for Planning Intervention. Gaithersburg, MD: Apsen, 1995.

47. Metropolitan Life Insurance Company. New weight standards for men and women. Stat Bull 40:1–4, 1959.

48. Metropolitan Life Foundation. 1983 Metropolitan height and weight tables. Stat Bull 64:2–9, 1983.

49. Dikovics A. Nutritional Assessment: Case Study Methods. Philadelphia: George F. Stickley, 1987.

50. Fidanza F. Nutritional Status Assessment: A Manual for Population Studies. New York: Chapman & Hall, 1991.

51. Kuskowska-Wolk A, Bergstrom R, Bostrom G. Relationship between questionnaire data and medical records of height, weight, and body mass index. Int J Obes 16:1–9, 1992.

52. Snetselaar LG. Nutrition counseling Skills: Assessment, Treatment, and Evaluation. Gaithersburg, MD: Aspen, 1989.

53. American Dietetic Association Public Health Nutrition Dietetic Practice Group. Quality assurance criteria for nutritional care of prenatal women and adolescents. Atlanta: US Dept of Agriculture, Public Health Service, Centers for Disease Control and Prevention, Division of Nutrition, 1993.

54. Trowbridge FL, Hiney CD, Robertson AD. Arm muscle indicators and creatinine excretion in children. Am J Clin Nutr 36:691–696, 1982.

55. Chen LC et al. Anthropometric assessment of energy-protein malnutrition and subsequent risk of mortality among preschool aged children. Am J Clin Nutr 33:1836–1845, 1980.

56. Mahan KL, Arlin M. Krause's Food Nutrition and Diet Therapy. 8th ed. Philapdelphia: Saunders, 1995.

Section VI

- ✦ Benefits and Risks Associated with Exercise
- ✦ Preliminary Screening
- ✦ Recommendations to Reduce the Incidence and Severity of Complications during Exercise
- ✦ Emergency Procedures and Exercise Safety
- ✦ Death and Cardiac Arrest
- ✦ Musculoskeletal Injury
- ✦ EXERCISE-RELATED INJURIES
- ✦ Injury Prevention
- ✦ Emergency Procedures
- ✦ Evaluation Skills
- ✦ Contraindicated and High-Risk Exercises

ACSM's Resources for the Personal Trainer

SAFETY, INJURY PREVENTION, AND EMERGENCY PROCEDURES

A. Benefits and Risks Associated with Exercise

This section discusses risks associated with exercise and exercise testing. Although the typical personal trainer will not supervise a client's exercise test, it is important for trainers to be aware of potential complications associated with testing.

Complications associated with exercise testing appear to be relatively low. The ability to maintain a high degree of safety depends on knowing when not to perform an exercise test, when to terminate the test, and being prepared for any emergency that might arise (1).

It remains difficult to identify persons who may be predisposed to cardiovascular complications during exercise. In general, the risk is lowest among healthy young adults and nonsmoking women, greater for those with symptoms and multiple risk factors, and highest in those with established cardiac disease. Although a profile of the "high risk" client has emerged, one or more of these widely varied characteristics may pertain to a significant number of cardiac patients who will never experience an exercise-related cardiovascular complication. Regardless of the presence or absence of heart disease, the overall absolute risk of cardiovascular complications during exercise is low, especially when weighed against the associated health benefits.

B. Preliminary Screening

Persons who are about to be exercise tested are usually required to be screened by a physician prior to the test. Lack of uniformity in guidelines and policies for exercise testing and participation has led to much discussion and concern among exercise program personnel. Issues of primary concern include who should be tested, physician attendance during the test, use of maximal versus submaximal testing, how to risk stratify individuals before and after testing, and defining the appropriate level of supervision for exercise training.

No matter how rigid or conservative guidelines and policies might be, due to the vagaries of the atherosclerotic process, the accuracy in predicting which persons will have a cardiovascular complication during exercise remains imperfect. Some data are available to estimate the likelihood of such an event, but clinical and legal judgment, as well as common sense, must be used to make policy decisions involving the safety of participants.

Exercise testing is performed in many settings for nondiagnostic purposes, such as worksite health promotion programs, YMCAs and YWCAs, Jewish Community Centers, health clubs, and other community recreation centers. This testing tends to be functional (in many cases the ECG is not monitored) and is aimed at assessing physical fitness, providing a basis for the exercise prescription, or monitoring progress in an exercise program.

The ACSM believes that this type of exercise testing is appropriate for fitness appraisal in conjunction with appropriate screening and when performed by qualified personnel. Such testing programs may be useful in educating participants about exercise and physical fitness and in helping to motivate sedentary individuals to exercise.

C. Recommendations to Reduce the Incidence and Severity of Complications during Exercise

Recommendations to reduce the incidence of musculoskeletal and cardiovascular complications during adult fitness and exercise-based cardiac rehabilitation programs include the following:

Ensure Medical Clearance and Follow-Up

Medical clearance and follow-up, including maximal exercise testing, are essential screening components in physical conditioning programs for older adults (men 45 years or older, women 55 years or older), those at increased risk for cardiovascular events (*e.g.,* two or more risk factors or one or more major signs or symptoms of coronary heart disease), and those with known cardiac, pulmonary, or metabolic disease, especially when vigorous exercise (more than 60% $\dot{V}O_{2max}$) is contemplated. Although routine exercise testing to forestall exercise-related cardiovascular complications has been questioned (2, 6), exercise testing clearly aids in identifying the individual who is at increased risk for symptomatic or asymptomatic myocardial ischemia, malignant ventricular arrhythmias, or both. Exercise testing has the greatest diagnostic impact in symptomatic persons and those with an intermediate likelihood of coronary artery disease (*i.e.,* a pretest probability of 10–90%).

Provide On-Site Medical Supervision, if Necessary

The degree of medical supervision should be linked inversely with the stability of the client. Although traditional, medically supervised group programs are associated with increased cost and extended travel time, such programs are more appropriate for the growing medical complexity of candidates who may be at increased risk for exercise-induced complications. Medically supervised programs that are equipped with a defibrillator and appropriate emergency drugs act to reduce complications during exercise therapy. Recent reports indicate that approximately 80% of all patients with cardiac arrest occurring under such conditions are successfully resuscitated (3). Moreover, one 16-yr experience (5) and the results of others (4) suggest that acute cardiac events can be treated successfully by nursing staff, assisted by exercise physiologists/technologists and emergency medical service backup, without direct gymnasium supervision by a physician (*i.e.,* in the exercise room).

Establish an Emergency Plan

Exercise program staff should be prepared to handle musculoskeletal and cardiovascular complications. This includes performing cardiopulmonary resuscitation (CPR), attending to orthopedic injuries (*e.g.,* having ice immediately available), and stabilizing the participant for transport to an emergency center, if necessary. To this end, emergency drills and CPR mannequin practice should be conducted regularly.

Cardiac rehabilitation programs should be medically supervised and equipped with a defibrillator and appropriate emergency drugs. The defibrillator should be charged and checked daily, and outdated drugs should be discarded and replaced. A "plan of action" should be established whereby specific responsibilities are assigned (*e.g.,* perform CPR, call emergency medical services, transport crash ["code"] cart and defibrillator to the victim, clear other participants from the immediate area, wait for and direct the emergency medical service to the victim). Finally, telephone numbers for emergency assistance should be clearly labeled on all telephones; if possible, a direct line (*e.g.,* "red phone") should be established.

Participant Education

Exercisers should know their prescribed heart rate range for exercise training, how to take their pulse accurately, and the work rates that are compatible with their aerobic requirements for training. Rating of perceived exertion is strongly recommended as a useful and important adjunct to heart rate as an intensity guide (7). Participants should be strongly encouraged to remain at or below the prescribed intensity and counseled to discontinue exercise and seek medical advice if they experience major warning signs or symptoms (*e.g.,* chest pain, light-headedness, abdominal discomfort, unusual fatigue or shortness of breath, palpitations)

that may suggest a deterioration in their clinical status or impending cardiovascular complications. They should be educated to alert staff as to changes in their medication regimen because an updated target heart rate may be warranted.

Initially Encourage Mild-To-Moderate Exercise Intensity

The lower the intensity, the less likely that an exercise-related complication will occur (3). Victims of exercise-related sudden cardiac death often have a history of poor compliance to the prescribed training heart rate range (*i.e.,* exercise intensity violators) (8, 9). These and other recent data suggest that unconventionally vigorous exercise is associated with an increased risk of musculoskeletal (10) and cardiovascular complications (11). The exercise leader should recognize that excessive frequency (5 d·wk^{-1}) and duration (45 min per session) of training offer the participant little additional gain in aerobic capacity, yet the incidence of orthopedic injury increases disproportionately (30). However, it appears that formerly overweight or obese clients may need to expend the caloric equivalent of more than 60 min of moderate-to-vigorous activity on most or all days of the week to maintain their weight loss.

D. Emergency Procedures and Exercise Safety

Although there is always risk with exercise programs, most health and fitness professionals believe the benefits outweigh the risks. However, vigorous exercise entails a variety of risks, including musculoskeletal injury and cardiovascular complications. The risk of injury and myocardial infarction associated with exercise and exercise testing can be reduced through appropriate screening and risk stratification procedures, exercise prescription techniques, and facility safety standards. Furthermore, rehearsing emergency procedures reduces the risk of serious complications in the event of an emergency. Staff training and client orientation sessions maximize safety and minimize liability. The information in this section is intended as a template for developing policies and procedures specific to facility, clientele, staff, and community medical resources. Numerous resources are available to assist in the development of safe and effective exercise programs for clientele and staff.

E. Death and Cardiac Arrest

Many researchers have investigated the incidence of sudden death and cardiac arrest during exercise. In cases of sudden cardiac death in persons under age 20, coronary artery disease is rare; congenital or other abnormalities such as hypertrophic cardiomyopathy, myocarditis, and conduction system abnormalities are often associated with these exercise-related deaths (12). Thompson et al. showed men 30–64 yr of age who jog at least 2 d·wk^{-1} had a yearly sudden death rate of 1/7620 (13).

Excluding men with known heart disease reduced the death rate to 1/15,200 joggers per year. The incidence of sudden cardiac death in women is lower at all ages (14). Studies report that the incidence of heart attack during exercise is less than 10/100,000 men per year (15). Many of these victims already had heart disease and were sedentary. The relative risk of heart attack is 5.9 times greater in men and women who are habitually inactive than in those who exercise regularly (16). As the frequency of regular, vigorous exercise increases, the risk of heart attack with exertion decreases significantly. These studies emphasize the need for risk factor stratification; appropriate medical screening, such as graded exercise tests; and a data-based exercise prescription to reduce the risk of complications and death.

Exercise-related risk should be examined relative to the risks associated with physical inactivity. Physical inactivity is a major risk factor for coronary artery disease. The average relative risk for coronary artery disease in inactive individuals is 1.9 times the risk for an active person (17). This is similar to the relative risk associated with smoking, hypertension, and hypercholesterolemia. Only modest amounts of regular activity are required for significant reductions in mortality rates from heart disease and cancer. Blair et al. reported that the greatest reduction (about 50%) in all-cause mortality rates occurred when an individual moves from the lowest level of fitness (6 METs) to the next lowest level (7 METs) (18). No additional reduction in mortality rate was associated with aerobic capacities greater than 9–10 METs. According to the Surgeon General's report, more than 60% of American adults and 50% of youth are not physically active on a regular basis; this exceeds the percentages of adults with risk factors for hypertension, hypercholesterolemia, or smoking, suggesting that physical activity should be vigorously targeted for intervention (18, 19). In view of this epidemiological evidence, the benefits of moderate exercise outweigh the risks in most individuals, assuming that ACSM guidelines for health screening, risk stratification, and exercise prescription are followed.

F. Musculoskeletal Injury

Epidemiological studies investigating the incidence of injury during vigorous activity provide valuable information for the selection of appropriate activities, based on health history and fitness evaluation. More epidemiological data are available for running than for other exercise. Studies investigating the incidence of running injuries report yearly rates of 24–77%, or 2.5–12 injuries per 1000 h of running; generally, lower rates are reported in recreational runners and higher rates in competitive athletes (20, 21). Differences in the definition of injury among studies also contribute to variation in the incidence of injury. Injury rates for other weight-bearing activities, such as aerobic dance classes, are approximately 45% for students (1/1000 h of aerobic dance) and 75% for instructors (22–24). Most of the classes studied were high-impact and many of the reported injuries resulted in discomfort, but little alteration in participation. During the late 1980s, low-impact and high–low-impact classes replaced many of the traditional high-impact classes. A more recent study reported an injury rate of 35% for students and 53% for instructors; injury rates for low-impact (24%) were lower than for high-impact (38%) aerobics (25). Studies investigating injury rates associated with other types of popular group exercise classes, such as kickboxing, yoga, Pilates, resistance training, and indoor cycling are lacking. The injury rates are lower in non–weight-bearing activities, such as swimming (26).

Risk Factors for Musculoskeletal Injury

Risk factors associated with injury can be classified as environmental, individual, or program factors. With regard to distance running, the most consistent predictors of injury are previous injury, high weekly mileage, lack of experience, and running to compete (20, 27–29). Pollock et al. reported that the incidence of injury in 70 men 20–35 years of age increased as the frequency and duration of training increased (30). The incidence of injury was 22%, 24%, and 54% in the 15, 30, and 45 min per session groups, respectively; incidence of injury was 0%, 12%, and 39% for the 1, 3, and 5 d·wk^{-1} groups, respectively. Training intensity was 85–90% of maximal heart rate for all groups. This study suggests that the incidence of injury in novice runners increases significantly with more than 30 min of exercise or more than 3 d·wk^{-1}. With regard to aerobic dance, factors such as a history of orthopaedic problems, type of class (high versus low impact), use of upper body weights, and frequency of participation (four or more classes a week) were associated with increases in injury rates (22–25).

Table 6.1 – Acute Responses for Common Injuries/Emergencies

INJURY OR EMERGENCY	SIGNS AND SYMPTOMS	ACUTE CARE
Closed skin wounds (blisters, corns)	Pain, swelling, infection	Clean with antiseptic soap; apply sterile dressing, antibiotic ointment
Open skin wounds (lacerations, abrasions)	Pain, redness, bleeding, swelling, headache, mild fever	Apply pressure to stop bleeding; clean with soap or sterile saline; apply sterile dressing; refer to physician for stitches, tetanus toxoid
Contusions (bruises)	Swelling, local pain, loss of function if severe	RICES; apply padding if necessary for protection
Strains[a]		
Grade I	Pain, local tenderness, tightness	RICES
Grade II	Loss of function, hemorrhage	RICES, refer for physician evaluation if impaired function
Grade III	Palpable defect	Immobilization, RICES, immediate referral to physician
Sprains[a]		
Grade I	Pain, point tenderness, strength loss, edema	RICES
Grade II	Hemorrhage, measurable laxity	RICES, evaluation by a physician
Grade III	Palpable or observable defect	Immobilization, RICES, evaluation by a physician
Fractures		
Stress	Pain, point tenderness	Evaluation by a physician, rest, non–weight-bearing activities
Simple	Swelling, disability, pain	Immobilize with splint; evaluation by a physician; radiography
Compound	Bleeding, swelling, pain, disability	Immobilize; control bleeding; apply sterile dressing; immediate evaluation by a physician
Dizziness, syncope	Disoriented, confused, pale skin	Determine responsiveness; place supine with legs elevated; administer fluids if conscious; begin emergency ventilation and/or compressions as needed
Hypoglycemia	Profuse sweating, tachycardia, hunger, double vision, tremors, headache, disorientation, seizure	Administer 10–30 g carbohydrate (regular soda, orange juice, or 3 glucose tablets) if conscious; follow with protein; if recovery requires more than 1–2 min, activate EMS; if unconscious, place sugar granules under tongue and activate EMS
Hyperglycemia	Lethargy; weakness; confusion; nausea; headache; sweet, fruity breath; thirst; abdominal pain and vomiting; hyperventilation	Activate EMS; administer fluids if conscious; turn head to side if vomiting
Hypothermia	Shivering, but may stop with extreme drops in core temperature; loss of coordination, muscle stiffness, lethargy	Activate EMS and transport to hospital; remove wet clothing; replace with dry, warm clothing
Hyperthermia		
Heat cramps	Involuntary isolated muscle spasms	Administer fluids with electrolytes; apply direct pressure to spasm and release; massage cramping area with ice
Heat exhaustion	Profuse sweating; pale, clammy skin; multiple muscle spasms; headache; nausea; loss of consciousness; dizziness; tachycardia; hypotension	Move to cool area; place supine with feet elevated; remove clothes; cool with fans, cold water, or ice but avoid chilling the victim; administer fluids; monitor body temperature; refer for evaluation by a physician
Heat stroke	Hot, dry skin, but can be sweating; dyspnea; confusion; unconsciousness common	Activate EMS and transport to hospital immediately; remove clothing; douse with cool water (ice water baths preferred) or wrap in cool wet sheets; administer fluids if conscious
Exertional rhabdomyolysis	Muscle pain, swelling and weakness, dark urine	Activate EMS and transport to hospital immediately; cool and administer fluids if conscious
Angina	Pain or pressure in the chest, neck, jaw, arm and/or back; sweating; denial of medical problem; nausea; shortness of breath	Stop activity; place in seated or supine position (whichever is more comfortable), activate EMS if pain is not relieved
Sudden cardiac arrest	No breathing or pulse	If AED is immediately available, defibrillate if appropriate; if not, activate EMS, begin CPR as needed
Dyspnea, labored breathing	Hyperventilation, dizziness, wheezing, coughing, loss of coordination	Maintain open airway; administer bronchodilator if prescribed; try pursed lip breathing; if no relief, activate EMS and transport

[a] Signs and symptoms for each grade include those for grades below the one listed: grade II includes those of grade I; Grade III includes those of grades I and II.

G. Exercise-Related Injuries

Exercise-related injuries fall into two categories, traumatic and overuse. Traumatic injuries usually occur in a single violent event. Injuries such as strains, sprains, tears, and fractures are considered traumatic injuries. Conversely, overuse injuries are caused by chronic, repetitive submax- imal forces leading to inflammation and pain (31). Common overuse injuries include tendonitis, strains, shin splints, stress fractures, and blisters. Acute treatments for common injuries are outlined in Table 6.1.

Treatment for Exercise-Related Injuries

Standard treatment is divided into initial (first

aid) and follow-up treatment. Initial treatment for acute musculoskeletal injuries is designated by the acronym RICES (41, 42). Initial treatment should be administered for the first 24–72 h, depending on the severity of the injury. The purpose of RICES is to limit the amount of secondary hypoxic injury, control edema, and aid physiology of the inflammatory response.

Rest

Rest allows time to control the effects of trauma and to avoid additional tissue damage. Rest is a continuum ranging from complete rest to restricted activity (relative rest). The approximate rest time is relative to the severity of the injury. Rest can be accomplished by immobilization or with assistive devices such as a cane or crutches. Premature movement may increase hemorrhage and the extent of injury, thus prolonging recovery time. Generally, pain and swelling should guide treatment, and excessively painful movements should be avoided.

Ice

The application of ice is the first step in treatment. Ice or some form of cold application lowers the temperature of tissue, slowing cell metabolism. Subsequent metabolic demands are reduced, which enables healthy surrounding tissue to survive diminished blood flow and hypoxia. This in turn decreases secondary hypoxic injury and edema formation (42). Cold applications also are beneficial for reducing pain and muscle spasm that accompany musculoskeletal injury.

Ice is usually applied in a plastic bag, but commercial ice bags, chemical cold packs, and reusable ice packs are appropriate. An ice bag should be applied for 20–30 min approximately every 2 h during the day. This procedure should be followed for the first 24 h (42).

Compression

Compression controls edema and prevents fluid from accumulating in the injured area by creating a pressure gradient that facilitates the resorption of fluid. In addition, the support offered by a compression wrap decreases unwanted movement and may help relieve pain. Compression is accomplished with an elastic wrap or bandage.

Elevation

Elevation of the injured area above the level of the heart (when possible) limits swelling and increases venous return by lowering capillary hydrostatic pressure and decreasing capillary filtration pressure. Controlling edema associated with injury also decreases tissue damage, resulting in a smaller area of damaged tissue to be repaired.

Stabilization

Muscular spasm (termed muscle guarding) and pain, both undesirable responses to injury, often result from an attempt to protect the injured area. Muscle spasm increases pressure on nerve endings, which increases pain, which in turn can lead to more spasm. This vicious circle is commonly called the pain–spasm cycle. Stabilization supports the injured area so surrounding muscles can relax. Early stabilization through the use of braces and splints allows the muscle to relax, thus decreasing the pain–spasm cycle.

Specific Injuries/Conditions

Skin Wounds

Skin wounds, including blisters, corns, abrasions, lacerations, punctures, sunburn, and infections, are caused by mechanical trauma, environmental factors, or transmission of infectious organisms. Blisters are caused by friction between the surface of the skin and athletic wear or equipment, resulting in fluid accumulation. The blister itself provides a protective dressing and should be covered with a sterile dressing, which promotes rapid healing and reduces the risk of infection (31). Blisters often rupture because of their location in areas such as feet or require drainage for other reasons. Properly fitting sport-specific socks, gloves, and shoes help prevent blisters.

Bleeding open skin wounds, such as lacerations, may require direct application of pressure and elevation to stop bleeding. It is important to prevent the transfer of bloodborne pathogens during cleaning of the wound. Medical evaluation is indicated for deep or large wounds or if signs of infection, such as swelling, redness, or pain, are present.

Contusions

Contusions are bruises with intact skin. Common in contact sports, muscle contusions incite an inflammatory response and may cause formation of a hematoma. The treatment of choice is rest, ice, compression, elevation, and stabilization (RICES) (Table 6.2). A physician should evaluate severe, painful contusions, especially when accompanied by hematoma formation.

Strains and Sprains

Strain is stretching or tearing of the musculotendinous unit, and sprain is injury to a ligament. Strains and sprains are classified as grade I, II, or III, depending on the severity of tissue tearing. Grade I strains and sprains are stretching or minor tearing of connective tissue. Grade II strains and sprains result from partial tearing; grade III strains and sprains involve extensive tearing or complete rupture of tissue and generally require surgery. The RICES protocol is appropriate for acute strains and sprains.

Following joint injury, proprioception, or the ability to perceive position in space and respond,

Table 6.2 – RICES Protocol for Acute Injuries

TREATMENT	PURPOSE	APPLICATION
Rest	Pain control, prevention of reinjury	Complete rest, immobilization, or reduction in training intensity, duration, frequency; or non–weight-bearing activities, depending on severity of injury
Ice	Reduction of pain, swelling, inflammation and bleeding	Immediately post-injury, 2–4 times daily, 20–30 min: plastic bag filled with crushed ice and secured with an elastic bandage; ice massage for small areas, such as tendons and strains, for 10–20 min
Compression	Reduction of swelling	Elastic wrap or compression sleeve
Elevation	Reduction of swelling	Elevate extremity above heart level
Stabilization	Reduce muscle spasm	Use of brace, splint, wrap to stabilize area around joint injury

is often affected; mechanoreceptor function and proprioceptive feedback to the brain are decreased (31). Therefore, proprioceptive exercises should be included in the rehabilitation program to restore kinesthetic awareness, coordination, and agility in addition to flexibility and strength.

Fractures

Fractures include three types: stress, simple, and compound. Stress fractures, or microfractures in the bone surface, are caused by repetitive stress. The bone remains within the skin in simple fractures, while compound or open fractures involve external exposure of bone, increasing the risk of infection. Common in runners, stress fractures are often related to sudden increases in running distance and/or intensity (32). Point tenderness and pain with weight bearing are characteristic of stress fractures, which may not appear on radiographs. Non–weight-bearing and partial weight-bearing activities, such as swimming and bicycling, are recommended for maintenance of cardiovascular fitness until pain-free activity is possible.

Dizziness and Syncope (Fainting)

Dizziness or syncope (temporary loss of consciousness) during exercise may be caused by hyperventilation, cardiac arrhythmias, heat stress, cardiomyopathy, aortic stenosis (narrowing of aortic valve), anomalous coronary arteries, or coronary artery disease (31). Acute care should always include evaluation of the airway, breathing, and pulse if the individual is unresponsive. Cessation of exercise is paramount, and evaluation by a physician is essential to determine whether an underlying condition is present.

Hypotension can also cause dizziness and fainting. Postexercise hypotension occurs when blood pools in the lower extremities because of inadequate cool-down. A 5–10-min low-intensity cool-down using large muscle groups is effective in preventing postexercise hypotension. Antihypertensive medications may exacerbate postexercise hypotension, necessitating a longer cool-down period. Orthostatic hypotension, a drop in blood pressure with changes in posture, may occur when moving from lying to standing. Gradual movement with momentary sitting often prevents orthostatic hypotension.

Plasma volume depletion caused by dehydra-

tion or diuretic medication is also a causative factor in hypotension; adequate hydration should always be encouraged.

Hypoglycemia and Hyperglycemia

Hypoglycemia is low blood glucose. Symptoms may occur at various blood glucose levels, especially in insulin-dependent diabetics (33). Hypoglycemic reactions, which may occur during or after exercise in diabetics, are associated with strenuous exercise, inadequate caloric intake, and inadequate adjustment of insulin dosage (34). Hypoglycemia may occur in nondiabetic individuals who are not eating appropriately, especially with respect to activity level.

Hypoglycemia and hyperglycemia are medical emergencies that, if not treated immediately, may lead to seizures, coma, or death. Signs and symptoms of hypoglycemia and hyperglycemia may be similar; however, symptoms of hypoglycemia develop rapidly, while signs and symptoms associated with hyperglycemia are slower to manifest.

Angina

Pain or discomfort in the chest, jaw, neck, arms, or other areas during exercise that is not altered by movement of the involved areas or extremity may require immediate medical attention. Individuals with angina-type of discomfort should discontinue exercise immediately and rest sitting or recumbent until the discomfort is resolved. Individuals with medication for angina symptoms should be encouraged to carry the medication at all times and use it as directed.

Sudden Cardiac Arrest

Sudden cardiac arrest, caused by factors such as heart disease and rhythm and congenital abnormalities, results in 250,000 deaths annually (36). During sudden cardiac arrest, the victim usually develops an abnormal heart rhythm called ventricular fibrillation, causing the heart to beat in an uncoordinated fashion. Since blood is not effectively pumped, the pulse and subsequently the breathing stop. If the heart is electrically shocked soon thereafter, normal rhythm may be restored. Cardiopulmonary resuscitation (CPR) alone can add only a few minutes to the time available for successful defibrillation. However, when defibrillation is performed during the first 3 min after collapse, survival rates can be as high as 70–80%; for every minute that defibrillation is delayed, there is a 7–10% reduction in the chance of survival (37). The automated external defibrillator (AED) is a portable device that identifies heart rhythms amenable to defibrillation, uses audiovisual prompts to direct the correct response, and delivers the appropriate shock. Even children can be trained to operate AEDs safely and effectively (38). Courses that incorporate AED training into traditional CPR training are available to the public. The Cardiac Arrest Survival Act extends Good Samaritan protections to AED users. The limited number of trial court verdicts on AEDs suggests that organizations adopting AED programs have a lower risk of liability than those who do not.

Dyspnea

Dyspnea (abnormal shortness of breath or labored breathing) may occur in response to bronchospasm, which can be triggered by allergens, cold air, airborne irritants, and respiratory infection. Prescription bronchodilators are often used to resolve such episodes.

H. Injury Prevention

Many injuries occurring in the fitness setting can be prevented with regular maintenance of equipment, training of personnel, and formal member orientations regarding equipment use, weight room etiquette, and safety policies. Outlined hereafter are precautions to ensure members' and employees' safety. ACSM's Health/Fitness Facility Standards and Guidelines contains a detailed list of guidelines (39).

The following recommendations for maintenance and safety apply to fitness facilities of many types:

1. Free-weight exercises, such as squats and bench presses, should be performed with a properly trained spotter. Two spotters are recommended for heavily loaded free-weight exercises.
2. The buddy system is ideal for resistance training. One individual monitors form and biomechanics and provides feedback to the partner. In the event of an emergency, a rapid response is ensured.
3. Routine inspection and maintenance of resistance and cardiovascular equipment are necessary to reduce risk of injury resulting from equipment malfunction.
4. Passageways between equipment should be sufficient (approximately 3 ft) to allow safe movement at all times (39).
5. Weights and other accessories (pads, attachments, collars, and pins) must be racked or properly stored after use.
6. Members should be oriented to equipment, including proper lifting technique, controlled speed of movement, adjustments required for proper alignment, appropriate amount of weight, and number of sets and repetitions.
7. Weight room etiquette should be shared with members to facilitate courteous flow of members through the weight room. Allowing others to rotate in during the rest period, racking weights, and wiping equipment with towels to decrease the risk of transmitting viral or bacterial infections are examples of such courtesy.
8. Staff should clean all pads daily with antifungal and antibacterial agents.
9. Equipment should be arranged in a manner consistent with the appropriate order of training.

I. Emergency Procedures

All facilities should have a written emergency plan for medical complications. This plan should list specific responsibilities of each staff member, required equipment, and a predetermined contact for emergency response. Emergency plans including telephone numbers for EMS, police, and fire should be posted next to all telephones. First aid kits, first responder bloodborne pathogen kits, latex gloves, AED, CPR mouthpieces, and resuscitation bags must be readily available and transportable. The areas where first aid equipment is stored should be clearly labeled and supplies checked monthly. Regular periodic review of the emergency plan by a medical professional is recommended to ensure that all appropriate steps are outlined.

The plan should be practiced with both announced and unannounced drills on a quarterly basis. Strategies for coping with potential and common injuries in the exercise and fitness testing setting should be rehearsed. Completion of a written report, including an evaluation of the drill and recommendations for any necessary changes, should follow each emergency drill.

Emergency plans specific to both minor and major medical incidents are required. Minor medical events are not life- or limb-threatening and can be initially managed within the facility, but may be referred to a medical resource. Major medical emergencies require an initial response by the staff followed by immediate transport to a medical facility. Since a medical emergency may arise at any time and any location, all employees, including secretarial, janitorial, and child care staff, should be certified in CPR and first aid. *ACSM's Guidelines for Exercise Testing and Prescription*

Figure 6.1 – Common high-risk exercises and recommendations for alternative exercises. Adapted with permission from Frankel, VH, Hang YS. Recent advances in the biomechanics of sports injuries. Acta Orthop Scand 46:484, 1975, and Wendell L, Haydu T, Phillips D. Questionable Exercises. President's Council on Physical Fitness and Sports Research Digest 3:8, 1-8, 1999.

CONTRAINDICTATED/HIGH-RISK EXERCISE		ALTERNATIVE EXERCISE
Straight leg or bent knee full sit-ups with hands behind neck 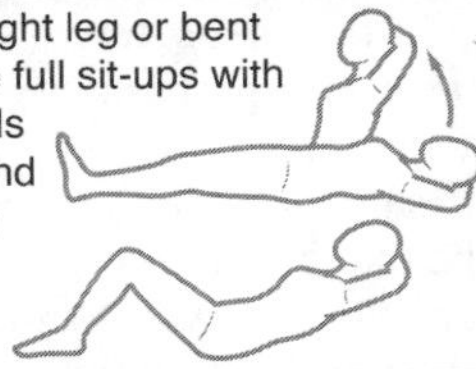	Risk: Stress on low back places high compressional forces on spinal discs, exercise primarily targets hip flexors, loaded neck flexion can sprain cervical ligaments and damage discs	Curls, Hands Under Lumbar Region, Lift Shoulder Blades but not Low Back off Floor 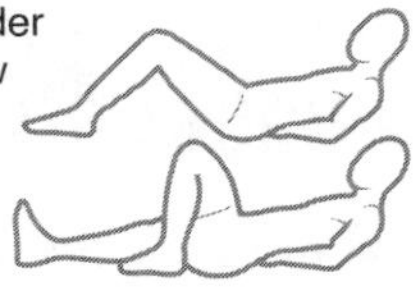
Double Leg Raises 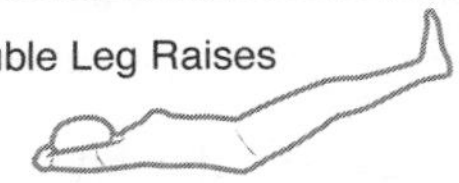	Risk: Hyperextends low back due to utilization of hip flexors with origin in the lumbar spine	Single Leg Raises- Opposite Knee Flexed 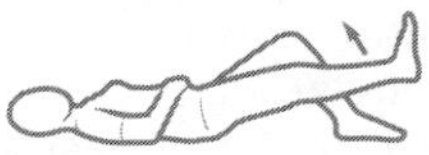
Full Squats 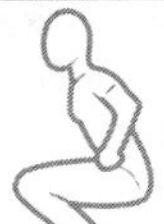	Risk: Patellar tendon forces during deep knee bending are 7.6 times body weight increasing the risk of chondromalacia and meniscal tears;	Squats to 90 Degrees of Knee Flexion-Knee Over Ankle 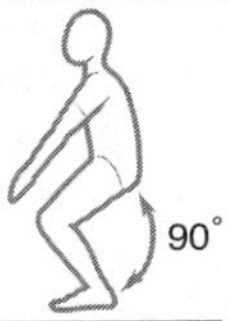 — 90°
Hurdler's Stretch for quadriceps (leaning backwards) 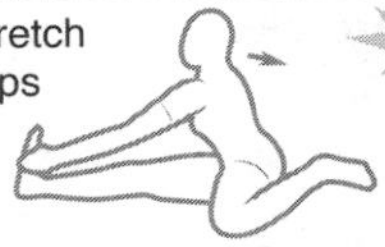	Risk: Knee flexion at end range of motion with rotational forces on hinge joint may stress the medial collateral ligament and menisci, also hyperextension of lumbar spine	Standing Quadricep Stretch, with Torso Upright; Hold Ankle, not Foot, with Opposite Hand; Avoid Hip Abduction 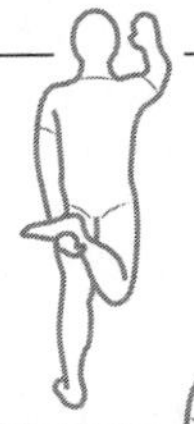
Standing quadricep stretch (same arm to ankle with hip abducted 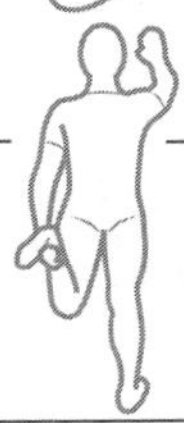	Risk: Hip abduction places rotational forces on knee and stresses the medial collateral ligament and menisci	Standing Quadricep Stretch, with Torso Upright; Hold Ankle, not Foot, with Opposite Hand; Avoid Hip Abduction 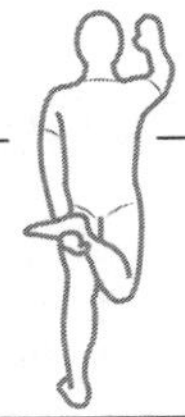
Hurdler's Stretch for hamstrings 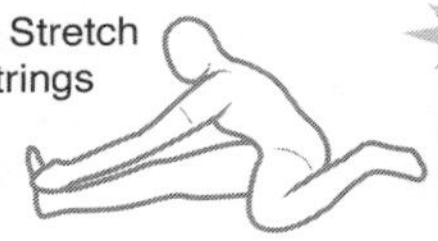	Risk: Knee flexion at end range of motion with rotational forces on hinge joint may stress the medial collateral ligament and menisci	Seated Hamstring Stretch, Back Flat with One Knee Flexed, Arms Behind Back 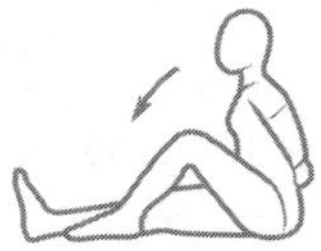
Plough 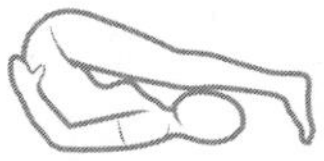	Risk: Loaded neck flexion can sprain cervical ligaments and damage discs, especially in those with spinal osteoporosis and arthritis	Double Knee to Chest 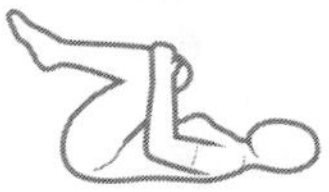
Back Hyperextension to increase strength 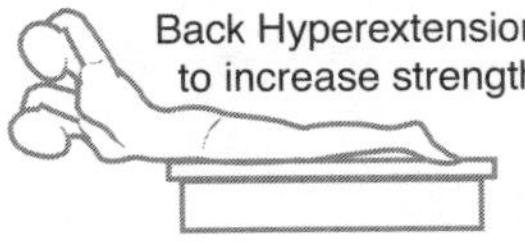	Risk: Uncontrolled, ballistic hyperextension of the lumbar spine can damage the vertebrae and spinal discs	Controlled Lumbar Extension to Normal Standing Lumbar Lordosis 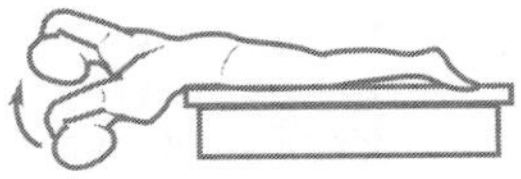
Full neck rolls 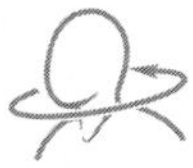	Risk: Compression of nerves and vessels which can lead to dizziness, disc damage	Slow, Controlled Lateral and Extension Neck Stretches Performed Separately 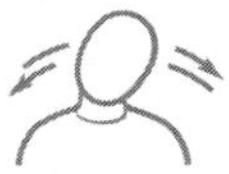
Loaded spinal flexion with rotation 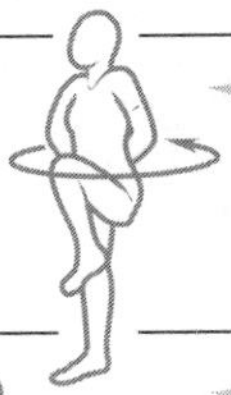	Risk: Loaded spinal flexion with rotation increases pressure and shear forces on spinal discs, common cause of low back injuries	Supine Crunches with Flexion followed by Rotation 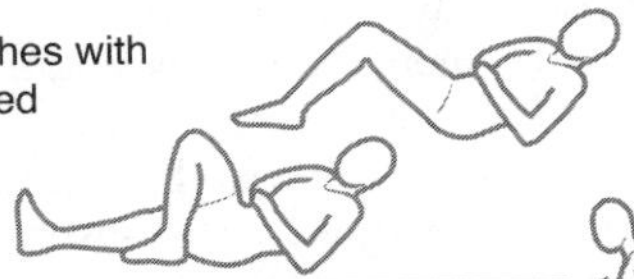
Standing toe touch 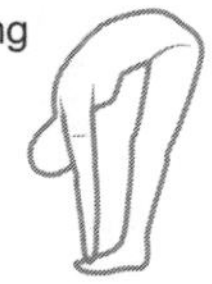	Risk: Increases pressure in lumbar disks and overstretches lumbar ligament	Standing Hamstring Stretch with Foot at a Height that Allows Maintenance of Flat Back as Hip is Flexed, Arms Behind Back 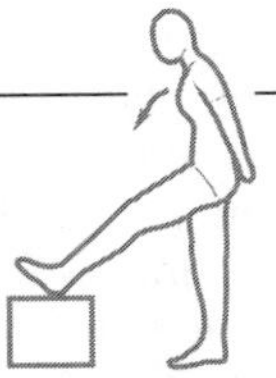

detail emergency plans for nonemergency and life-threatening situations (40). Emergency plans may vary according to the facility size, staff, and local emergency response.

J. Evaluation Skills

A critical responsibility of the exercise professional is evaluation of technique and body position during resistance, flexibility, and cardiovascular training. Early recognition and correction of poor technique may help reduce the risk of injury and ensure that the client receives the maximum benefit possible. Participants are usually appreciative and respectful if approached in a friendly, knowledgeable manner. The utmost concern for client safety and science-based information should be emphasized when correcting form or technique. Clients should be discouraged from selecting high-risk exercises.

When selecting exercises appropriate for the group or individuals, the following evaluation is recommended; a "yes" answer to all questions is required to maximize participants' safety.

- Is the exercise safe for all participants based on age and health status?
- If the exercise is safe, are the participants able to perform the exercise properly?
- Is this exercise an effective way to increase flexibility, strength, coordination, balance, or cardiovascular endurance?

If any questions are answered with a "no," replace the activity with a safe exercise that is more effective in achieving the ultimate goal.

The personal trainer or fitness instructor working one-on-one has to make decisions regarding the safety and effectiveness of exercises for only one client at a time. This task is easier than evaluating a group exercise class; however, the same procedure should be used.

K. Contraindicated and High-Risk Exercises

Much controversy surrounds the decision to label specific exercises as contraindicated or inappropriate for everyone. Factors such as age, flexibility, strength, type of exercise, pre-existing orthopaedic problems, and individual ability to perform an exercise properly make it difficult to label exercises as acceptable or unacceptable for all persons. Therefore, the term "high risk" may be more appropriate than contraindicated, since an exercise may be appropriate for an athlete in sports requiring high-risk movements, such as gymnastics but inappropriate for the general fitness setting. Figure 6.1 is a list of commonly performed high-risk exercises and some alternatives.

In a group exercise setting when all individuals are performing the same exercise, caution in selecting appropriate exercises for all ages, disabilities, and skill levels is crucial. Demonstration of a modified form of an exercise is always appropriate in a group, since individuals in advanced classes may exhibit high levels of cardiovascular fitness, but poor levels of flexibility, agility, strength, and/or muscular endurance. Since many popular group exercise classes (*e.g.,* kickboxing, boot camp) involve high-intensity ballistic movements that require above-average flexibility and agility, the fitness professional should provide a mechanism for screening participants prior to participation. Selection of the most effective and safe exercises is important, as most exercise classes attempt to provide multiple fitness components within a limited (45–60 min) time.

SECTION VI References

1. Fuller T, Movahed A. Current review of exercise testing: application and interpretation. Clin Cardiol 1987;10:189–200.

2. Malinow MR, McGarry DL, Kuehl KS. Is exercise testing indicated for asymptomatic active people? J Cardiac Rehabil 1984;4:376–379.

3. Haskell WL. The efficacy and safety of exercise programs in cardiac rehabilitation. Med Sci Sports Exerc 1994;26:815–823.

4. Vongvanich P, Paul-Labrador MJ, Merz CNB. Safety of medically supervised exercise in a cardiac rehabilitation center. Am J Cardiol 1996;77:1383–1385.

5. Franklin BA, Bonzheim K, Gordon S, et al. Safety of medically supervised outpatient cardiac rehabilitation exercise therapy: a 16-year follow-up. Chest 1998;114:902–906.

6. Thompson PD, Stern MP, Williams P, et al. Death during jogging or running: a study of 18 cases. JAMA 1979;242:1265–1267.

7. Borg G. Borg's Perceived Exertion and Pain Scales. Champaign, IL: Human Kinetics, 1998.

8. Mead WF, Pyfer HR, Trombold JC, et al. Successful resuscitation of two near simultaneous cases of cardiac arrest with a review of fifteen cases occurring during supervised exercise. Circulation 1976;53:187–189.

9. Hossack KF, Hartwig R. Cardiac arrest associated with supervised cardiac rehabilitation. J Cardiac Rehab 1982;2:402–408.

10. Kilbom A, Hartley L, Saltin B, et al. Physical training in sedentary middle-aged and older men. I. Medical evaluation. Scand J Clin Lab Invest 1969;24:315–322.

11. Friedwald VE Jr, Spence DW. Sudden cardiac death associated with exercise: the risk-benefit issue. Am J Cardiol 1990;66:183–188.

12. Drory Y, Turetz Y, Hiss Y, et al. Sudden unexpected death in persons less than 40 years of age. Am J Cardiol 68:1388–1392, 1991.

13. Thompson PD, Funk EJ, Carleton RA, Sturner WQ. Incidence of death during jogging in Rhode Island from 1975 through 1980. JAMA 247:2535, 1982.

14. Cupples LA, Gagnon DR, Kannel WB. Long- and short-term risk of sudden coronary death. Circulation 85:I11–I18, 1992.

15. Nieman DC. Exercise Testing and Prescription. 4th ed. Mountain View, CA: Mayfield, 1999

16. Mittleman MA, Maclure M, Tofler GH, et al. Triggering of acute myocardial infarction by heavy physical exertion: Protection against triggering by regular exertion. N Engl J Med 329:1677–1683, 1993.

17. Powell KE, Thompson PD, Caspersen CJ, Kendrick JS. Physical activity and the incidence of heart disease. Ann Rev Publ Health 8:253–287, 1987.

18. Blair SE, Kohl HW, Paffenbarger RS, et al. Physical fitness and all-cause mortality: A prospective study of health and unhealthy men. JAMA 262:2395–2401, 1989.

19. U.S. Dept. of Health and Human Services. Physical Activity and Health: A Report of the Surgeon General. Atlanta: National Center for Chronic Disease Prevention and Health Promotion, 1996.

20. Caspersen CJ. Physical inactivity and coronary heart disease. Phys Sportsmed 15:11, 43–44, 1987.

21. Pate RR, Macera CA. Risk of exercising: Musculo-skeletal injuries. In: Bouchard C, Shephard RJ, eds. Exercise, Fitness, and Health: A Consensus of Current Knowledge. Champaign, IL: Human Kinetics, 1994.

22. Van Mechelen W. Running injuries: A review of epidemiological literature. Sports Med 14:320, 1992.

23. Garrick JG, Requa RK. Aerobic dance: A review. Sports Med 6:169–179, 1988.

24. Richie DH, Kelso SF, Bellucci PA. Aerobic dance injuries: A retrospective study of instructors and participants. Physician Sportsmed 13:130–140, 1991.

25. Rothenberger LA, Chang JI, Cable TA. Prevalence and types of injuries in aerobic dancers. Am J Sports Med 16:403–407, 1988.

26. Janis LR. Aerobic dance survey: A study of high-impact versus low-impact injuries. J Am Podiatr Med Assoc 80:419–423, 1990.

27. Baxter-Jones A, Maffulli N, Helms P. Low injury rates in elite athletes. Arch Dis Child 68:130–132, 1993.

28. Hoeberigs JH. Factors related to the incidence of running injuries: A review. Sports Med 13:408–422, 1992.

29. Van Mechelen W. Can running injuries be effectively prevented? Sports Med 19:161–165, 1995.

30. Pollock ML et al. Effects of frequency and duration of training on attrition and incidence of injury. Med Sci Sport Exerc 9:31-36, 1977.

31. Grana WA, Kalenak A, eds. Clinical Sports Medicine. Philadelphia: Saunders, 1991.

32. McKeag DB, Dolan C. Overuse syndromes of the lower extremity. Phys Sportsmed 17:108, 1989.

33. Skinner JS. Exercise Testing and Exercise Prescription for Special Cases. Philadelphia: Lea & Febiger, 1987.

34. Konick-McMahan J. Riding out a diabetic emergency. Nursing 29(9):34–39, 1999.

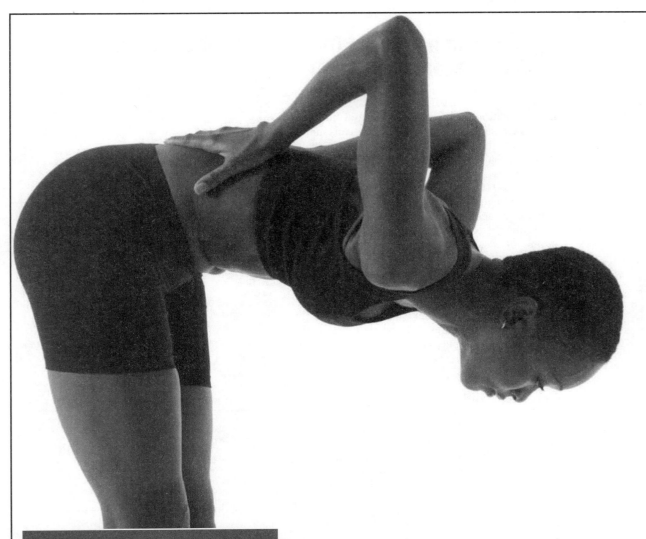

Section VII

- ✦ Choosing a Healthy Diet May Prevent Disease
- ✦ Specifics on Weight Management

ACSM's Resources for the Personal Trainer

NUTRITION AND WEIGHT MANAGEMENT

A. Choosing a Healthy Diet May Prevent Disease

The foods we eat affect our health throughout life. In addition to providing essential nutrients for growth and development, foods can supply substances that either contribute to or protect against chronic disease. Diseases such as cancer, osteoporosis, diabetes, hypertension, coronary heart disease (CHD), and obesity can be profoundly affected by diet.

Even though the typical personal trainer will not routinely counsel exercise participants with chronic disease, many current dietary recommendations have come about because of what we know about eating and disease risk. Table 7.1 lists dietary guidelines recommended by the American Heart Association (1).

Note that the Step I Diet was developed for the general U.S. population and that the Step II diet was developed for persons with a history of CHD or high cholesterol.

American Heart Association Recommendations

The American Heart Association (AHA) and the National Cholesterol Education Program (NCEP) have made specific recommendations for a heart-healthy diet, including limiting total fat intake to less than 30% of total calories; limiting saturated fat to less than 10% of total calories, with polyunsaturated fat providing no more than 10% of total calories and the remainder of the fat intake provided by monounsaturated fat (2, 3). The AHA also recommends limiting cholesterol to less than 300 mg·d^{-1}.

These recommendations for healthy individuals over age four do not limit total caloric intake. However, they are easily incorporated into a weight loss plan by specifying a number of grams of fat for dietary intake. Decreased fat is usually compensated for by increased intake of carbohydrates. Tables 7.2 and 7.3 illustrate details of the NCEP recommendations (3). The categories of naturally low-fat foods, such as grain products, fruits, and vegetables, allow more latitude with serving sizes, depending on caloric needs.

American Diabetes Association Recommendations

The American Diabetes Association (ADA) has also made dietary recommendations that can be used for weight loss (4). Although they were designed for individuals with diabetes mellitus, they present a healthy eating plan for all individuals. This eating plan, commonly known as the exchange system, is also the basis of many commercial weight loss plans. Food is divided into six

Table 7.1 – Recommended Intake as a Percent of Total Calories

NUTRIENT	STEP I DIET	STEP II DIET
Total fat	30% or less	30% or less
Saturated fatty acids	8–10%	7% or less
Polyunsaturated fatty acids	Up to 10%	Up to 10%
Monounsaturated fatty acids	Up to 15%	Up to 15%
Carbohydrate	55% or more	55% or more
Protein	Approximately 15%	Approximately 15%
Cholesterol	Less than 300 mg per day	Less than 200 mg per day
Total Calories	To achieve and maintain desired weight	

Table 7.2 – National Cholesterol Education Program Diet Therapy Recommendations

NUTRIENT	RECOMMENDED INTAKE (% TOTAL CALORIES) STEP I DIET	STEP II DIET
Total fat	30% of total calories	
Saturated FA	8–10%	7%
Polyunsaturated FA	Up to 10% of total calories	
Monounsaturated FA	Up to 15% of total calories	
Carbohydrates	≥ 55% of total calories	
Protein	Approximately 15% of total calories	
Cholesterol	< 300 mg/day	< 200 mg/day
Total calories	To achieve and maintain desirable weight	

FA, fatty acids.

Table 7.3 – NCEP General Recommendations for Food Choices

Six or more servings per day of breads, cereals, pasta, potatoes, rice, dried peas, and beans
Two or three servings per day of low-fat dairy products
Up to 5–6 oz per day of lean meats, poultry, and fish
No more than 6–8 teaspoons per day of fats and oils, including fats and oils used in food preparation
Five or more servings per day of fruits and vegetables
No more than 4 egg yolks per week on Step I and no more than 2 per week on Step II

groups (starches, milk, meat, fat, fruits, and vegetables) based on carbohydrate, protein, and fat content. Within each group, a serving size for each food that yields similar calories and macronutrients is determined. These exchanges can be switched with foods in another group. As a result, these foods can be used interchangeably in creating a meal plan. The number of servings from each group is based on caloric requirements for weight loss. The exchange system encourages a wide selection of food from different food groups and offers the advantage of providing an easy way to substitute one food for another while remaining within a caloric limit.

Counting Fat Grams

Counting fat grams has become an accepted method for weight loss. The basis is restriction of fat intake, which also helps limit total caloric intake. Fruits and vegetables are not limited, but foods high in fats (e.g., meats, cheeses, snack foods) are limited by a daily fat allowance. Although the literature supports reduced fat intake without additional caloric restriction, epidemiological data demonstrate that Americans continue to get fatter even as the percentage of total calories provided by fat decreases (5). Total caloric intake remains the most important aspect of a weight loss plan.

Counting Calories

Calorie counting may again emerge as an acceptable method of weight loss, since individuals continue to gain weight as fat intake is reduced. A detailed calorie book and attention to the new food labels may allow individuals to count total calories. This may result in lower fat intake as it becomes clear to the individual that foods high in fat are also high in calories. This method allows the individual to consume favorite foods as long as the intake of other calories is reduced proportionally. The disadvantage of calorie counting is that the nutritional quality of the diet may be inadequate if the individual fails to select from a variety of food groups.

High-Protein Diets

High-protein diets with reduced fats and carbohydrates are usually associated with a low-calorie or very low calorie diet. They are based on the premise that high protein intake preserves lean body mass during rapid weight loss. Examples of commercial variations of the high-protein diet are Medifast, Optifast, New Direction, and Health Management Resources (HMR).

The nutrient profiles of high-protein diets differ by the amount of carbohydrate and fat they contain. Some are very low in carbohydrates; the high protein–low carbohydrate profile results in mild ketosis. This type of diet, referred to as ketogenic, should contain 1–1.5 g of protein per kilogram of ideal body weight to preserve lean body mass and should be supervised by a physician (6).

High-protein diets provide safe, rapid weight loss with dramatic improvements in many cardiovascular risk factors. However, for the weight loss to be maintained, the programs must provide intensive behavioral counseling, exercise guidelines, and nutrition education. High-protein diet plans that limit carbohydrates until the evening meal are controversial and should be used with great caution.

General Recommendations

Health professionals should assist clients in choosing a safe and realistic weight loss plan that fits into the lifestyle of the individual. Healthy nutrition management is more than an eating plan; it requires changes in other behaviors as well. Most successful weight management programs include behavioral management in addition to a healthy eating plan. A program with record keeping, exercise, and social support would be preferred.

Weight-Loss Program Guidelines

Selecting an appropriate weight-loss program is difficult for the average consumer, given the myriad of diet and lifestyle books that promise great recipes, easy instructions, and fast results. Furthermore, there are no regulations regarding weight loss programs, although the Food and Nutrition Board recently issued guidelines to help health professionals and consumers evaluate them (6). A primary goal of the document is to shift the concern from simply weight loss to weight management and improved health. The suggested means of accomplishing this change of attitude is by emphasizing significant improvements in health and the reduction of risk factors that result from modest weight loss, especially if the loss is maintained. Three categories of weight management programs were presented:

- Do-it-yourself programs
- Nonclinical programs
- Clinical programs

Do-It-Yourself Programs

This category includes individual or group efforts to lose weight. They include Overeaters Anonymous, Take Off Pounds Sensibly (TOPS), and the use of Richard Simmons' Deal-A-Meal Plan, among others. Books, tapes, and work site programs are included in this category. The distinguishing feature of these programs is a lack of individual attention by a professional.

Nonclinical Programs

This category includes many commercial programs. The program, calorie levels, and educational materials are established by a parent company and are consistent at all company locations. Examples of nonclinical programs include Weight Watchers, Jenny Craig, Diet Centers, and Nutri-System. Educational materials and program guidelines are commonly written by health care professionals, but the personnel delivering the program are trained by the program as group leaders or counselors.

Clinical Programs

Clinical programs and services are provided by a licensed professional who may or may not have special training in the treatment of obesity. The program may be offered by a single health care professional or by a multidisciplinary team who coordinate the care. This team may include a physician, an exercise physiologist, a registered or licensed dietitian, a nurse, and a behavioral counselor. They may use a moderately reduced calorie diet, a very low calorie diet, exercise, psychological counseling, drugs, surgery, or combinations of these modalities to achieve weight loss and maintenance.

Appropriate Weight-Loss Methods

Despite efforts to the contrary, fitness professionals often find that exercisers do not adhere to safe, proven practices for losing body fat and gaining lean body mass. In a recent position stand, the American College of Sports Medicine recommended that the combination of reduced energy intake and increased energy expenditure, through structured exercise and other forms of physical activity, be the major focus of weight loss intervention programs.

An energy deficit of 500–1000 kcal·d^{-1} achieved through reductions in total caloric intake is recommended. Moreover, it appears that reducing dietary fat intake to less than 30% of total caloric intake may facilitate weight loss by reducing total caloric intake. Although there may be advantages to modifying protein and carbohydrate intake, the optimal doses of these macronutrients for weight loss have not been determined.

With respect to exercise, it has been found that significant health benefits can be recognized with participation in a minimum of 150 min (2.5 h) of moderate intensity exercise per week. Overweight and obese adults should progressively increase to this initial exercise goal. There may also be advantages to progressively increasing exercise to 200–300 min (3.3–5 h) of exercise per week, as recent scientific evidence indicates that this level of exercise facilitates the long-term maintenance of weight loss.

The addition of resistance exercise to a weight-loss intervention will increase strength and function but may not reduce the loss of fat-free mass typically observed with reductions in total caloric intake and loss of body weight. When medically indicated, pharmacotherapy (drugs) may be used for weight loss, but pharmacotherapy appears to be most effective when used in combination with modifications of both eating and exercise behaviors (7).

Ergogenic aids

Ergogenic aids consist of any number of legal or illegally obtained substances taken most often by athletes hoping to improve sport performance. In fact the word "ergogenic" refers to the "work producing" effect that athletes of every ability hope to achieve. In a joint position stand with the American Dietetic Association, and Dieticians of Canada, the American College of Sports Medicine concluded that in general, no vitamin and mineral supplements should be required if an athlete is consuming adequate energy from a variety of foods to maintain body weight. Although vitamin and mineral supplements may very well be appropriate for some athletes, it is unlikely that these supplements will enhance exercise and sport performance in those already eating a balanced diet. For example, if an athlete is ill, recovering from injury, or has a specific micronutrient deficiency, a multivitamin/mineral supplement may be appropriate.

No single nutrient supplements should be used without a specific medical or nutritional reason (e.g., iron supplements to reverse iron deficiency anemia). This holds true for other substances often consumed for their ergogenic value such as caffeine, creatine monohydrate, herbal supplements, or synthetic hormones (steroids). Athletes should be counseled regarding the use of ergogenic aids. They should only be used with caution and only after careful evaluation of the product for safety, efficacy, potency, and legality (8).

B. Specifics on Weight Management

Approximately one-third of American adults are overweight (9). Obesity is associated with several chronic diseases, such as diabetes mellitus, hypertension, hyper-cholesterolemia, hyperinsulinemia, and hypertriglyceridemia, all of which increase the risk of cardiovascular disease (10). Severe obesity may limit the ability to exercise because of a low tolerance for activity or perhaps musculoskeletal problems. For individuals with severe obesity, exercise complements caloric restriction and may promote a more rapid weight loss. It can also facilitate an improvement in blood lipid profiles (11).

Exercise professionals who work in nutrition and weight management programs should understand the concepts of healthy nutrition and provide support for the behavioral changes necessary for successful weight management.

A vital role for the exercise professional is to assist in the evaluation of programs to determine which are most likely to help the individual meet the weight management goals. The exercise professional should consult the state dietetic association to determine regulations regarding nutrition counseling and the practice of dietetics.

Setting A Weight Goal

The Expert Panel on Healthy Weight recommends that adults maintain a BMI of less than 25 (12). Persons with a BMI above 25 should develop a healthier weight goal, equivalent to a loss of approximately 2 BMI units (approximately 10 lb) and maintain that weight loss six months before further weight loss. Obese individuals with chronic disease or who are at risk for chronic disease should consult a health care professional for weight reduction recommendations. These recommendations are suggested as an initial point for achieving goal weight. Intermediate goals for those with more ambitious objectives may prevent discouragement and failure in reaching the goal weight.

Energy Balance

Weight loss generally occurs when energy expenditure exceeds energy intake, that is, when a negative energy balance is achieved. It is generally accepted that weight loss of 1 lb·wk^{-1} requires a negative energy balance of about 3500 Kcal/week, or 500 Kcal/day. This can be accomplished by the following:

- Reducing daily intake by 500 Kcal
- Reducing daily intake by 250 Kcal and increasing daily energy expenditure by 250 Kcal, or some other combination of decreased intake and increased expenditure equal to a loss of 500 Kcal/day
- Increasing caloric expenditure (physical activity) by 500 Kcal/day

The last option may be the most difficult for most obese individuals, who may not be able to tolerate the frequency, duration, or intensity of exercise needed to achieve this level of energy expenditure. A combination of moderate caloric restriction and moderate exercise is perhaps most likely to achieve the best result.

To improve compliance, the caloric restriction should be moderate, avoiding hunger and deprivation of favorite foods. The exercise component helps reduce stress, anxiety, and depression, which may trigger overeating. Exercise and activity can literally get you out of the kitchen or any location that contributes to unstructured eating. Individuals who exercise and conform to moderate caloric restriction achieve greater loss of fat mass and preserve lean body mass (13).

Exercise also establishes the types of behaviors required for weight maintenance. Research has shown that the best predictor of weight maintenance is continued regular exercise (14). Individuals can lose weight successfully without exercise, but successful weight maintenance without regular exercise is difficult.

How Should Individuals Determine Caloric Needs?

Current energy intake requirements can be determined in a number of ways, including dietary intake records and formulas that estimate daily caloric expenditure requirements for activity level and gender. Table 7.4 contains a list of factors that can be helpful in determining a person's daily energy requirements (15). Daily energy balance for weight loss can be determined using the estimated daily energy requirement, then increasing caloric expenditure (i.e., increasing physical activity) and/or reducing caloric intake proportionally.

The arbitrary assignment of caloric restriction

Table 7.4 – Estimation of Daily Energy Allowances at Various Levels of Physical Activity for Men and Women Aged 19-50

LEVEL OF ACTIVITY	ENERGY EXPENDITURE (KCAL/KG PER DAY)
Very light	
Men	31
Women	30
Light	
Men	38
Women	33
Moderate	
Men	40
Women	47
Heavy	
Men	50
Women	44

Very light activity is defined as mostly seated and standing activities such as driving, typing, ironing, cooking, and playing cards.
Light activity is defined as walking on a level surface at 2.5–3 mph, such as house cleaning, child care, golf, restaurant trades.
Moderate activity is defined as walking 3.5–4 mph, weeding and hoeing, cycling, skiing, and dancing.
Heavy activity is defined as walking with a load or uphill, heavy manual labor, basketball, climbing, football, and soccer.
Reprinted with permission from Food and Nutrition Board. Recommended Dietary Allowances, 10th ed. Washington: National Academy Press, 1989.

is a third technique for meeting caloric requirements during weight reduction (16). Caloric ranges of 1200–1500 for women and 1800–2000 for men are common recommendations. Adjustments are generally made after some weeks, depending on compliance and results.

Caloric restriction plans of 1200 Kcal or above are considered moderate calorie restriction programs, or balanced calorie deficit diets. A 1200 Kcal diet is believed to be the minimum level at which the recommended amounts of essential vitamins and minerals can be obtained without supplementation.

Greater caloric restriction requires vitamin and mineral supplementation. Diet plans that provide 800–1200 Kcal are considered low-calorie diets; plans that provide less than 800 Kcal are considered very low calorie diets and should not be undertaken without medical supervision (17).

A 1200 Kcal diet, though considered moderate for many individuals, is a very low calorie diet for the morbidly obese. For someone consuming 3500 Kcal/day, the 1200 Kcal plan provides a 2300 Kcal deficit. This individual can be expected to demonstrate metabolic responses (i.e., decreased thyroid hormone activity, increased diuresis, and decreased blood pressure) similar to those of a normal or thin individual on a very low calorie diet. The resulting rate of weight loss is rapid and requires medical supervision. A weight loss of 1–2 lb·wk^{-1} after the first 2 weeks is considered safe. A faster rate of weight loss should be monitored by a health care professional, even when the calorie intake is considered safe.

Eating Plans

While there are many guidelines for optimizing the diet, the operational foundation of any meal plan should be the Dietary Guidelines for Americans, fourth edition (1996), which includes the Food Guide Pyramid. The Dietary Guidelines encourage variety in intake and moderation in fat, sugar, and alcohol consumption. The Food Guide Pyramid recommends a variety of foods with particular emphasis on grains, fruits, and vegetables. To incorporate these guidelines into a weight loss program, special attention must be paid to serving size and choosing mainly from food groups appearing in the lower half of the Food Guide Pyramid.

Finally, fitness professionals should assist clients in choosing a safe and realistic weight loss plan that fits into the lifestyle of the individual. Healthy nutrition management is more than an eating plan; it requires changes in other behaviors as well. Most successful weight management programs include behavioral management in addition to a healthy eating plan.

Calculation of Energy Cost

Energy expenditure values can be expressed in kilocalories per kilogram of body weight per hour, kilocalories per minute, kilocalories per hour, or kilocalories per 24 hours. The most accurate way to determine the kilocalorie energy cost of an activity is to measure the kilocalories expended during rest (i.e., the RMR) and multiply that value by the MET values listed below. Because RMR is fairly close to 1 kcal·kg^{-1} body weight·h^{-1}, the energy cost of activities may be expressed as multiples of the RMR (18). By multiplying the body weight (kg) by the MET value and duration of activity, it is possible to estimate a kilocalorie energy expenditure that is specific to a person's body weight. For example, bicycling at a 5-MET value expends 5 kcal·kg^{-1} body weight·h^{-1}. A 60-kg individual bicycling for 40 min expends the following: (5 METs × 60 kg body weight) × (40 min/60 min) = 200 kcal. Dividing 200 kcal by 40 min equals 5 kcal·min^{-1}. However, it is important to note that to the extent the RMR is not equal to 1 kcal·kg^{-1} body weight·h^{-1} for individuals, the estimates of energy expenditure that include weight will more closely reflect body weight than the metabolic rate (19). See table 7.5 for the METs of selected activities.

Eating Disorders

While it is often emphasized that healthy body composition involves low body fat percentages, it is also important for fitness professionals to recognize that eating disorders and distorted perceptions of body image are common in the general public. Among the recognized disorders in the field of weight management are anorexia nervosa and bulimia nervosa, although there is now a wide range of recognized eating disorders (20–23).

Anorexia Nervosa

Anorexia nervosa is synonymous to self-starvation and involves a refusal to maintain a minimally normal body weight. In severe cases, anorexia can be life-threatening. The main feature of anorexia involves dramatic weight loss, sometimes achieved by self-induced vomiting, abuse of laxatives, use of diuretics or exercise. It is also not uncommon for affected individuals to exhibit an intense fear of gaining weight, a negatively altered body image, menstrual changes in women or the absence of menstruation, fatigue, and depression.

Bulimia Nervosa

Bulimia nervosa is often confused with anorexia nervosa but is usually characterized by repeated

Table 7.5 – Energy Expenditure (METs) of Selected Activities[1]		
METS USED	**ACTIVITY CLASS**	**SPECIFIC ACTIVITY**
5.0	Conditioning exercise	Bicycling, stationary, general
8.0	Conditioning exercise	Circuit training, general
2.5	Home activities	Putting away groceries (e.g., carrying groceries, shopping without a grocery cart)
6.0	Home activities	Moving furniture, household
1.8	Miscellaneous	Sitting-in class, general, including note-taking or class discussion
8.0	Running/jogging	Running/jogging 5 mph (12 min·mile^{-1})
3.0	Sports	Frisbee playing, general
5.0	Sports	Skateboarding
7.0	Walking	Backpacking, general
3.5	Walking	Walking, for pleasure, work break, walking the dog

[1]Ainsworth BE, Haskell WL, Leon AS, et al. Compendium of Physical Activities: classification energy costs of human physical activities. Med Sci Sports Exerc 1993;1: 71–80.

episodes of binge eating, followed by ways of trying to purge the body of the food or of expected weight gain. People can have this condition and be of normal weight. Although complications associated with bulimia are not as serious as those for anorexia, they often include teeth and gum problems, low potassium levels, and digestive problems all of which occur as the result of excessive vomiting.

While the suspicion or discovery of an eating disorder can be alarming to the personal trainer, it is important to recognize that experts disagree about the exact causes of eating disorders. It appears that many factors are involved, including genetics, family behavior and culture. In some instances, the biological systems in the brain that govern mood and appetite go awry. As a result, the U.S. National Institute of Mental Health reminds concerned professionals that people with eating disorders often do not recognize or admit that they are ill. As a result, they may strongly resist getting and staying in treatment. Fitness professionals or other trusted individuals can be helpful in ensuring that the person with an eating disorder receives attention in the form of a referral to a physician, psychologist, or other qualified professional for proper treatment (20–23).

Female Athlete Triad

The female athlete triad is a serious syndrome among girls and women consisting of disordered eating, amenorrhea (loss of menstrual function), and osteoporosis. Disordered eating refers to the harmful and ineffective eating behaviors described above used in attempts to lose weight or achieve a lean appearance. Alone or in combination, female athlete triad disorders can decrease athletic performance and cause disease or death (23).

Section VII References

1. He J, Ogden L, Vupputuri S, et al. Dietary sodium intake and subsequent risk of cardiovascular disease in overweight adults. JAMA 282:2027–2033, 1999.
2. Chait A et al. Rationale for the Diet-Heart Statement of the American Heart Association. Report of the nutrition committee. Circulation 88:3008, 1993.
3. National Cholesterol Education Program. Second report of the Expert Panel on Detection, Evaluation, and Treatment of High Blood Cholesterol in Adults. (Adult Treatment Panel II). Circulation 89:1329, 1994.
4. Maximizing the Role of Nutrition in Diabetes Management. Arlington, VA: American Diabetes Association, 1994.
5. Allred J. Too much of a good thing? An overemphasis on eating low fat foods may be contributing to the alarming increase in overweight among US adults. J Am Diet Assoc 95:417, 1995.
6. Weighing the options: Criteria for evaluating weight management programs. Washington: National Academy Press, 1994. (Summary available in J Am Diet Assoc 95:96, 1996.)
7. ACSM Position Stand: Appropriate Intervention Strategies for Weight Loss and Prevention of Weight Regain for Adults, December 1, 2001.
8. ACSM Joint Position Statement: Nutrition and Athletic Performance, December 1, 2000.
9. Kuczmarski R, Flegal K, Campbell S, et al. Increasing prevalence of overweight among US adults. JAMA 272:205, 1994.
10. Pi-Sunyer FX. Health implications of obesity. Am J Clin Nutr 53:1595S, 1991.
11. Katzel L, Bleecker E, Colman E, et al. Effects of weight loss vs. aerobic exercise training on risk factors for coronary heart disease in healthy, obese, middle-aged and older men. JAMA 274:1915, 1995.
12. Meisler J, St. Jeor S. Summary and recommendations from the American Health Foundation's Expert Panel on Healthy Weight. Am J Clin Nutr 63:474S, 1996.
13. Svendson O et al. Effect of an energy restrictive diet, with and without exercise, on lean tissue mass, resting metabolic rate, cardiovascular risk factors, and bone in overweight postmenopausal women. Am J Med 95:131, 1993.
14. Kayman S, Bruvold W, Stern J. Maintenance and relapse after weight loss in women: Behavioral aspects. Am J Clin Nutr 52:800, 1990.
15. Food and Nutrition Board. Recommended Dietary Allowances. 10th ed. Washington: National Academy Press, 1989.
16. Lichtman S, Pisarka K, Berman E, et al. Discrepancy between self-reported and actual caloric intake and exercise in obese subjects. N Engl J Med 327:1893, 1993.
17. National Task Force on the Prevention and Treatment of Obesity. Very low calorie diets. JAMA 270:967, 1993.
18. Taylor H, Jacobins DR Jr., Schucker B, et al. A questionnaire for the assessment of leisure time physical activities. J Chronic Dis 1978;31:741–755.
19. Blair SN, Haskell WL, Ho P, et al. Assessment of habitual physical activity by a 7-day recall in a community survey and controlled experiment. Am J Epidemiol 1985; 122:794–804, 1985.
20. MayoClinic.com. Eating disorders, 03/19/04. Retrieved 09/06/04.
21. http://www.mayoclinic.com/invoke.cfm?objectid=D95D8CE6-D330-4647-896530535E892A08&dsection=1.
22. National Institutes of Mental Health. Eating Disorders: Facts About Eating Disorders and the Search for Solutions, NIH Publication No. 01-4901, 2001.
23. ACSM Position Stand: The Female Athlete Triad, May 1, 1997.

Section VIII

✦ Equipment
✦ Legal and Business
✦ Health and Fitness Programming:
   Development, Implementation,
   and Evaluation

ACSM's Resources for the Personal Trainer

PROGRAM ADMINISTRATION, QUALITY ASSURANCE, AND OUTCOME ASSESSMENT

A. Equipment

Whether an independent contractor, sole proprietor, or employed by a large chain of fitness facilities, most personal trainers will be involved at some point with selecting and maintaining exercise equipment.

Equipment Selection

New equipment may be requested for several reasons:
- Long waiting lines at existing equipment
- High repair costs of outdated equipment
- Member requests
- An intriguing piece seen in a trade journal
- Improved ergonomic and biomechanical design

In any case, it is vital to make an informed decision without allowing emotions to lead to a costly mistake (Table 8.1).

Need

Before purchasing any equipment, the first step is to confirm the need. Ask the following questions:
- Is this equipment necessary?
- Is the product in question a legitimate option or a fad?
- Is the equipment suited for the demographics of membership?
- Is it affordable?

Space

Evaluate availability of space by examining dimensions of the equipment and the available space. For example, a treadmill may not be the best choice if the space is narrow or near a walkway. A climber, because of the small space requirements, may be more desirable. Equipment layout is another factor that must be considered, including the location of the appropriate electrical outlets. It is also important to allow for traffic flow and to avoid blocking access to an emergency exit. Refer to *ACSM's Health/Fitness Facility Standards and Guidelines* for additional information regarding spacing of equipment.

Gathering Information

Gathering product information is the next step. Review and compare as many equipment choices as possible. Trade magazines, trade shows, and equipment vendors are excellent sources of this information. Trade magazines and journals provide reader service cards and often publish an annual guide listing names and numbers for all equipment manufacturers. In addition to advertisements featuring a variety of brand names, monthly issues also have an advertising index in each issue.

Attendance at trade shows also facilitates gathering information. The differences between brands are more obvious and choices become clearer and narrow quickly when direct comparison is possible.

Table 8.1 – Equipment Selection Checklist

Date	Equipment	Serial No.	Problem	Date Repaired	Order #	Cost

Cardiovascular Equipment

Cardiovascular equipment is no longer limited to bikes, treadmills, and rowers. Each has advantages and disadvantages, and there is no best choice for every environment or situation.

Treadmills

Treadmills are consistently among the favorites in fitness settings. Treadmills have distinct advantages. Most people do not require time to learn the activity because walking and running are natural activities. Walking is a weight-bearing activity, and the large muscles of the leg require significant energy production for exercise, so heart rate can be raised and maintained in the target range, leading to sustained training for an increased length of time without extensive local fatigue. Intensity of exercise can be changed easily by increasing speed or elevation. Treadmills also have some disadvantages. Weight-bearing exercise may be difficult for those with weight problems or orthopedic injury. In these cases, non–weight-bearing exercise may be more appropriate. Also, treadmills take up considerable space. Finally, treadmills are the most expensive type of cardiovascular equipment.

Stationary Bikes

The stationary bicycle is popular and time tested. Among its advantages:

- Cycling is a motion that most people are comfortable performing.
- Little time is required for habituation.
- It is non–weight bearing and therefore non-impact.

A stationary bicycle can be an ideal mode of exercise in rehabilitative settings. However, because of lack of habituation, fatigue of leg muscles may cause difficulty achieving and maintaining a target heart rate for those using a bicycle ergometer.

Recumbent Bikes

Recumbent and semirecumbent bicycles are popular and have become standard in many facilities. The seat is more comfortable than traditional bicycle seats. These bicycles may be beneficial for special populations because they give back support. Safety is increased because of the wide base of support and the ease of mounting and dismounting. The disadvantages are similar to those of other stationary bicycles. Maintaining target heart rate may be more difficult than on upright bicycles because of the supine position. Local fatigue can also be a consistent problem on these bicycles.

Stair Climbers

Stair climbers, or stair steppers, are another popular cardiovascular exercise option. The advantages of stair climbers include the following:

- The motion of stepping or climbing is famil-

iar, making it easy to learn.
- It is weight bearing, which makes it relatively easy to maintain target heart rate.
- It is low impact.
- Climbers occupy less space than many other types of equipment.

Elliptical Trainers

Elliptical trainers are the newest type of cardiovascular machines in the industry, but they are already a popular piece in most health and fitness environments. As with stair climbers, they have the advantage of being weight-bearing and nonimpact. Their perceived benefit is the elliptical movement of the pedals, attempting to mimic the natural movement of the lower body. Some also have variable elevations, further enhancing the resistance options. Like treadmills, elliptical trainers are large, so they are space intensive, and they are relatively expensive.

Rowers

Though a legitimate form of cardiovascular exercise, rowing machines have never enjoyed the popularity of most other modalities and have decreased in popularity recently. Rowing uses large muscles of the legs as well as the large upper body muscles of the arms and back; raising and sustaining target heart rate is relatively easy. Rowing is a nonweight-bearing, nonimpact exercise. On the negative side, the rowing motion is unfamiliar to most users, making it more difficult to learn. Emphasis on proper instruction is required. Also, rowers require significant floor space (especially in length) and may require specially shaped space.

Cross-Country Skiers

Cross-country ski machines have become commonplace in fitness centers. Skiers offer some advantages. Large muscle mass (upper and lower body muscle groups are used) is used during exercise, and therefore target heart rate range is easily reached and sustained. Though it is weight-bearing, cross-country skiing is nonimpact. Most people are unaccustomed to this activity and have difficulty learning the skill. Despite the disadvantage, ski machines enjoy a great deal of positive press as well as very effective marketing. Consequently, many exercisers try skiers more than once in an attempt to learn the skill.

Resistance training equipment

In recent years, resistance training has become one of the most popular forms of exercise. This growing popularity has compelled manufacturers to extend the market and types of equipment. Where there was once a single multistation unit with one exercise option per muscle group, there are now multiple machines and free weights, offering several exercise options for each muscle group. Expanding demographics of the exercising population have caused manufacturers to change the appearance of equipment, creating broader market appeal.

Types of Equipment

Manufacturers of resistance training equipment offer three types: 1) isotonic, 2) variable resistance, and 3) isokinetic. Isotonic resistance training, in which the resistance remains constant throughout the range of motion, is performed using free weights and some machines. Variable resistance machines, by changing the radius of a cam, increase the resistance through part of the range of motion coinciding with the biomechanics of contraction. Isokinetic machines increase resistance at the point of maximum force while controlling the speed of contraction. This is accomplished through the use of systems including hydraulics or motors.

Resistance training machines come in a variety of styles and shapes. Although the majority are "selectorized" (using a weight stack), some manufacturers offer plate-loaded equipment with manually placed weight plates instead of weight stacks. In many cases this plate-loaded equipment looks and feels similar to the selectorized counterparts. This type of machine can be purchased at a much lower cost than selectorized machines.

Although the increased popularity of variable resistance machines has diminished, the demand for free weight training, barbells and dumbbells continues to increase. Most recently, developers have added dual-axis machines, which offer resistance in multiple planes. This type of exercise is consistent with natural movement patterns.

Safety Considerations

Safety has primary importance in selection of fitness equipment. Health and fitness facilities are legally obligated to provide a safe exercise environment.

1. Ensure that all electrical plugs are secured, grounded, and covered or removed in all traffic areas.
2. Treadmills should have easily accessible emergency cutoff switches.
3. Mount safety instructions on all equipment.
4. Ensure that equipment accommodates various body sizes and types. Adjustable seats, back pads, and leg pads should be available.
5. The machines must restrict joint movements beyond normal range of motion.
6. Back pads should never force loss of the natural curve of the spine.
7. Bench width should provide support without restricting the movement of the upper arm in supine exercises.

8. Free weight racks must be wide enough to accommodate the width of an Olympic bar, decreasing the risk of pinching a hand when reracking a weight. The apparatus must be constructed properly to sustain adequate amounts of weight.

Equipment trials in the fitness center may be important to the decision-making process. Purchasing equipment based on advertisements is not recommended. Direct experience to determine workmanship, comfort, and biomechanical appropriateness is imperative. An exercise session on the equipment provides an accurate feel for the machine.

Decision-Making Factors

Once needs are determined and product information has been gathered, evaluation begins. Factors in evaluation include cost, aesthetics, references, warranty, support and training, and maintenance.

Cost

The cost of a product is often the first question. If the product costs more than the budget allows, buying the equipment is not feasible. However, though cost is a major factor, it should not be the only one, and purchasing a piece of equipment because it is the least expensive may be a mistake. Many factors determine cost, including quality of the materials used, manner of assembly, and sales volume.

Aesthetics

Appearance of equipment is rightfully a consideration. It is important that all equipment fit with the desired look of a facility. Beyond decor, some equipment may particularly appeal to certain demographic groups. For example, large, high-profile pieces of weight-lifting equipment might appeal to members interested and skilled in weight lifting but may intimidate members of a wellness facility.

References

When considering any exercise equipment, request references from current owners, including familiar companies if the product in question is unfamiliar or new to the facility. An equipment manufacturer may make quality treadmills but inferior bicycle ergometers.

Warranty

Manufacturer's warranty is another important issue. The length and terms of the warranty (exactly what is covered) are important considerations. Most manufacturer warranties on strength equipment place a different warranty period on moving parts and upholstery than on metal frames. One way to determine practical life of any piece of equipment prior to need for replacement, repair, or refurbishing is to determine the warranty period.

Support and Training

Many companies provide a representative to help set up equipment and train staff and members on proper usage. Amount, speed, and quality of support provided are also important. Some equipment may require minimal support after installation and training, while other types (e.g., computer-based or automated equipment) may require continued support. For some types of equipment, these may be critical factors in purchasing.

Maintenance

All equipment requires maintenance. Determining the level of local service is a concern. Most major companies train local technicians to service and stock parts. Review the local company and obtain references.

Demonstration Period

Some equipment manufacturers offer trial periods or demonstrations. In these situations, facilities may allow members to assist in the decision, although some managers believe this is undesirable, as some members may become attached to a piece of equipment that ultimately is not purchased.

After potential suppliers are identified, request a bid and layout. At this point, with a narrowed field, a decision may be based on cost. Bids may be formal or informal and may involve some negotiating. A minimum of three bids should be obtained for all purchases.

Equipment Purchasing Options

Before making a final decision, some purchasing options should be considered: buying new, buying used, or leasing.

Buying New Equipment

The first option is buying new equipment outright. Although payment structures can be negotiated, most manufacturers require 50% down and the balance at installation. It is important to know whether freight and installation are included in the purchase price. Some facilities withhold 10% of the cost for 30 days to ensure satisfactory installation, training, and support.

Buying Used or Refurbished Equipment

A second option is buying used or refurbished equipment. Many equipment dealers specialize in refurbished and used equipment. They resell at prices of up to 30–50% less than new equipment. This is a good option, especially for resistance equipment which is well made and sturdy; many used pieces are considered as good as new. The

same is generally not true of cardiovascular equipment. The warranty on most cardiovascular equipment is two years, as opposed to 10 or more for resistance equipment. Most fitness facilities maintain resistance equipment at least that long. Older equipment is considered outdated and is likely to have excessive wear and tear.

Leasing

Leasing equipment may be a consideration if funds to buy the equipment outright are not available. Some manufacturers work through leasing companies to make this possible. Leasing requires a smaller initial cash outlay, allowing the organization to acquire more equipment. Leasing to own often provides better selection, better warranty, and sometimes buyback options. In addition, tax credits may be available for leased equipment. However, leasing is usually considered high risk, and interest rates may be high.

Equipment Maintenance

A maintenance program can extend the life of equipment. Some facilities have knowledgeable and experienced staff specifically for repairing equipment or dedicated to maintenance. Others use the services of an outside person or company for preventive maintenance and repair. The advantage of on-staff employees to service equipment is that response time is shorter. The disadvantage is that a staff maintenance worker, because of lack of training on intricacies of equipment, may misdiagnose a problem and delay the repair. In addition, facilities rarely stock adequate parts and must order them, resulting in more delay. Regardless of the approach, exercise equipment must undergo regular preventive maintenance to extend life and save repair costs.

Table 8.2 – Cardiovascular Equipment Checklist

Treadmills
   Check tension and alignment of walking belt monthly
   Check speed calibration monthly
   Check grade calibration monthly
   Lube drive belt monthly
   Lube elevation gears monthly
   Wax walking deck semiannually
Bicycles
   Lube chain semiannually
   Check crank bearings monthly
   Check seat monthly
   Check tension and RPM sensor monthly
   Lube pedals bimonthly
Steppers
   Lube pivots quarterly
   Grease sprockets quarterly
   Lube chains quarterly
   Check chain tension quarterly
   Tighten drive belt quarterly
Rowers
   Oil chains quarterly
   Check RPM sensors quarterly
   Inspect seat bearings quarterly

In addition, it is important that all pieces be cleaned throughout each day to remove perspiration, dust, dirt, and other elements that may come into contact with equipment and people.

Internal Maintenance

While some maintenance is suited for a trained professional, designated staff can regularly perform other tasks that reduce cost. This is internal maintenance. Much of internal maintenance is cleaning, which is the single most effective means of preventing premature breakdown. Some claim that cleaning can double the life of a piece of cardiovascular equipment. A preventive maintenance program can cut expenses as much as 50%; therefore, an effective internal maintenance program is critical. The checklist in Table 8.2 is an example of an effective maintenance schedule.

Upholstery

Upholstery on resistance training equipment is one of the most important parts of the equipment because it is the point of contact between the user and the equipment. Regular disinfecting is essential. Some forms of herpes skin virus have been shown to survive on a warm, moist surface for up to 6 h. Regular cleaning also prevents drying and cracking caused by oils and salts from perspiration. The most common areas for cracking are the points at which the head and elbows are supported. Another cause of upholstery damage is the buckles of weight-lifting belts. The use of belts on this equipment should be avoided. It is easy and cost-effective to replace upholstery on high-use areas. Other steps that can prolong the life of the equipment are listed in Table 8.3.

With good records, the upkeep cost of each piece of equipment can be determined. One commonly accepted rule of thumb can help determine when to replace equipment that requires constant and costly upkeep. If the cost of repair over two years is greater than the cost of a new unit or if a single repair costs 50% of the cost of a new unit, replace the unit.

After it is determined that a single piece or an entire line of equipment is too costly to maintain, there are two options: replace or refurbish. Refurbishing is a viable alternative to replacing equipment because of the cost savings, although it is not always the best decision. Refurbishing cardiovascular equipment may not be a good decision because life span is comparatively short. However, refurbishing resistance training equipment, especially free weight and plate-loaded equipment, is a good investment because of the long life span. Another consideration is the amount of structural damage sustained. If the frame has been exposed to large amounts of rust or heat (*e.g.,* from a fire), refurbishing is not a good idea. High levels of rust or heat can weaken stress joints and make a unit unstable.

B. Legal and Business Considerations

Legal considerations constitute an important dimension of service for those administering fitness evaluations and exercise tests, engaging in physical activity counseling and exercise prescription, or providing fitness programs for apparently healthy adults or individuals with stable chronic diseases. One area of paramount concern to exercise leaders, fitness instructors, rehabilitation specialists, and program administrators is the professional–client relationship and activities performed within the confines of that relationship. Other considerations with special significance in law include the physical setting and areas in which program activities are conducted, the specific purpose for which exercise services are performed, the equipment used, and the techniques employed with the exerciser.

The law influences exercise professionals in each of these domains and in others. Furthermore, expectations are substantially affected by the exercise environment—recreational, commercial, or clinical—and by the type of clientele being served. Regardless of the situation, sensitivity to issues of law and rigorous application of risk management principles may enhance the quality of service and client satisfaction. Moreover, practicing with a risk management perspective may reduce service-related injuries, the likelihood of personal injury litigation, and the extent of damage to the provider in the event of claim and lawsuit.

Laws affecting these matters vary considerably from state to state. Nonetheless, certain legal principles have broad application to preexercise screening, exercise testing, prescription, and activ-

Table 8.3 – Resistance Training Equipment Checklist

General
  Wax upholstery with a hard floor wax monthly.
  Remove pads at first sign of cracking.
  Stock backup pads.
Frames
  Inspect for cracks in welds monthly.
  Apply factory touch-up paint to chipped areas to prevent spreading as needed.
  Inspect for loose nuts and bolts monthly.
  Clean chrome parts with a chrome polish monthly. Household cleaners will fade the finish.
  Apply car polish to painted surfaces quarterly.
  Remove rust with fine steel wool and apply polish to surface as needed.
  Replace worn or missing warning decals.
Replace worn hand grips and seat belts.
Moving parts
  Inspect all parts and connections monthly.
  Replace any worn, stretched, or frayed cables, belts, or chains.
  Lubricate bearings and bushings with a Teflon type-lubricant when metallic dust or shavings or when squeaking or grinding sounds appear.
  Lubricate chains with chain lubricant monthly.
Weight Stack
  Clean guide rods with an aerosol cleaner that leaves no residue weekly.
  Apply a light coating of a Teflon lubricant to the guide rods weekly.
  Clean chrome weight stacks with a chrome polish weekly.

ity supervision. All exercise program personnel should know these principles, endeavor to develop practices aimed at reducing risks of negligence litigation, and maintain safe care of clients.

Legal Terminology and Concepts

Generally, claims against exercise professionals center on alleged violations of either contract or tort law. These two broad concepts, along with written and statutory laws, define and govern most legal relationships between individuals, including activities of exercise professionals with clients.

Contract Law

A contract is simply a promise or performance bargained for and given in exchange for another promise or performance, all of which is supported by adequate consideration (i.e., something of value). In examining exercise testing and prescription activities, the law of contracts affects the relationship between exercise professionals and clients. The client may receive physical fitness information and recommendations on exercise training. Likewise, the professional may perform exercise testing in exchange for payment, or some other consideration of value. This contract relationship also encompasses any related activities that occur before and after exercise testing, such as health screening prior to testing, exercise prescription, and first aid and basic emergency care that arises from exercises temporally associated with on-site provider services. If expectations during this relationship are not fulfilled, lawsuit for breach of contract may be instituted. Such potential suits allege nonfulfillment of certain promises or a breach of alleged warranties that the law sometimes imposes on many contractual relationships. Apart from the professional–client relationships, contract law also has implications for interprofessional relations, such as those with equipment companies, independent service contractors, and employees.

Informed Consent

Aside from breach of contract claims arising from a lack of promise fulfillment, claims against exercise professionals can be based upon a type of breach of contract for failure to obtain adequate informed consent from exercise participants. Although claims based on lack of informed consent, founded upon contract principles, are somewhat archaic, suits based upon such failures are still put forth in some jurisdictions. More frequently today, however, such claims are brought forth in connection with negligence actions rather than breach of contract suits. Before an exercise professional subjects a client to a specific exercise procedure both properly and lawfully, the client must give informed consent to the procedure. Informed consent is intended to ensure that the

client entered into the procedure with full knowledge of the material, relevant risks, any alternative procedures that might satisfy certain of the objectives, and the benefits associated with that activity. This consent can be express (written) or implied by law simply as a function of how the two parties to the procedure conducted themselves. To give valid consent to a procedure, the person must be of age, not be mentally incapacitated, know and fully understand the importance and relevance of the material risks and benefits, and give consent voluntarily and not under any mistake of fact or duress (1). Written consent is certainly preferable to any oral or implied form of consent; it expressly demonstrates the process should questions arise later as to whether that was the case.

In many states, adequate information must be provided to ensure that the participant knows and understands the risks and circumstances associated with the procedure before informed consent can be given. In such states, a so-called subjective test is used to determine whether that person understood and comprehended the risks and procedures associated with the matter at hand. Although some states do not require the use of informed consent for non-surgical procedures or when a test is performed for health care–related purposes, adherence to the process is a desired approach. Examples of informed consent documents for exercise testing and training programs are available elsewhere (1–4).

Suits arising from alleged deficiencies in the informed consent process related to testing, exercise prescription, or physical activity have become more commonplace. The law is moving toward a broadening requirement for disclosure of risk to participants. Some courts have even gone so far as to require the disclosure of all possible risks as opposed to those that are simply material (5). Such a requirement imposes unusual burdens on programs and raises substantial medicolegal concern (6). These concerns require individual analysis and response.

One element of the informed consent process relates to confidentiality and disclosure of personal and sensitive information that may be gathered from the client in the course of evaluating health status or delivering services. Provision should be made in the informed consent or other documentation to secure the written authorization to disclose specific test results, exercise progress reports, and so on, to health care professionals who have a need to know, such as a primary care physician. Written authorization may also be secured from clients if there is an intent to use data in reporting group statistics for program evaluation or research purposes, even when such information is only to be presented in ways not identifiable with the client. Many states and the federal government have promulgated privacy statutes that may affect the release of personally identifiable material regarding a program participant. The application of these laws to a program and rights to release information will depend on a variety of factors that only a local counsel can properly address.

Negligence

Although negligence has no precise definition in law, it is regarded as failure to conform one's conduct to a generally accepted standard or duty. A legal cause of action based on claims of negligence may be established given proof of certain facts, specifically that one person failed to provide due care to protect another to whom the former owed some duty or responsibility and that such failure proximately caused some injury to the latter person (1). Thus, the validity of negligence claims is typically established through a specific process that examines certain facts and establishes whether:

- A defendant owed a particular duty or had specific responsibilities to some person who has issued a claim of negligence
- One or more failures (breaches) occurred in the performance of that duty, as compared to a particular set of behaviors that were expected (due care, standard of care)
- The injury or damage in question was attributable to the established performance failure or failures; that is, they were the proximate cause of the injury or damage

When negligence claims arise, whether an exercise professional provided due care is critically important. Once a duty is established, the nature and scope of expected performance are usually determined by reference to published standards and guidelines from peer professional associations. Standards of care are discussed in a different section of this chapter. Ultimately, the most effective shield against claims of negligence may be the daily pattern of adhering to and documenting compliance with the most rigorous published guidelines that are relevant.

Malpractice

Malpractice is a specific type of negligence action involving claims against defined professionals. Malpractice actions generally involve claims against professionals who have public authority to practice (arising from specific state statutes) for alleged breaches of professional duties and responsibilities toward clients or other persons to whom they owed a particular standard of care or duty (1). Historically, malpractice claims have been confined to actions against physicians and lawyers. By statute or case law, however, some states have expanded this group to include nurses, physical therapists, dentists, psychologists, and other health professionals. In 1995, Louisiana became the first state to pass legislation to license and regulate exercise practitioners who work under the authority of physicians with patients in cardiopulmonary rehabilitation treatment programs (7, 8). The Louisiana State Board of Medical Examiners now provides regulatory management for this practitioner group. As yet, no published reports have addressed the effect of this relatively new public regulation on cardiac rehabilitation professionals in Louisiana. The more obvious possibilities of effect include level of autonomy in practice, changes in provisions of liability insurance, costs of such insurance, and exposure to claims of malpractice.

Standards of Practice

Standards of practice (or care) express how contemporary services should be delivered to give reasonable assurance that desired outcomes will be achieved in a safe manner. In most professions, such standards are developed and periodically revised by consensus among professionals or national associations of providers. Standards documents address what are considered to be benchmark methods, procedures, processes, and so on, that are applied in almost all settings regardless of location, resources, or training of the provider.

In reality, the national standard of practice at any time typically is influenced by a variety of sources, including published statements from professional associations, government policies, state and national government regulations, and so on. In recent years, the promulgation of standards for fitness and health care has increased dramatically. This circumstance mandates that professionals stay abreast of new pronouncements and regulations. Without knowledge of the most relevant and current standards and incorporation of those tenets into the operating protocols and records of service fulfillment, the individual practitioner becomes vulnerable to damage and loss in the event of legal challenges arising from personal injury lawsuits.

Several organizations have published documents that influence the standard of care in the health and fitness and exercise rehabilitation fields, although these documents vary in scope and applicability. Professionals should carefully examine services, uses of technologies and procedures, and clientele before deciding which standards and guidelines are most applicable.

Forms also may be developed for staff to use routinely in ensuring standardization in areas in which injury and/or legal risks are considered significant. Examples of these situations include forms for pre-exercise screening and consultation, instruction of new clients in exercise routines, specific cautions for avoidance of injury to the client, and staff inspection of equipment and facilities. Effective forms demonstrate how a facility has linked an important standard to a critical area of service. Use of such forms along with routine annotation of client records shows consistency of fulfillment.

Ethics

Generally, ethics can be described as standards of conduct that guide decisions and actions, based on duties derived from core values. Specifically, core values are principles that we use to define what is right, good, and/or just. When a professional demonstrates behavior that is consistent, or aligned, with widely accepted standards in their respective industry, that professional is said to be behaving "ethically." On the other hand, "unethical" behavior is when a professional demonstrates behavior that is not consistent with industry-accepted standards. As a fitness professional, you have an obligation to stay within the bounds of the defined scope of practice for a certified Personal Trainer, as well as to abide by any and all industry-accepted standards of behavior at all times. Furthermore, as a certified or registered professional through ACSM, it is your responsibility to be familiar with all aspects of the ACSM's Code of Ethics, listed below:

Code of Ethics for ACSM Certified and Registered Professionals

Purpose

This Code of Ethics is intended to aid all certified and registered American College of Sports Medicine Credentialed Professionals (ACSMCP) to establish and maintain a high level of ethical conduct, as defined by standards by which an ACSMCP may determine the appropriateness of his or her conduct. Any existing professional, licensure or certification affiliations that ACSMCPs have with governmental, local, state or national agencies or organizations will take precedence relative to any disciplinary matters that pertain to practice or professional conduct.

This Code applies to all ACSMCPs, regardless of ACSM membership status (to include members and non-members. Any cases in violation of this Code will be referred to the ACSM Committee on Certification and Registry Boards (CCRB).

Responsibility to the Public

- ACSMCPs shall be dedicated to providing competent and legally permissible services within the scope of the Knowledge, Skills, and Abilities (KSAs) of their respective credential. These services shall be provided with integrity, competence, diligence, and compassion.
- ACSMCPs provide exercise information in a manner that is consistent with evidence-based science and medicine.
- ACSMCPs respect the rights of clients, colleagues, and health professionals, and shall safeguard client confidences within the boundaries of the law.
- Information relating to the ACSMCP–client

relationship is confidential and may not be communicated to a third party not involved in that client's care without the prior written consent of the client or as required by law.
- ACSMCPs are truthful about their qualifications and the limitations of their expertise and provide services consistent with their competencies.

Responsibility to the Profession

- ACSM cPTs maintain high professional standards. As such, an ACSM cPT should never represent him/herself, either directly or indirectly, as anything other than an ACSMCP unless he/she holds other license/certification that allows him/her to do so.
- ACSMCPs practice within the scope of their knowledge, skills, and abilities. ACSMCPs will not provide services that are limited by state law to provision by another health care professional only.
- An ACSMCP must remain in good standing relative to governmental requirements as a condition of continued Credentialing.
- ACSMCPs take credit, including authorship, only for work they have actually performed and give credit to the contributions of others as warranted.
- Consistent with the requirements of their certification or registration, ACSMCPs must complete approved, additional educational course work aimed at maintaining and advancing their knowledge, skills and abilities.

Principles and Standards for Candidates of the Certification Exam

Candidates applying for a Credentialing examination must comply with candidacy requirements and to the best of their abilities, accurately complete the application process.

Public Disclosure of Affiliation

Any ACSMCP may disclose his or her affiliation with ACSM Credentialing in any context, oral or documented, provided it is currently accurate. In doing so, no ACSMCP may imply College endorsement of whatever is associated in context with the disclosure, unless expressively authorized by the College. Disclosure of affiliation in connection with a commercial venture may be made provided the disclosure is made in a professionally dignified manner, is not false, misleading or deceptive, and does not imply licensure or the attainment of specialty or diploma status. ACSMCPs may disclose their credential status. ACSMCPs may list their affiliation with ACSM Credentialing on their business cards without prior authorization (ACSM Health/Fitness Director®, ACSM Health/Fitness Instructor®, ACSM Group

Exercise Leader®, ACSM Program Director℠, ACSM Exercise Specialist®, ACSM Exercise Test Technologist®, ACSM Registered Clinical Exercise Physiologist®, ACSM certified Personal Trainer™). ACSMCPs and the institutions employing an ACSMCP may inform the public of an affiliation as a matter of public discourse or presentation.

Discipline

Any ACSMCP may be disciplined or lose his or her certification or registry for conduct which, in the opinion of the Executive Committee of the ACSM Committee on Certification and Registry Boards, goes against the principles set forth in this Code. Such cases will be reviewed by the ACSM Committee on Ethics and Professional Conduct, which will include a liaison from the ACSM Committee on Certification and Registry Boards as appointed by the Chair of the Committee on Certification and Registry Boards. The ACSM Committee on Certification and Registry Boards will make an action recommendation to the Executive Committee of the ACSM Committee on Certification and Registry Boards for final review and approval.

Business Models

In addition to familiarity with the legal considerations of the fitness industry, the fitness professional should understand the various models for organizing and managing a business. The influence of taxes and personal risk weigh heavily in the process of deciding which type should be used. Some examples follow.

Sole Proprietorship

The name defines the sole proprietorship: a single person owns the business. This is the simplest, least expensive form of business to start. Often, only a license or registration is required to begin operation. Few government regulations apply, and earnings are subject to personal income tax. A major disadvantage is the difficulty in obtaining significant capital to start or expand such a business. Also, the personal liability for debt is extensive.

Independent Contractor

An independent contractor is usually someone who performs specific services for others. Many personal trainers operate as independent contractors, where a member of a facility pays the facility for personal training services, and then the club pays the personal trainer. Usually, you are an independent contractor if you work at multiple facilities, provide your own equipment, are paid by the session, set your own work hours, and control how you provide your services.

Partnership

A partnership can be either an informal agreement or a formal written document filed with the state government. Partnerships have limited governmental constraints, and the partners are personally taxed in proportion to their share of ownership. This form of business can consolidate the skills and resources of each partner, but transfer of ownership or the death of a partner can cause problems. Partnership does carry financial liability, including exposure to risk of loss of personal assets if other partners cannot meet obligations.

Corporation

The corporation is a formal establishment and is heavily influenced by laws, regulations, and stockholders, who are free from debt liabilities. The charter and bylaws govern the operations of a corporation. The risk to owners is limited, and a wide variety of investors may be attracted to the business. Transfer of ownership is easier than with either a partnership or a sole proprietorship. The corporation is a legal entity that is completely separate from managers and owners. Changes in management and ownership do not affect the charter or bylaws.

Subchapter S Corporation

The subchapter S corporation, or S corporation, is a hybrid of a partnership and corporation. At times, a small business with grand growth plans begins as an S corporation. This entity combines the advantages of the sole proprietorship, the partnership, and the corporation without the accompanying disadvantages. There is limited risk and exposure of personal assets, and partners cannot be taxed twice on salary and business income. A partner is free to distribute dividends, avoiding the complexities of a partnership.

C. Health and Fitness Programming: Development, Implementation, and Evaluation

One of the greatest challenges for the health and fitness manager is to offer a wide menu of programs and services that is consistent with the business objectives of a particular organization and able to meet the specific demands of diverse client populations. This chapter presents an overview of typical business objectives for health and fitness organizations and methods for determining the needs of specific client populations. In addition, systems for program development, delivery, and evaluation are presented and discussed. Because of the dynamic nature of the health and fitness industry, emphasis has been placed on providing a systematic approach to programming that can be used across many types of facilities and population groups.

Programming Based on Organizational Objectives

As the health and fitness industry has matured over the past decade, facilities have become more similar with respect to general design characteristics and types of equipment. It is likely, for example, that a prospective participant will find a similar range of cardiovascular equipment (treadmills, stair machines, bicycles, and rowers) available at both community and commercial fitness facilities. As a result of this lack of differentiation with regard to facilities and equipment, health and fitness programming has become the primary product that differentiates organizations in the marketplace. Therefore, it is important that the menu of programs offered by a health and fitness facility be carefully designed to match specific facility and program goals and objectives.

The following section outlines four general categories of organizational settings in the health and fitness industry. A description of typical business objectives in each of these categories has been presented to provide the health and fitness manager with a point of reference. In reality, regardless of the category, there is likely to be a combination of objectives within the business plan of a given organization. It is the responsibility of the health and fitness manager to identify clearly the specific objectives of the facility. The four general categories of organizational settings in the health and fitness industry are commercial, community, work site, and clinical.

Commercial Settings

Commercial health and fitness organizations are usually operated with the intention of generating a profit. Private health and fitness clubs, country clubs, and spas are examples of commercial organizations. Health and fitness programming contributes to the profitability of commercial organizations in several ways. Programs can generate revenue directly through assessment of fees for specific services (fee-for-service programs). These fees are often charged in addition to the fees that are collected monthly or annually for use of the facility. Personal fitness training is an example of a highly profitable revenue-generating program that is popular in many commercial organizations. In addition to fee-for-service programs, complimentary programs also contribute to the profit-generating objectives of a commercial organization.

Complimentary programs are often packaged into the general membership fees that participants are charged for use of the facility. In many cases, participants make decisions to join facilities based on the types of complimentary programs and services offered. In addition, the decision to continue paying dues is based largely on individual assessment of the value received for the money expended. A client who uses the facility and participates regularly in the programs and services offered is likely to meet individual goals and perceive membership as having value. Programs that encourage regular participation and effective facility use can improve member retention and therefore profitability.

Community Settings

The objective of most community health and fitness organizations is to provide services to the members of a specific community group. YMCAs, Jewish Community Centers, community recreation centers, and university recreation centers are examples. Health and fitness programs in these organizations typically target a specific market and attempt to provide services to as many members of that market as resources will allow. Most community organizations receive some level of outside funding and are classified as not-for-profit organizations. These favorable financial circumstances can allow community organizations to offer programs at low cost, increasing access for many segments of a given community. It is fairly common for some programs in a community organization to be offered on a for-profit basis as a way of generating revenue to deliver other programs at little or no cost to participants. In many YMCAs, for example, fitness memberships are sold to the public as a way to generating revenue to offset the cost of non–profit-generating programs such as children's summer camps, senior exercise classes, and programs for individuals with special needs.

Work Site Settings

Work site health and fitness organizations typically are intended to reduce health care costs and/or increase productivity, morale, and recruitment. Work site settings may include traditional fitness facilities or may simply be health and fitness programs in existing space at the work site. Health and fitness programs in these settings can be funded entirely by the company, but in various models individual employees share at least a portion of the program costs. The programs provided in work sites are quite broad. Wellness-oriented programs (e.g., health education classes, smoking cessation, nutrition, stress management) are often given emphasis equal to that of fitness programs. Outdoor activities, such as walking, running, and cycling, are also popular programs that can be offered at the work site without the benefit of additional facilities. Programs offered in the work site are often directly tied to the objective of creating a healthier employee population.

Clinical Settings

Clinical health and fitness organizations are a broad category of businesses that operate with many objectives. Examples of clinical organizations include health and fitness facilities at hospitals, satellite clinics, physical therapy offices, and chiropractic offices. If a clinical health and fitness organization operates as a for-profit business, programs are conducted with similar objectives to those in a commercial setting. If the business model is not-for-profit, objectives are more similar to those of a community or work site setting. As an example, a hospital may operate a work site business for its employees in an attempt to control health care costs and to improve productivity and morale. The facility may also operate as a community business for health insurance subscribers with the objective of helping clients maintain healthy lifestyles and reduce use of medical services. Finally, the hospital may operate commercially, offering health and fitness programs as a way to position itself as a wellness-oriented health care provider, thus improving health insurance sales to subscribers and increasing profitability.

As can be seen from these examples, it has become increasingly difficult to define an appropriate menu of health and fitness programs for an organization based solely upon business setting (*e.g.,* commercial, community, work site, or clinical). The business objectives of an organization provide important guidance, but for programming to be successful, the specific needs of individual participants must also be considered.

Programming Based on Participant Goals

Regardless of the organizational setting, each individual participant has specific needs (goals) related to health and fitness. Understanding and identifying the range of goals within the target population for a particular organization is an essential step in programming. The following section describes three categories of goals for individuals who are considering participation in a health and fitness program. Participant goals are rarely limited to a single category, however, and often change over time. It is important to identify the range of participant goals in a particular setting and offer a variety of programs and services to address as many of these goals as possible without compromising quality for quantity. In this manner, as the goals of individuals change over time, the organization will adjust programs and services so as to continue to address participants' goals. Individual goals related to health and fitness programs can be categorized as wellness goals, physical health and fitness goals, and performance goals.

Wellness Goals

People often consider participation in a health and fitness program as a way of improving the overall feeling of wellness. Wellness is an expanded idea of health that goes beyond physical fitness or absence of disease. Wellness is a feeling of optimal health and vitality that encompasses physical, emotional, intellectual, social, mental, and spiritual dimensions (9). Health and fitness settings offer numerous opportunities for wellness programming. Classes directed at lifetime learning, social interaction, travel adventures, relaxation, and meditation are several examples of programs that can help participants meet wellness goals. In addition, educational programs can be offered to assist individuals with achieving positive health behavior changes such as quitting smoking, changing nutritional habits, or beginning an exercise program.

In the case of a participant who is new to exercise, initial assessments, such as health risk appraisals, provide important information about health status and risk of chronic disease. Fitness assessments can also provide valuable information regarding baseline fitness levels. As with any exercise program design, recommendations with the beginning exerciser should be provided in three distinct phases: the initial phase, improvement phase, and maintenance phase. The initial phase is a gentle introduction to activity emphasizing regular participation and proper technique. The improvement phase is a progressive increase in frequency, intensity, and duration of the activity. The maintenance phase includes variations in program design in a manner that maintains the level of fitness and assists in long-term adherence. Beginning exercisers may need to spend considerable time in the initial phase before proceeding to the improvement phase. Incentive programs may also prove helpful for beginning exercisers, particularly when they have reached the maintenance phase of a program.

Physical Fitness Goals

Many people participate in health and fitness programs to accomplish specific physical fitness goals such as losing weight or getting in shape. Programming opportunities for physical fitness goals are numerous and new ideas are continually emerging. Group exercise classes, personal fitness training, cardiovascular equipment, weight training machines, free weights, stretching programs, yoga, and martial arts are just a few examples of popular programs that can help individuals meet physical fitness goals.

Regardless of initial fitness levels, all participants with physical fitness goals should have a complete health screening prior to initiating a program. Fitness assessments can also provide baseline information for each component of fitness. Programming for this population should involve individualized exercise prescriptions based on the participant's specific goals. Emphasis is placed on the improvement phase of exercise programming.

Performance Goals

In addition to wellness and physical fitness, people participate in health and fitness programs to achieve specific performance goals. Participants may desire to improve ability in a specific sport or type of activity. The range of abilities and skill levels among individuals with performance goals is broad. Some individuals may wish to learn techniques that allow them to take part in a new sport, such as tennis or golf. Others may wish to achieve a high level of performance in a particular competition. Still others may be looking to rehabilitate from an injury and reach a performance goal of getting back to a particular baseline of physical ability. Programming opportunities are very broad in this category. Examples of programs that can be offered at health and fitness facilities include sport technique training, such as tennis, fly-fishing, or golf; specialty conditioning classes, such as ski conditioning, rowing, or swimming; and educational classes on topics such as nutrition and advanced exercise program design. Specific exercise prescription with frequent reevaluation is necessary when working with individuals who have performance goals. Measuring outcomes is essential to assess the effectiveness of the programs being offered.

Effective Program Planning Models

Developing a menu of programs to meet the specific goals of a particular client population is a four-step process that involves needs assessment, program planning, program implementation, and program evaluation.

The Needs Assessment

The purpose of the needs assessment is to determine the specific goals and interests of the client population. This information, combined with industry trends and organizational objectives, can help define an appropriate menu of programs and services. Options for conducting the needs assessment include the following.

Target Market Surveys

The purpose of a target market survey is to determine levels of interest among prospective participants. The target market survey should be conducted early in the planning process. Surveys can be administered through personal distribution of questionnaires, mailing surveys to homes, or interviewing individuals by telephone. Questions must be carefully constructed and sample groups must be selected at random to obtain accurate and relevant information. In the case of a start-up operation, with which initial programming decisions may have a significant financial influence on facility design, facilities should consider hiring a professional consultant for a thorough market analysis. Consultation fees may seem high initially, but the relative cost of renovating a facility to accommodate programming needs that were not initially discovered usually justifies the investment.

Focus Groups

Focus groups are informal discussions conducted with small groups of participants. The group is usually selected according to common characteristics, such as age, sex, or previous participation. A skilled facilitator who tries to obtain information on participants' reactions or attitudes to specific topics typically leads focus group discussions. Before designing a health and fitness facility, focus groups can be an effective way to obtain detailed information regarding prospective participants' interests. Focus groups can also be used to obtain information regarding appropriate pricing, scheduling, and other details related to specific program plans. In an existing facility, focus groups can be used to learn about current programs and clients' interests for expansion. The involvement of a third party in the interview can make participants more comfortable and less reluctant to express their views.

Participant Surveys

If new programming is being considered in an existing facility, a survey of current participants can provide valuable insight. These surveys can be distributed through billing statements, at specific programs, or as part of registration for other activities in the facility. Regardless of the method used, participation is likely to increase if an incentive is offered for completion of the survey. It is important to recognize that any programming changes in a facility affect all other programming. If scheduling changes are involved, some participants will be displaced. If a new program is added, some participants will switch activities and may leave another program undersubscribed.

Evaluation of Current Programs

As part of complete program delivery, evaluations of all programs offered within a facility should be conducted from time to time (see next section for further details). These program evaluations provide valuable information regarding adaptations of existing programs and can detect opportunities for new program development. This process should be ongoing and should include budgetary analysis of revenue and expenses, attendance records, participants' satisfaction, and attainment of program goals and objectives.

Surveys of Staff, Management, and Advisory Committees

Input from staff, management, and other experts can provide important insight for program development. In addition, these individuals can provide an important base of support for marketing during the implementation phase of the program. Individuals who are involved in the planning phase of a program are likely to feel a sense of ownership and high level of support and excitement. Staff members who have direct contact with participants can often provide the most insightful feedback regarding participant needs. These staff members are regularly exposed to informal suggestions and complaints, many of which never are written down or placed on survey questionnaires. Managers often have important input as well regarding operational issues and financial considerations related to overall business objectives. Finally, expert advisers from the community provide an unbiased outside perspective.

Health Screening and Fitness Assessment

Establishing specific program goals and objectives is an essential step in programming. Health appraisal questionnaires and fitness assessment tests can provide specific and detailed information on the baseline status of a given population group. As an example, a specific work site may implement an employee exercise program as a way to lower the incidence of hypertension and obesity in the population. Initial testing for resting blood pressure, body mass index, and body composition could provide important baseline data by which this program could be monitored and evaluated in the future. Initial health risk appraisals can also be used as a way to identify program priorities for the population.

Health Care Usage Reports

Reports on health care usage can also assist an organization in identifying priorities for health and fitness programming. For example, a health insurance company may identify a particular work site that has a large number of claims related to back pain and injury. In this particular facility, educational programs, stretching classes, and ergonomic workstation adjustments may be identified as priority areas of health and fitness programming.

Community Agency Data

Organizations and agencies such as the American Heart Association, American Lung Association, American Red Cross, Centers for Disease Control, and local public health departments provide a wealth of information regarding prevalence of specific diseases and risk factors in the population. In addition, these agencies can provide a wealth of resources, such as written materials, Web Sites, programs, and consultants.

Program Planning

Once the needs assessment phase has been completed and program needs have been clearly defined, the second phase of program development begins. Program planning is the phase of development in which program details are clearly defined and put into operation. All program plan-

ning should include a long-term vision so that short-term planning becomes a means by which the long-term vision is achieved. The following steps should be included in the planning process.

Defining the Target Market

The first step in the program planning phase is to define the target market for the specific program under consideration. Needs assessment data should be used to identify the specific characteristics of people who are likely to participate. In addition, this information can help to determine whether the market size is adequate to meet the specific program objectives.

Identifying Program Goals and Objectives

The next step is to define the specific goals and objectives for the program. Clearly defined goals and objectives provide the foundation for all future planning decisions. In addition, program objectives provide a basis for program evaluation. Examples of program goals for a health and fitness facility include the following:
- Generating net revenue
- Acquiring new participants
- Improving participant retention
- Providing community service
- Program objectives are more specific than program goals. Examples of program objectives:
- Decreasing the average body fat level of program participants from 32% to 28% as measured by skinfold caliper tests
- Increasing program participants' knowledge of general nutritional guidelines as measured by change in scores on a nutritional knowledge test
- Reducing cardiovascular risk factors among exercise program participants at a work site as measured by scores on a health risk appraisal instrument

Developing Program Content

Once program goals and objectives are established, specific program content can be developed. Program content decisions include the identification of specific materials, equipment, documents, and reference materials to be used and the specific knowledge and skills to be presented. In addition, program content should clearly identify any procedures that are required before participation, such as health screenings, informed consent, and signatures on waivers. The amount of time available, participants' initial knowledge and skill, facility resources, budgetary guidelines, and staff qualifications are among the many issues that must be considered when planning program content.

Establishing a Delivery Model

The delivery model for a program includes decisions related to the location, time of day, duration of sessions, length of the program, number of participants, and instructional techniques to be used. These decisions depend on the specific goals and objectives for the program, characteristics of the target market, projected number of participants, availability of qualified staff, and program budget.

Location: The location must be accessible and convenient for the target market. In addition, the facility must be appropriate for the program content.

Scheduling: The program must be scheduled at a time that is convenient for participants and consistent with the overall business objectives of the facility. Consider scheduling of other programs that serve this target market, including programs and events outside of the facility, such as school vacations and public holidays.

Staff-to-participant ratio: Establishing these ratios in advance allows for establishing enrollment limits, accurate budgeting, and identification of facility requirements. These limits ensure that the program content can be effectively delivered.

Developing Marketing and Sales Plans

The marketing plan defines the message that will be communicated to potential participants about the program. The marketing plan also identifies the specific methods that will be used to inform potential participants about the program. The sales plan outlines the direct action that will be taken to get participants to sign up for the program. Since marketing and sales activities have serious financial implications for the success or failure of a program, it is especially important that the target market be clearly identified and understood in advance. Typical marketing activities include newsletter articles, e-mail messages, voice mail messages, brochures, fliers, bulletin board displays, posters, information sessions, program demonstrations, and direct staff interaction with potential participants. Sales activities involve instructing staff on effective communication techniques. This can be accomplished through role playing and the use of scripts. These activities can help staff gain confidence and be more effective communicating program benefits and registering participants.

Developing a Budget and Establishing Pricing

Once program planning is complete, specific pricing and budgets can be established. Typical program expenses include salaries, payroll taxes and benefits, marketing expenses, sales commissions, program materials, equipment, and facility use charges. Pricing is typically established through consideration of a number of factors. It is essential to consider the general program objectives (*e.g.,* profit, overall retention, improved health status of participants) and the projected number of participants. If the program has been

designed with the objective of generating a profit, it is important that minimum and maximum participant numbers be projected and program fees established at a level that adequately covers program costs. Sometimes it is appropriate to offer a program at a loss initially as a way of building a base of support, refining program content and delivery issues, and marketing the program for the future. In such cases, however, it is important to have established timelines and target dates for programs to reach profitable levels. To conduct programs within established budgetary guidelines, revenues and expenses should be reviewed throughout all phases of program delivery, not just at the completion of the program.

Program Implementation

Program implementation entails hiring staff, implementing marketing and sales plans, registering participants, and finally, delivering the program components as planned. The implementation phase is a dynamic process that continually rolls back into small planning phases as new needs of participants are identified. The most effective programs are created with enough flexibility to make immediate changes in the delivery model as new needs are identified.

Program Evaluation

Program evaluation should be conducted throughout the implementation phase (process evaluation) and immediately upon conclusion of the program (impact evaluation). In some cases, long-term follow-up is also appropriate (outcome evaluation). Process evaluations provide insight into delivery. Process evaluations can demonstrate whether procedures were followed and whether they are appropriate and effective. Impact and outcome evaluations assess effectiveness by measuring whether goals and objectives have been met.

Process Evaluation

Process evaluation is the assessment of the ability to carry out specific components of the program. Process evaluation should be conducted throughout the implementation phase. Techniques for process evaluation include direct supervision, soliciting participants' suggestions (Fig. 8.1), surveys of staff members, and tracking of daily participation levels. Once needs are identified, changes in delivery should be made immediately. Waiting until the next session to implement changes may drive away current participants and preclude recruitment of new ones.

Impact and Outcome Evaluation

The first step in evaluating the outcome of a program is to refer to the original program goals and objectives. Goals and objectives provide the standard for measuring success. Table 8.4 illustrates examples of goals and objectives and appro-

Figure 8.1 – Sample Participant Questionnaire

Please help us evaluate the effectiveness of this program by completing the following questions:

Name of program: _____   **Date:** _____
Instructor: _____

How did you hear about this program? _____

Circle the appropriate number:
1   Strongly disagree
2   Disagree
3   No opinion
4   Agree
5   Strongly agree

1)	This program met my expectations	1	2	3	4	5
2)	The facility location was appropriate and convenient	1	2	3	4	5
3)	The time allowed for this program was appropriate	1	2	3	4	5
4)	The program was scheduled at a convenient time	1	2	3	4	5
5)	The instructor was an effective communicator	1	2	3	4	5
6)	The instructor allowed time for participant questions	1	2	3	4	5
7)	I would recommend this program to other potential participants	1	2	3	4	5

Comments: _____
_____
_____
_____

Optional:

Name: _____   Phone #: _____

Table 8.4 – Program Evaluaton

Evaluation of program goals	
Generate net revenue	Financial analysis of revenues and expenses
Improve client retention	Analysis of length membership in the facility for program participants vs. nonparticipants
Acquisition of new clients	Questionnaire that gathers information on reasons given by clients for joining the facility
Provide community service	Track the number of participants served by the program and their satisfaction levels
Evaluation of program objectives	
Improving performance	Pre/post measurements of performance on specific tasks
Improving fitness level	Pre/post fitness measures
Increasing knowledge	Pre/post knowledge assessments
Decreasing risk factors	Pre/post health risk appraisals and screenings

priate methods of evaluation. A cost–benefit analysis can also be conducted as a method of evaluation. This process requires identification of all expenses and assignment of a dollar value to all benefits. The overall cost, savings, or profit that a program produced can then be calculated.

Specific Program Planning

The following section provides an overview of some common programs that are found in health and fitness settings. This list is by no means exhaustive. Program offerings in health and fitness facilities are continually in transition. As new information is made available, programs must be adjusted. As clients become complacent, creative strategies must be developed. The purpose of this section is to highlight some of the programs that have been successful at meeting specific program objectives.

Health Screening and Fitness Assessment

Individualized health screenings and fitness assessments should be made available to participants in all health and fitness facilities. There are a variety of options for screening and assessment programs. Protocol selection should be based on the target population and the specific objectives for the program. The most basic screening tool is the PAR-Q (Physical Activity Readiness Questionnaire), a self-administered questionnaire designed to detect medical contraindications to exercise. Customized questionnaires and health risk appraisal instruments can provide more detailed information regarding risk factors, personal medical history, family history, lifestyle factors, and exercise history. Fitness assessment can provide more detailed information regarding the specific components of fitness: aerobic capacity, muscular strength and endurance, body composition, and flexibility. This information can provide an important foundation for other individual and group exercise programs offered in the facility.

Health screenings and fitness assessments can be offered free or for a fee. This decision should be based on the specific objectives of the program. Objectives for screenings and assessments include revenue production, client safety, and client retention. In addition, assessments can identify contraindications to exercise, establish baseline fitness levels, and assist in evaluating program effectiveness. Only experienced health and fitness professionals should conduct screenings and assessments. These professionals must be able to obtain accurate results, recognize abnormal responses, adapt tests for specific participants' needs, properly interpret data, and communicate effectively with clients. It is important for a program manager to interview and screen these professionals, validate the accuracy of data collection techniques, and ensure consistency with other staff members. It is also important to establish policies and procedures that ensure confidentiality.

Personal Fitness Training

Offering fitness professional services on a fee-for-service basis has grown into a significant revenue-generating business for many health and fitness facilities. Most facilities have a staff of fitness professionals who are available to participants on a complimentary basis for introductory appointments and basic fitness information. A second group of staff members are usually designated as personal fitness trainers. These staff members are for hire on a fee-for-service basis.

There are several models for personal training programs in health and fitness facilities. Some facilities pay trainers a percentage of the revenue generated by the services they deliver. Other facilities hire personal trainers as full-time salaried employees with designated work shifts and pay the trainers an additional commission for services rendered. Individual salaries or commission rates for trainers are often determined by specific evaluation criteria, such as education, certification,

experience, seniority, job performance, and volume of revenue produced. Regardless of the type of employee compensation model, it is important that all program costs be considered during planning. Additional costs for marketing, administrative support, meetings, uniforms, payroll taxes, liability insurance, and continuing education can dramatically affect the profitability of the personal training program.

Skills required for the position of personal trainer are similar to those required for other health and fitness professionals. Emphasis should be placed on communication and leadership skills. A strong knowledge base in health screening, fitness assessment, and exercise program design for all population groups is essential. Successful trainers typically have strong business skills in sales, marketing, administration, and time management. Facilities should require all trainers to be certified by a nationally recognized organization, such as those certifications offered by the American College of Sports Medicine. Other national organizations offer more specialized certification programs that may be appropriate for specific population groups. It is the responsibility of the health and fitness manager to know about various certifications and decide which are appropriate for their particular facility.

Wellness Education Programs

Most fitness facilities offer a variety of programs to enhance knowledge on a range of health topics. The range of wellness programs offered in health and fitness facilities is broad. Programs may address any of the various dimensions of health, namely, physical, emotional, intellectual, spiritual, and social. Examples of wellness education programs include cardiopulmonary resuscitation and first aid, stress management and relaxation, smoking cessation, nutrition, back care, injury prevention, relationships, and a variety of other social, family-oriented, and personal development programs. Depending on the topic, programs can be offered in a variety of formats, such as single-session lectures, ongoing workshops, and off-site retreats. Programs offered with the objective of improving participant retention and adherence are usually presented free or at a minimal cost to cover expenses. Programs offered with the objective of revenue production are usually presented on a fee-for-service basis with pricing based on projected expenses and desired profit margins.

An advisory board of wellness professionals from the community can assist in identifying appropriate topics, approving content, and recommending instructors. Many community agencies and private businesses are willing to trade services for the opportunity to market products and services to the members.

Nutrition and Weight Management

Scientifically based nutrition and weight management programs are important programs for most health and fitness facilities, since many participants have specific weight loss goals. Weight management programs should be consistent with the ACSM position statement "Proper and Improper Weight Loss Programs" (10). Emphasis should be placed on education, the development of lifetime habits, and the benefits of exercise.

Nutrition programs vary in size and scope depending on facility and staff resources. A number of programming models are available for nutrition programs in health and fitness facilities. Many facilities have a registered dietitian as an independent contractor. The facility provides office space and other administrative resources and in exchange is able to offer nutritional services to participants without making a large financial investment. The registered dietitian typically charges fees for services rendered and is paid a commission on the revenue that is generated. If a registered dietitian is contracted, it is important to interview and screen this individual carefully to ensure that his or her philosophy is consistent with the philosophy of the facility and other professional staff.

There are also a number of models for weight management programs in health and fitness facilities. One popular model provides options for participants to purchase a number of related programs and services, including nutrition consultations, dietary analysis, fitness assessments, exercise prescriptions, educational lectures, grocery shopping trips, healthy cooking demonstrations, and personal fitness training sessions. Services can be offered à la carte or in structured packages. A typical package may include a 12-wk program with before-and-after fitness assessments, access to the related services, and weekly group exercise training sessions. Such programs require detailed planning and coordination. Planning this kind of specialized program requires an advisory board of wellness professionals.

Other models for nutrition and weight management programs include the sale of food and nutritional supplements. These programs are popular in many fitness facilities because they have the potential to produce large amounts of revenue. It is important that a health and fitness manager fully investigate these products prior to the implementation of such a strategy. It is imperative that all product claims be accurate and that all products be safe and effective.

Group Exercise Classes

Group exercise classes can add an important dimension to health and fitness programming in a facility. Group exercise classes allow facilities to provide instruction, motivation, and guidance to participants at a relatively low cost. Most health and fitness facilities have an extensive menu of group exercise classes that include traditional aerobics classes and aerobics classes that use equipment such as steps and bikes. Other popular program offerings include resistance training, body sculpting, flexibility, sport-specific conditioning, prenatal and postnatal programs, programs for children and older adults, martial arts, yoga, and various types of dance.

Program schedules vary with the facility's resources and the number of participants. For example, small facilities may offer a limited number of the most popular group exercise classes during prime hours. A larger facility with several studios may offer a wider variety of programs concurrently. The health and fitness manager must stay current on programming trends by attending conferences, reading journals, and attending continuing education programs. Successful group exercise programs regularly survey participants to assess satisfaction levels, interest areas, and appropriateness of scheduling.

Skills required for the position of group exercise instructor are similar to those for other exercise professionals. Emphasis is placed on strong group leadership qualities. Instructors should know about health risk factors, be able to conduct appropriate screenings, and design programs that meet the needs of members. The ability to modify programs for special populations is also essential. Facilities should require group exercise instructors to hold appropriate certifications from nationally recognized organizations. As with the personal training staff, the health and fitness manager is responsible for being informed about various certifications and deciding which will be required or accepted by the organization.

Section XIII References

1. Herbert DL, Herbert WG. Legal Aspects of Preventive and Rehabilitative Exercise Programs. 3rd ed. Canton, OH: Professional Reports Corporation, 1993.
2. American College of Sports Medicine. ACSM's Guidelines for Exercise Testing and Prescription. 6th ed. Philadelphia: Lippincott Williams & Wilkins, 2000.
3. American College of Sports Medicine. ACSM's Health/Fitness Facility Standards & Guidelines. 2nd ed. Champaign, IL: Human Kinetics, 1997.
4. American Association for Cardiovascular and Pulmonary Rehabilitation. Guidelines for Cardiac Rehabilitation and Secondary Prevention Programs. 3rd ed. Champaign, IL: Human Kinetics, 1998.
5. Hedgecorth v. United States. 618 F. Supp.627 (E.D. Mo, 1985).
6. Herbert DL. Informed Consent Documents for Stress Testing to Comport With Hedgecorth v. United States. Exerc Stand Malpract Rep 1:81, 1987.
7. Louisiana licenses clinical exercise physiologists! Exerc Stand Malpract Rep 9:56 (editorial) 1995. (Reproduction of the licensing act included.)
8. Herbert WG. Licensure of clinical exercise physiologists: Impressions concerning the new law in Louisiana. Exerc Stand Malpract Rep 9:65, 1995.
9. Greenberg, J. Health and wellness: A conceptual differentiation. Health Educ 16:4–6, 1985.
10. American College of Sports Medicine. Proper and Improper Weight Loss Programs. Med Sci Sports Exerc 15:ix–xiii, 1983.

Section IX

+ Coronary Artery Disease (CAD) Risk Factors
+ Basic Principles of Electrocardiography (ECG)
+ Lung Diseases
+ Orthopaedic and Musculoskeletal Conditions Seen in Clients
+ Medications

ACSM's Resources for the Personal Trainer

CLINICAL AND MEDICAL CONSIDERATIONS

A. Coronary Artery Disease (CAD) Risk Factors

Cardiovascular disease is the leading cause of death in developed countries and is a major component of the global burden of disease, accounting for 45.6% of deaths (1). In the United States, 13.5 million people have a history of myocardial infarction or angina, and many times that number are at risk for developing coronary heart disease (2). However, the age-adjusted rate of cardiovascular mortality has decreased by 40% in the past 30 years. This decline is attributable to better treatment options and more effective primary and secondary prevention strategies (3).

Coronary atherosclerosis is related to many factors. The process begins in childhood and results from clustering of several genetic, biological, behavioral, and environmental factors collectively known as coronary risk factors. The term *risk factor*, proposed by the Framingham investigators, came with the realization that no known single factor causes coronary atherosclerosis, but a combination of factors can be correlated with the development of coronary heart disease (4). The second important consideration is the greater the number of risk factors, the greater the level of risk. For example, a smoker with modest elevation of cholesterol or hypertension is at much higher risk for developing coronary heart disease than a non-smoker with severe hypertension and high cholesterol. Therefore, a comprehensive risk evaluation of an individual is an essential prerequisite to developing strategies for primary prevention of coronary heart disease. Risk factors for coronary heart disease are classified as shown in Table 5.3 in the health appraisal section of this manual.

CAD Causal Risk Factors

The major causal risk factors for CAD are cigarette smoking, elevated cholesterol (or low levels of low-density lipoprotein [LDL] cholesterol), decreased levels of high-density lipoprotein (HDL), hypertension, and diabetes.

Cigarette Smoking

Cigarette smoking is the most preventable cause of death in the United States (5). Autopsy studies have shown that the extent of atherosclerosis (accumulation of fatty plaque on the artery walls) is linearly related to the number of cigarettes smoked (6). The risk also increases in accordance with the number of years of smoking and the depth of inhalation. Nearly 40% of cardiovascular deaths are attributable to cigarette smoking. Smokers have twice the risk of developing coronary heart disease and a twofold to fourfold increased risk of sudden death.

The bad effects of smoking are particularly noteworthy in the young. In myocardial infarction (heart attack) survivors under age 40, the most common accompanying risk factor is cigarette smoking. As in men, women who smoke are at increased risk for coronary artery disease (7). Risk doubles in women who smoke as few as one to four cigarettes per day.

Acutely, cigarette smoking increases risk by elevating the myocardial (heart muscle) oxygen demand (through increases in heart rate and blood pressure), reducing oxygen transport, increasing susceptibility to heart arrhythmias, predisposing the coronary artery to spasm, and increasing platelet adhesiveness. There is overwhelming evidence that stopping smoking reduces the cardiovascular risk substantially. On an average, the rate can be reduced by 50% within one year of stopping of smoking (8). Finally, it has been estimated that approximately 50,000 deaths per year in the United States are caused by passive (second-hand) smoke. Most of these deaths are due to cardiovascular disease (9).

Cholesterol and Low-Density Lipoproteins

Scientific studies clearly show that high blood cholesterol is a major cause of coronary heart disease and that lowering cholesterol level reduces the risk (11). About 38 million Americans are estimated to have total cholesterol levels of at least 240 $mg \cdot dL^{-1}$ (2). Cholesterol circulates in the plasma (liquid part of blood) in three sizes of lipoprotein particles, very low density lipoprotein (VLDL) cholesterol, LDL cholesterol, and HDL cholesterol. Total cholesterol is equal to the sum of these three components. Coronary heart disease is directly and linearly related to the levels of total cholesterol and LDL cholesterol and inversely related to the levels of HDL cholesterol. Most of the risk attributed to total cholesterol is explained by the LDL cholesterol concentration (40). Oxidized LDL cholesterol is considered to be a major factor in the pathogenesis of atherosclerosis. The National Cholesterol Education Program Adult Treatment Panel (NCEP-ATP) sets a high priority on LDL cholesterol management (12). In the MRFIT Trial, for each 50 $mg \cdot dL^{-1}$ increase in total cholesterol above 200 $mg \cdot dL^{-1}$, coronary heart disease rates doubled (13). Framingham risk prediction model uses total cholesterol (not LDL cholesterol) and HDL cholesterol along with other major risk factors in estimating the risk of coronary events in the asymptomatic individual (14). Several large studies have proved the benefit of reducing blood cholesterol (15–19).

High-Density Lipoprotein Cholesterol

A low level of serum HDL cholesterol is an important predictor of coronary heart disease. Several large studies suggested that for each 1 $mg \cdot dL^{-1}$ increase in HDL cholesterol, a 2% decrease in coronary heart disease risk is noted in men and 3% decrease in women (20). The Framingham risk prediction model incorporates HDL cholesterol as a negative risk factor. Furthermore, a low LDL cholesterol level did not eliminate the risk imparted by low HDL cholesterol, while a high HDL cholesterol seemed to offset some of the risk of high LDL cholesterol (21). HDL cholesterol plays a critical role in reverse cholesterol transport (22). In addition, HDL cholesterol may slow plaque formation through prevention of LDL cholesterol oxidation and monocyte adhesion to endothelial cells (23). Therapeutic options to increase HDL cholesterol levels include exercise and moderate alcohol use, and pharmacological agents, including niacin, gemfibrozil, 3-hydroxy-3-methyglutaryl-coenzyme A (HMG-CoA) reductase inhibitors and hormone replacement therapy. The recently published Veterans Affairs High Density Lipoprotein Cholesterol Interventional Trial reported that in men with coronary heart disease and an HDL cholesterol level less than 40 mg·dL^{-1}, gemfibrozil resulted in a significant 24% reduction in death, nonfatal myocardial infarction, and stroke (24).

Hypertension

Nearly 50 million adult Americans have high blood pressure (≥140/90 mm Hg; Table 9.1) (25). Data from numerous studies indicate a continuous relationship between blood pressure and cardiovascular risk, with lowest risk for adults with systolic blood pressure below 120 mm Hg and diastolic blood pressure below 80 mm Hg (26). The Framingham risk prediction model incorporates systolic blood pressure as a major risk factor in the occurrence of major coronary events. Elevation of blood pressure causes vascular endothelial dysfunction and injury leading to increased migration of atherogenic elements, including LDL, monocytes, and macrophages. A meta-analysis of the major randomized trials of antihypertensive therapy demonstrated a 42% reduction in the incidence of stroke and 14% reduction in coronary heart disease events (27). Isolated systolic hypertension, defined as systolic blood pressure at least 140 mm Hg and diastolic blood pressure less than 90 mm Hg, is common in men and women over age 65 years and is an independent risk factor for coronary heart disease. A recent meta-analysis suggests that one coronary or cerebral vascular event would be prevented for every 18 patients treated (28). The Joint National Commission–VI (JNC-VI) guidelines recommend a very aggressive approach in the treatment of hypertension, especially in the presence of target organ damage, diabetes, or clinical cardiovascular disease (25).

Lifestyle modification, including weight reduction, increased physical activity, and moderation of dietary sodium and alcohol intake, are recommended both as definitive and adjunctive therapy for hypertension (25). If blood pressure remains at

Table 9.1 – Classification of Blood Pressure for Adults Age 18 years and older*

CATEGORY	SYSTOLIC (MM HG)	DIASTOLIC (MM HG)
Normal[b]	< 130	< 85
High normal	130–139	85–89
Hypertension[c]		
STAGE 1 (mild)	140–159	90–99
STAGE 2 (moderate)	160–179	100–109
STAGE 3 (severe)	180–209	110–119
STAGE 4 (very severe)	≥ 210	≥ 120

[a] Not taking antihypertensive drugs and not acutely ill. When systolic and diastolic pressures fall into different categories, the higher category should be selected to classify the individual's blood pressure status. For instance, 160/92 mm Hg should be classified as stage 2, and 180/120 mm Hg should be classified as stage 4. Isolated systolic hypertension (ISH) is defined as SBP ≥ 140 mm Hg and DBP < 90 mm Hg and staged appropriately (e.g., 170/85 mm Hg is defined as stage 2 ISH).
[b] Optimal blood pressure with respect to cardiovascular risk is SBP < 120 mm Hg and DBP < 80 mm Hg. However, unusually low readings should be evaluated for clinical significance.
[c] Based on the average of two or more readings taken at each of two or more visits following an initial screening.
Note: In addition to classifying stages of hypertension based on average blood pressure levels, the clinician should specify presence or absence of target-organ disease and additional risk factors. For example, a patient with diabetes and a blood pressure of 142/94 mm Hg plus left ventricular hypertrophy should be classified as "stage 2 hypertension with target-organ disease (left ventricular hypertrophy) and with another major risk factor (diabetes)." This specificity is important for risk classification and management.

least 140/90 mm Hg despite 3–6 months of lifestyle modification, drug therapy should be initiated. This is especially important in individuals with target organ disease and/or other known coronary artery disease risk factors (25). A variety of factors, including other diseases, demographic characteristics, the use of accompanying drugs that may lead to drug interactions, cost of medication, and metabolic and subjective side effects should be considered in the selection of antihypertensive drugs (Table 9.1) (25).

Diabetes

Coronary heart disease is also the most common cause of death in clients with type II diabetes, and it contributes significantly to the mortality in type I diabetes. One-fourth of myocardial infarctions occur in clients with diabetes (29). Diabetes is considered a major coronary risk factor, especially in women. Vascular diseases are strongly associated with diabetes and appear to be major components of the onset of atherosclerosis in diabetics. The diagnostic criteria for diabetes include a fasting blood sugar level above 126 mg·100 mL^{-1} and a 2-h postprandial glucose level above 200 mg·dL^{-1} (30). Diabetes is associated with a low level of HDL cholesterol and increased levels of VLDL cholesterol and triglycerides. There also appears to be a clustering of other risk factors, including hypertension, obesity, and abnormal blood lipids, in diabetics. Women with diabetes partially or completely lose their gender-related protection from coronary artery disease (31). The term *syndrome X* is used to describe a cluster of conditions, namely glucose intolerance, abnormal blood lipids, hypertension, central obesity, and insulin resistance.

The importance of diabetes as a major coronary risk factor is further recognized by the JNC-VI guideline on the management of hypertension, which considers the presence of diabetes equal to the presence of clinical cardiovascular disease (25). Furthermore, death from coronary heart disease in clients with type II diabetes may be as high as that in nondiabetic individuals with previous myocardial infarction (heart attack) (32).

CAD Conditional Risk Factors

Conditional risk factors are those that are associated with an increased risk of coronary heart disease but whose causal link has not been proved with certainty. The possible reasons causal link is uncertain include the following:

- Compared to the causal risk factors, the atherogenic potential may be weak.
- The prevalence of these risk factors may not be enough to detect a significant independent effect in epidemiological studies.

The conditional risk factors include elevated triglyceride level and a group of novel or emerging risk factors, including lipoprotein-a, homocysteine, coagulation factors, such as fibrogen and plasminogen activator inhibitor-1, and C-reactive protein.

In considering the clinical utility of a new marker for coronary heart disease and risk assessment, three important issues must be considered. First, there must be a reliable assessment technique for the marker of interest. Second, there must be consistency in the prospective epidemiological studies, indicating that the novel marker of interest can be detected in the individual before the onset of clinical disease. Third, there must be evidence that assessment of the new risk factor adds to the ability to predict the risk independent of conventional risk factors. Another issue to be considered in the evaluation of novel risk factors is modifiability. To date there is no conclusive evidence that modifying these new risk factors improves outcomes in primary or secondary prevention scenarios.

Triglycerides

The importance of triglycerides as a coronary risk factor remains speculative. The correlation between plasma triglyceride level and coronary heart disease tends to weaken or disappear when adjusted for HDL cholesterol levels.

Homocysteine

Homocysteine is an amino acid formed during methionine metabolism. In the normal individual, fasting plasma homocysteine level is 5–15 $\mu mol \cdot L^{-1}$. Homocysteine levels increase with aging; menopause; chronic renal insufficiency; vitamin B_6, B_{12}, and folate deficiency; and cardiac transplantation (33). Increased homocysteine levels seem to predict death in clients with known coronary artery disease (34). The clinical usefulness of measuring homocysteine levels as part of cardiovascular risk evaluation is uncertain because of nonstandardized assessment techniques, inconsistent epidemiological studies, and lack of additive value to total and HDL cholesterol.

Fibrinogen

Elevated levels of fibrinogen have been shown to correlate with myocardial infarction (heart attack) and stroke, probably as a result of enhanced blood viscosity (thickness) and increased blood clot formation. Fibrinogen levels are generally higher in men than women and smokers than nonsmokers (33). Physical inactivity and elevated triglycerides are also associated with increased fibrinogen levels (56). Nonetheless, the assessment techniques for fibrinogen levels are not standardized, and the clinical utility of measuring fibrinogen levels as part of risk factor screening is unproved.

Tissue Plasminogen Activator

Increased levels of tissue plasminogen activator (t-PA) and plasminogen activator inhibitor-1 have been associated with increased risk of coronary artery disease. Insulin resistance and hypertriglyceridemia are also associated with increased plasminogen activator inhibitor levels. For t-PA and plasminogen activator inhibitor, nonstandardized assessment techniques and lack of independent prognostic value beyond total cholesterol and HDL levels limit the clinical utility (33).

C-Reactive Protein

C-reactive protein is a marker for inflammation and is related to plaque build-up in the artery walls. Several studies have shown a large correlation between C-reactive protein, atherosclerosis, and coronary heart disease risk (36).

CAD Predisposing Risk Factors

Obesity, physical inactivity, various behavioral characteristics, poor socioeconomic status, male gender, family history of premature coronary artery disease, postmenopausal status, and aging are considered predisposing risk factors. This classification is the result of either their effect on causal or conditional risk factors or their as yet unrecognized independent effect on the development of coronary heart disease. Clearly, the presence of some predisposing risk factors intensifies certain causal risk factors; for example, obesity worsens insulin resistance and thereby increases the risk of vascular disease. However, modification of risk factors such as obesity and physical inactivity may reduce the coronary heart disease event rate, although again, it is uncertain whether the beneficial effects are independent of favorable influences on causal or conditional risk factors.

Obesity

The prevalence of obesity in the United States appears to have increased substantially during the past decade, and one in three adults is now considered overweight (37). Obesity contributes to many adverse health outcomes, and obesity-related conditions are estimated to contribute to 300,000 deaths annually in the U.S. (38). Obesity is associated with an accentuated risk of cardiovascular disease. Analysis of the relationship between obesity and coronary artery disease is difficult because of its association with other risk factors, in particular physical inactivity, hypertension, abnormal blood lipids, and diabetes. However, recent reports from the Framingham Heart Study support the independence of obesity as a risk factor for coronary artery disease (39). In syndrome X, central abdominal obesity, high triglyceride levels, low HDL cholesterol levels, insulin resistance, and hypertension are metabolically linked. This form of obesity is relatively common and is associated with a markedly increased risk of coronary artery disease.

No studies have specifically evaluated the effect of weight loss on coronary artery disease events. Comprehensive programs that incorporate behavioral modalities to increase physical activity and improve diet have been shown to induce weight loss sufficient to produce significant cardiovascular health benefits in many obese individuals. In this respect, even modest weight loss of 5–10% of initial body weight has positive benefits on coronary artery disease risk factors, and weight loss of this magnitude may be realistic for many individuals (40).

Unfortunately, improvements in coronary artery disease risk factors are not maintained if weight is regained, and most of those who lose a significant amount of weight regain the lost weight within a relatively short time. Recognition of the need for long-term and perhaps lifelong treatment has led certain experts to embrace the concept of long-term drug therapy, as is used in other chronic diseases. A national task force on the prevention and treatment of obesity, however, recently concluded that until more long-term data are available, pharmacotherapy cannot be recommended for routine use in obese individuals, although it may be helpful in carefully selected patients (41).

Physical Inactivity

Epidemiological (study of disease epidemics) criteria have been used to establish a relationship between physical activity and coronary artery disease. However, the precise mechanism by which physical inactivity predisposes persons to coronary artery disease has yet to be fully clarified.

Regarding the beneficial effect on other coronary artery disease risk factors, regular physical activity has been shown to lower resting systolic and diastolic blood pressure, reduce serum triglyceride levels, increase serum HDL cholesterol levels, and enhance glucose tolerance and insulin sensitivity (42, 43). However, despite this evidence, millions of U.S. adults remain essentially sedentary. Indeed, the number of individuals who are inactive is substantially greater than the number who smoke cigarettes, have high cholesterol, or have high blood pressure. Thus, the overall effect of stimulating Americans to lead a more physically active lifestyle could lower coronary artery disease rates more than by reducing any other single risk factor (44).

Behavioral Characteristics

The psychosocial factors associated with risk of coronary artery disease include the so-called type-A personality, hostility, depression, chronic stress produced by situations with high demand and low control, and social isolation (45). Psychosocial factors are postulated to accentuate the risk via two major mechanisms. First, they may exert a detrimental influence by direct mechanisms such as changes in catecholamine and serotonin levels. Second, they may indirectly modify risk by influencing adherence to lifestyle recommendations and compliance with drug therapy. Interventions of potential benefit include behavior modification, biofeedback, meditation, exercise, and when indicated, pharmacotherapy.

Postmenopausal Status

Coronary artery disease manifests itself approximately a decade later in women than in men. Nevertheless, it remains the leading cause of death among women in the United States. The role of hormone replacement therapy in postmenopausal women is uncertain. The postmenopausal estrogen–progesterone intervention trials have established the efficiency of hormone replacement therapy in raising HDL cholesterol levels and decreasing levels of LDL cholesterol, total cholesterol, and fibrinogen (46). Nonetheless, beneficial effects on coronary heart disease end points have not been found (47).

CAD Unmodifiable Risk Factors

Male gender, family history of premature coronary artery disease, low socioeconomic status, and age are risk factors that are not amenable to intervention. Recognition of them is nonetheless important for helping to reduce the risk of future cardiac events and should be considered when attempting to match the level of management with the level of risk (48).

B. Basic Principles of Electrocardiography (ECG)

Electrocardiography (ECG) is the study of the electrical events that occur in the heart. Despite the development of newer techniques that assist doctors in evaluating cardiac disorders, the ECG has remained an invaluable diagnostic tool. By careful assessment of the ECG tracing, one may obtain information about the heart rate and rhythm, any chamber enlargement and conduction abnormalities, evidence of acute or previous myocardial infarctions (heart attacks), myocardial ischemia (lack of oxygen to the heart), drug and metabolic effects, and much more. The monitoring of the ECG during exercise is a valuable means of evaluating patients with chest pain (see figure 9.1 for a normal rhythm strip).

One of the most prevalent uses of electrocardiography is the identification of patients with myocardial infarction or myocardial ischemia. Monitoring the electrocardiogram (ECG) during exercise testing is a commonly used technique to assess whether myocardial ischemia is the cause of chest discomfort. Myocardial infarction results when blood flow to a region of heart muscle is interrupted by total occlusion of a coronary artery. ECG changes occur as a result of the impairment of flow to the myocardium. Myocardial ischemia occurs when the supply of blood flow is inadequate to meet the demands of the myocardium. The patient often has chest pain with exertion. ECG changes include ST segment depression and/or inversion of the T waves.

Although much information can be obtained from ECG, it has limitations. A patient may have ECG abnormalities and have no underlying heart disease or exhibit a normal ECG in the setting of significant cardiac disease. It is therefore important to interpret the ECG in the context of the history and physical examination findings.

Electrical Activity of the Heart

The impulse that drives electrical depolarization of the heart originates in the sinoatrial (SA), or sinus node. This area is located in the right atrium near the superior vena cava. The wave of activity initially spreads in a radial fashion through the right atrium and subsequently the left atrium. The impulse reaches the atrioventricular (AV) node, an ovoid structure that lies at the base of the intra-atrial septum. The impulse takes approximately 100 ms to traverse the AV node and depolarize the bundle of His. In the normal heart, the AV node and the His bundle are the only point of connection between the atria and ventricles. The bundle of His extends through the fibrous skeleton of the heart into the superior portion of

the intraventricular septum and divides into right and left bundles. The right bundle is quite discrete and travels down the right side of the interventricular septum and through the moderator band, beyond which it branches into the right ventricle. The left bundle divides into anterior and posterior divisions; in reality, these divisions are more complex and diffuse as they fan out into the left ventricle. The bundle branches terminate in Purkinje fibers (specialized cells that spread the electrical activity rapidly through the myocardium). The depolarization wave stimulates myocardial cells to contract by initiating a series of events referred to as excitation–contraction coupling.

Action Potentials

Electrical events occur because of the movement of ions across the membrane of the cell. In the resting phase, cardiac muscle cells have a greater number of negatively charged ions within the cell, which results in a voltage difference across the cell membrane. This difference is called the transmembrane potential and is approximately −80 to −90 mV. When the cell is stimulated, channels in the cell membrane open and allow positively charged sodium ions to enter the cell, causing depolarization. Depolarization occurs during phase 0 of the action potential. The depolarization of one cell leads to the depolarization of neighboring cells; in this fashion an impulse (phase 1) is propagated through the heart. Once a cell depolarizes, it cannot depolarize again until repolarization has occurred. The time during which the cell cannot depolarize is termed the refractory period. Repolarization, the restoration of transmembrane potential, occurs during phases 2 and 3 of the action potential. Phase 4 is a quiescent phase for most cardiac cells. However, in certain cells, such as those at the sinus node, ions travel across the membrane during phase 4, resulting in a gradual decrease of the membrane potential. Once the voltage reaches a threshold level, depolarization occurs. Cells that possess this property of automaticity include the sino-atrial (SA) node, atrioventricular (AV) node, and His-Purkinje fibers. The SA node possesses the most rapid phase 4 depolarization, causing it to depolarize first and thereby function as the pacemaker of the heart. The rate of phase 4 depolarization may be delayed by certain classes of medications, namely beta blockers and some calcium channel antagonists, resulting in a slowing of the heart rate. Exercise, via enhanced sympathetic nervous system stimulation and elevated circulating catecholamines, increases the phase 4 depolarization rate, elevating the heart rate.

ECG measures the action potentials of the cardiac cells. The P wave records atrial stimulation. The QRS wave represents the electrical activity of the stimulation of the ventricles. Finally, the T wave represents the repolarization of the ventricles so they may be stimulated again (Figure 9.1).

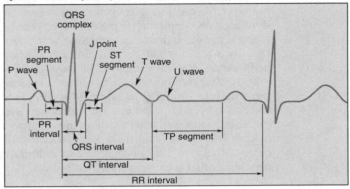

Figure 9.1 – A normal rhythm strip

C. Lung Diseases

Chronic Obstructive Pulmonary Disease (COPD)

COPD is a common disorder characterized by progressive expiratory flow obstruction, labored breathing on exertion, and some degree of reversible airway hyper-reactivity (49). Symptoms develop insidiously over years to decades. Many such patients are chronic cigarette smokers. There are two main syndromes: chronic bronchitis and emphysema.

Chronic Bronchitis

Chronic bronchitis is characterized by a chronic cough that produces substance (sputum). The main sign of chronic bronchitis is enlargement and overabundance of mucous glands in the walls of large lung airways. The airway wall thickens, and the surface becomes irregular. Inflammation may reduce airway diameter. These changes are made worse by bacterial growth in the airway associated with episodes of acute bronchitis.

Narrowing of large bronchi produces a marked increase in airflow resistance, while intrathoracic pressure generated by muscular effort and lung elastic recoil is normal. Expiratory flow rates may improve after inhaled bronchodilators. Chronic bronchitis leads to lack of oxygen in the blood (hypoxia). Hypoxemia, a potent stimulus of smooth muscle constriction in pulmonary arterioles and venules, leads to increased pulmonary vascular resistance, pulmonary arterial hypertension, and right ventricular strain.

In chronic severe disease, heart failure eventually develops. Hypoxemia stimulates the production of erythropoietin (EPO), resulting in excessive blood volume, hemoglobin concentration, and hematocrit. This may lead to high blood viscosity (thickness), increasing flow resistance in blood vessels and potentially decreasing blood flow in small vessels of the brain and heart. Typical patients with severe chronic bronchitis are known as blue bloaters because they have a cyanotic coloration.

Emphysema

Emphysema is a disease of the lung tissue affecting small airways (50). It includes abnormal permanent enlargement of air spaces accompanied by destruction of alveolar walls. Destruction of lung tissue results. The main sign of emphysema is loss of lung elasticity and reduction of elastic recoil pressure due to accelerated alveolar (air sacs) destruction. Small airways become easily collapsi-

ble during expiration because intrathoracic pressure becomes greater. Patients with emphysema can expel a larger volume during a slow exhalation than during a maximal forced exhalation because intrathoracic pressure is lower and airway compression is minimized during a slow exhalation.

Emphysema is unresponsive to bronchodilators because the basis of obstruction is altered mechanical properties of the lung tissue. Patients can minimize air trapping and labored breathing by pursed-lip breathing, in which the lips are puckered during exhalation (51). Pursing the lips creates external resistance to flow and maintains a more positive intra-airway pressure during exhalation retarding small airway compression.

Small Airway Disease

Small airway disease is an early sign of the same processes that eventually lead to chronic bronchitis and/or emphysema. Cigarette smoking increases risk of small airway flow obstruction and loss of elastic recoil in a dose-dependent fashion. Objective abnormalities in small airway flow pattern can be demonstrated within 1–5 yr of smoking; in early stages, such abnormalities are largely reversible with stopping of smoking. Symptoms are usually mild in the absence of large airway involvement.

Management of COPD

The management of clients with these types of COPD generally includes the following strategies:

1. Identify and eliminate sources of inflammation (*i.e.*, cigarette smoking, inhaled irritants, recurrent respiratory infections).
2. Identify and treat reversible airway narrowing with inhaled or oral bronchodilators and corticosteroids.
3. Vaccinate against infectious agents, such as pneumococcus and influenza; by adequate respiratory hygiene; and in selected patients, by prophylactic administration of antibiotics.
4. Establish individualized rehabilitation programs for stable clients.

Rehabilitation programs generally have some

component of moderate physical and breathing exercises. Maximal oxygen uptake may improve if significant deconditioning is present. Selective respiratory muscle training can improve ventilatory capacity in patients with lung disease, and exercise performance may also improve in some patients (52). Neither cardiovascular nor selective respiratory muscle training significantly improves mechanical lung function or alveolar gas exchange. However, exercise training improves oxygen delivery and extraction; hence, overall efficiency of oxygen use is enhanced and endurance for submaximal exercise is improved (49).

Asthma

Asthma affects about 5% of the general population. It is characterized by increased airway reactivity to various stimuli, resulting in widespread reversible narrowing of airways (53, 54). The repetitive nature and reversibility of the narrowing are important features. It is sometimes possible to identify specific agents that bring about attacks (allergic asthma), such as pollens, dust mites, animal dander, drugs, foods, wine, fumes, and chemicals. Asthma attacks may also be induced by other factors such as emotional stress, exercise, exposure to cold, or a viral respiratory infection. Often no onset factors can be identified (perennial asthma). Asthma may be associated with allergies, nasal polyps, and aspirin sensitivity. Asthma may be hereditary (genetic).

An asthma attack causes airway smooth muscle constriction (bronchospasm). Physical stimuli, such as cooling and fluid evaporation across the airway during exercise or cold air exposure, may directly stimulate constriction (55). Prolonged bronchospasm leads to secondary mucosal edema and mucus accumulation. During an acute asthmatic attack, patients typically hyperventilate initially. Severe or prolonged attacks unresponsive to therapy may lead to respiratory failure with decreased oxygen and increased carbon dioxide in the blood.

Management of Asthma

Management of asthmatic patients generally includes the following strategies:

1. Identification and elimination of agents that seem to bring on an asthma attack.
2. Preventing and minimizing attacks by teaching the client to improve compliance with medication. Prevention via medications can be achieved by use of inhaled corticosteroids to reduce airway inflammation and inhaled cromolyn sodium to stabilize mast cells.
3. Establishing the best inhaled or oral bronchodilator therapy to achieve the maximal possible flow rates and maximal exercise tolerance.

Exercise-Induced Asthma (EIA)

Exercise-induced asthma (EIA) develops when strenuous exercise causes airway narrowing in people who have heightened bronchial reactivity. EIA is an airway obstruction that occurs during or after exercise. Symptoms include cough, wheezing, labored breathing, and/or chest tightness.

EIA can occur in otherwise apparently healthy nonasthmatic people. Exercise is the only stimulus for their asthma symptoms. However, EIA can also occur in people who have asthma. Because the treatments for EIA and asthma are different, it is crucial that every new client with asthma symptoms be assessed with baseline pulmonary function tests to determine whether they have asthma or EIA.

D. Orthopaedic and Musculoskeletal Conditions Seen in Clients

Osteoporosis

Osteoporosis is a disease of the skeleton characterized by low bone mass and deterioration of bone tissue leading to fragile bones and increased risk of fracture. It is estimated that more than 1.5 million osteoporotic fractures occur annually, which clearly establishes osteoporosis as a major public health care concern. Common fracture sites include the wrist, spine, and hip. Estimates of direct health care costs associated with these three types of fractures in white women over age 45 have been projected to be $45.2 billion over the next 10 years (56). Hip fractures will account for most of these expenses, and hip fractures have the most devastating personal consequences, such as loss of independence, prolonged immobility, and death. As with other chronic diseases, prevention of osteoporotic fractures is the focus of much research and debate (57).

As an osteoporosis prevention strategy, exercise has four main applications, to:

1. Increase bone mass during and just after periods of growth, thus improving peak bone mass;
2. Increase or maintain bone mass in early to middle adulthood;
3. Decrease rates of bone loss in older adults; and
4. Reduce falls.

In light of the principles of training and available research, weight-bearing modes of exercise that emphasize high force magnitude and encourage development of the muscular system are recommended for skeletal health. Deciding on an exercise mode requires consideration of the age and/or physical limitations of the group or individual. Certainly adolescents and younger individuals have more capacity to perform intensive activities, such as jumping, than do the frail elderly. Young and middle-aged adults can benefit from programs that include both impact and muscular development exercises, as this combination has been found effective for improving bone mass without consequent increases in joint injury (58, 59). Making 25–50 jumps in place at floor level 3 $d \cdot wk^{-1}$ has been well tolerated in healthy postmenopausal women without osteoporosis, and recent evidence suggests that older women who participate in long-term (5 yr) weighted vest exercise with jumping maintain hip bone mineral density (BMD) (60, 61, 62). In addition to maintaining hip BMD, jumping exercise improves most women's muscle power, which is an important determinant of functional ability in elderly women (63). In addition, strength training in men and women in their 50s and 60s has produced similar absolute increases in muscular strength and power as in subjects in their 20s (64). In the frail elderly, many weight-bearing exercise modes, including high-intensity weight training and exercise with free weights, have met with success (65). In epidemiological research, the amount of walking and the overall caloric expenditure are higher in those who do not fracture, and thus, these general markers of habitual physical activity consistently emerge as factors that reduce the risk of hip fracture (66). Further research is needed to determine the exercise mode that is most effective for reducing dangerous falls that result in hip fractures in the elderly.

Young bone is likely to respond more favorably to mechanical loading than old bone, and therefore, introduction of high mechanical loads during this stage of life may produce the best skeletal response. Prepubertal children tolerate and even enjoy a high degree of mechanical loading. Children in the second grade jumped from 24-inch boxes up to 100 times three times per week. Bone mass at the hip was 5% higher in jumpers than in controls at the end of the 8-month intervention (58). Achieving optimal peak bone mass at the end of longitudinal growth will afford skeletal protection by delaying the point at which BMD is critically reduced, fractures are more likely, and preventive measures are few. Interestingly, premenopausal and postmenopausal women completing the same jumping intervention had different bone mass responses: the premenopausal women increased BMD at the hip, but the postmenopausal women exhibited no consistent pattern, despite having controlled for estrogen replacement status (61). Calcium intake and self-reported physical activity were important contributors to increases in spine bone mass in women in the third decade

of life, a time at which bone mass may level off (67). The premenopausal years may therefore be a fruitful time to increase bone mass, especially if progressive training regimens (*i.e.,* impact exercise and/or free weight training) are used.

It is unlikely that dramatic increases in bone mass are attainable in the older skeleton. However, small improvements in, or maintenance of, bone mass can make a difference in the overall fracture risk profile. Resistance training that promotes functional ability may not elicit improvements in bone mass in all older persons, but the benefits of this training, such as reducing key indices of fall risk, are substantial. Weight training programs are therefore recommended for older adults, even for those who are frail. The frequency of training should be 2–3 times per week, with varying recommendations of the number of sets, repetitions, and intensity, depending on the characteristics of the target group. Impact exercise should not be performed by those with osteoporosis and/or other conditions (*i.e.,* osteoarthritis, urinary incontinence, severe dizziness) for whom the exercise may be contraindicated or otherwise objectionable. Other contraindicated activities for those with osteoporosis include exercises that place high compressive forces on the spine with trunk flexion as well as activities that result in quick trunk rotation. Standard screening practices should be followed, and older individuals with multiple risk factors for osteoporosis who have not been diagnosed should be treated conservatively.

Osteoarthritis

Osteoarthritis is a chronic disease involving the joints, especially those bearing weight. Osteoarthritis is characterized by destruction of articular cartilage, overgrowth of bone with lipping and spur formation, and impaired function. Overweight/obesity is a major risk factor for the development of osteoarthritis. Lifestyle modification such as regular physical activity and proper diet may help prevent or control osteoarthritis symptoms.

Rheumatoid Arthritis

Rheumatoid arthritis is an autoimmune disease where the body starts to degrade its own joint tissue. It is associated with inflammation of the joints, stiffness, swelling, cartilaginous hypertrophy, and pain.

Chronic Low Back Pain

Low back and abdominal exercises are prescribed for a variety of reasons, but primarily for rehabilitation of the injured low back, prevention of injury, and/or as a component of fitness training programs. The objective of exercise prescription is to stress both damaged tissue and other healthy supporting tissues to promote tissue repair while avoiding further excessive loading that can exacerbate existing structural weakness. While knowledge of tissue forces during exercise is important to avoid further injury, choosing the optimal load requires a blend of art and science. In general, the most effective exercise programs are designed to train the motor control system to activate the spine stabilizers, then progress to endurance training, and finally to initiate enhancement of strength and flexibility.

Exercise and Low Back Pain

Several hypotheses can be considered to explain the general role of exercise on maintaining low back tissue health and optimizing the repair process. Powerful evidence demonstrates that exercise does the following:

- Stimulates tissue hypertrophy
- Slows (possibly reverses) several degenerative conditions
- Enhances the nutritional benefit to the disc
- Is effective in treating the injured back compared to surgical intervention, bed rest, or simple flexibility programs (68–71)

In addition, the success of a carefully formulated exercise program that includes progressive stabilization exercise routines, emphasizing muscle contraction with the spine in a neutral posture, has been documented (72). While hip flexibility has been shown to be important, spine flexibility has never been shown to enhance the outcome of low back exercise programs for those with low back injury or to reduce the risk of future injury in healthy populations.

E. Medications

It is beyond the scope of practice of the ACSM certified Personal Trainer™ to prescribe or recommend the use of any medication to a client.

Several medications are available for treatment of joint and muscle inflammation and pain caused by direct trauma, overuse injury, and orthopaedic disease (74). Medications prescribed by the physician include aspirin, nonsteroidal anti-inflammatory drugs (NSAIDs), and newer immunosuppressive agents for the treatment of inflammatory rheumatic disease. In osteoarthritis and minor joint inflammations, NSAIDs and acetaminophen are often prescribed to manage stiffness and pain. Pharmacological management to control the discomfort associated with low back injuries includes the use of acetaminophen to manage pain, muscle relaxants, and NSAIDs.

The three nonprescription drugs most often used are aspirin, ibuprofen, and acetaminophen. Aspirin and ibuprofen are NSAIDs with analgesic, antipyretic, and anti-inflammatory properties. Aspirin, a salicylate drug, and ibuprofen, reduce pain, fever, and inflammation. Aspirin and various other NSAIDs have been associated with a variety of adverse reactions, including nausea, gastric discomfort, and decreased platelet aggregation. Although most individuals tolerate ibuprofen, gastric discomfort and stomach pains indicate poor tolerance. Acetaminophen has both analgesic and antipyretic effects but does not have significant anti-inflammatory properties. Aspirin-sensitive individuals should consult a physician before taking these pain relievers because they may encounter cross-reactivity with other medications.

Medications fulfill legitimate needs to relieve minor pain and discomfort. However, if dosage instructions are not followed, these products can be harmful. Use of nonprescription and prescription medications should be discussed with a physician or pharmacist. Individuals with persistent pain or injuries that do not resolve despite pharmacological intervention should consult a physician.

Classes af Medications

1. Antianginal—any drug used in the treatment of angina pectoris (chest pain), a symptom of ischemic heart disease. Beta blockers can fall under the category of antianginal, antihypertensive, and antiarrhythmic.
2. Antihypertensive—any drug used to reduce high blood pressure.
3. Antiarrhythmic—any drug used to prevent or control abnormal heart rhythms.
4. Bronchodilator—any drug that relaxes and dilates (widens) the bronchial passageways and improves the passages of air into the lungs. Example: albuterol.
5. Hypoglycemic—any drug that helps reduce blood sugar levels.
6. Psychotropic—any drug that affects behavior.
7. Vasodilator—any drug that causes blood vessels to become wider (dilate) by relaxing smooth muscle in the vessel wall. Reduced blood pressure might allow blood to flow around a clot.
8. Antihistamine—any drug which blocks the action of histamine, thus preventing symptoms of an allergic response.
9. Tranquilizer—any drug used to decrease stress or tension without reducing mental clarity.
10. Diet pills—any drug used to lose weight, typically they contain stimulants such as caffeine and or other potentially harmful substances.

11. Cold tablets—any drug used to alleviate the effects of the common cold. Often they contain decongestants and/or antihistamines. (Table 9.2 and Table 9.3).

Commonly Used Substances

Caffeine

Caffeine is the most widely consumed behaviorally active substance in the world. Implications/significance: Caffeine as an ergogenic aid (any substance thought to enhance performance) may extend endurance in moderately strenuous aerobic exercise. It may also improve performance in higher-intensity, shorter duration physical efforts. Taking caffeine prior to exercise seems to increase the breakdown of fat for energy and reduces carbohydrate metabolism, sparing muscle glycogen. The negatives of caffeine are many however: it is addictive, acts as a potent diuretic (substance that causes body fluid loss) potentially related to dehydration, stimulates the central nervous system, produces restlessness, headaches, insomnia, muscle twitching, decreases motor skill, elevates heart rate, increases blood pressure, and may contribute to premature heart contractions (PVCs). Also, high intakes of caffeine may contribute to bone density loss (73).

Alcohol and Other Substance Abuse

Implications/significance: Alcohol intake may elevate heart rate response to submaximal effort, impair exercise tolerance, promote dehydration, and increase risk of heart injury. Chronic high intakes of alcohol may also contribute to bone density loss and weight gain. Habit-forming drugs, such as cocaine, may accentuate risk of cardiac complications during exercise.

Nicotine

Implications/significance: Acute cigarette smoking may elevate heart rate, respiration, and blood pressure response to exercise, increase susceptibility toward heart arrhythmias, increase risk of producing excess blood clots, and increase likelihood of coronary artery spasm. Chronically, cigarette smoking increases the risk of atherosclerosis, coronary heart disease, several cancers including lung cancer, and many other harmful conditions/diseases.

Table 9.2 – Generic and Brand Names of Common Drugs by Class

Generic Name	Brand Name*
β-Blockers	
Acebutolol	Sectral
Atenolol	Tenormin
Betaxolol	Kerlone
Bisoprolol	Zebeta
Carteolol	Cartrol
Esmolol	Brevibloc
Metoprolol	Lopressor, Toprol
Nadolol	Corgard
Penbutolol	Levatol
Pindolol	Visken
Propranolol	Inderal
Sotalol	Betapace
Timolol	Blocadren
β-Blockers in Combinations With	
Diuretics	Inderide, Lopressor Hydrochlorothiazide (HCTZ), Tenoretic, Timolide, Ziac, Corzide
α- and β-Adrenergic Blocking Agents	
Carvedilol	Coreg
Labetalol	Normodyne, Trandate
α₁-Adrenergic Blocking Agents	
Doxazosin	Cardura
Prazosin	Minipress
Terazosin	Hytrin
Angiotensin-Converting Enzyme (ACE) Inhibitors	
Benazepril	Lotensin
Captopril	Capoten
Enalapril	Vasotec
Fosinopril	Monopril
Lisinopril	Zestril, Prinivil
Moexipril	Univasc
Perindopril erbumine	Aceon
Quinapril	Accupril
Ramipril	Altace
Trandolapril	Mavik
ACE Inhibitors + Diuretics	
Captopril and HCTZ	Capozide
Enalapril maleate and HCTZ	Vaseretic
Lisinopril and HCTZ	Prinzide, Zestoretic
Moexipril and HCTZ	Uniretic
Angiotensin II Receptor Antagonists	
Irbesartan	Avapro
Losartan	Cozaar
Valsartan	Diovan
Diuretics	
Thiazides	
Hydrochlorothiazide (HCTZ)	Esidrix
"Loop"	
Bumetanide	Bumex
Ethacrynic acid	Edecrin
Furosemide	Lasix
Potassium-sparing	
Amiloride	Midamor
Spironolactone	Aldactone
Triamterene	Dyrenium
Combinations	
Triamterene and HCTZ	Dyazide, Maxzide
Amiloride and HCTZ	Moduretic
Others	
Metolazone	Zaroxolyn
Antiarrhythmic Agents	
Class I	
IA	
Disopyramide	Norpace
Moricizine	Ethmozine
Procainamide	Pronestyl, Procan SR
Quinidine	Quinora, Quinidex, Quinaglute, Quinalan, Cardioquin

Table 9.2 continued – Generic and Brand Names of Common Drugs by Class

Generic Name	Brand Name*
Angiotensin-Converting Enzyme (ACE) Inhibitors	
Benazepril	Lotensin
Captopril	Capoten
Enalapril	Vasotec
Fosinopril	Monopril
Lisinopril	Zestril, Prinivil
Moexipril	Univasc
Perindopril erbumine	Aceon
Quinapril	Accupril
Ramipril	Altace
Trandolapril	Mavik
ACE Inhibitors + Diuretics	
Captopril and HCTZ	Capozide
Enalapril maleate and HCTZ	Vaseretic
Lisinopril and HCTZ	Prinzide, Zestoretic
Moexipril and HCTZ	Uniretic
Angiotensin II Receptor Antagonists	
Irbesartan	Avapro
Losartan	Cozaar
Valsartan	Diovan
Diuretics	
Thiazides	
Hydrochlorothiazide (HCTZ)	Esidrix
"Loop"	
Bumetanide	Bumex
Ethacrynic acid	Edecrin
Furosemide	Lasix
Potassium-sparing	
Amiloride	Midamor
Spironolactone	Aldactone
Triamterene	Dyrenium
Combinations	
Triamterene and HCTZ	Dyazide, Maxzide
Amiloride and HCTZ	Moduretic
Others	
Metolazone	Zaroxolyn
Antiarrhythmic Agents	
Class I	
IA	
Disopyramide	Norpace
Moricizine	Ethmozine
Procainamide	Pronestyl, Procan SR
Quinidine	Quinora, Quinidex, Quinaglute, Quinalan, Cardioquin
Antiarrhythmic Agents	
Class I	
IB	
Lidocaine	Xylocaine, Xylocard
Mexiletine	Mexitil
Phenytoin	Dilantin
Tocainide	Tonocard
IC	
Flecainide	Tambocor
Propafenone	Rythmol
Class II	
β-Blockers	
Class III	
Amiodarone	Cordarone
Bretylium	Bretylol
Sotalol	Betapace
Class IV	
Calcium channel blockers	

Table 9.2 continued – Generic and Brand Names of Common Drugs by Class

Antihyperlipidemic Agents

Atorvastatin	Lipitor
Cerivastatin	Baycol
Cholestyramine	Questran, Cholybar, Prevalite
Clofibrate	Atromid
Colestipol	Colestid
Fluvastatin	Lescol
Gemfibrozil	Lopid
Lovastatin	Mevacor
Nicotinic acid (niacin)	Nicobid, Nicolar, Slo-Niacin, Niaspan
Pravastatin	Pravachol
Simvastatin	Zocor

Sympathomimetic Agents

Albuterol	Proventil, Ventolin
Ephedrine	Primatene
Epinephrine	Adrenalin
Isoetharine	Bronkosol
Metaproterenol	Alupent
Terbutaline	Brethine

Others

Clopidogrel	Plavix
Dipyridamole	Persantine
Pentoxifylline	Trental
Warfarin	Coumadin

*Represent selected brands; these are not necessarily all-inclusive.

Table 9.3 – Effects of Medications on Heart Rate, Blood Pressure, the Electrocardiogram (ECG), and Exercise Capacity

Medications	Heart Rate	Blood Pressure	ECG	Exercise Capacity
I. β-Blockers (including carvedilol, labetalol)	↓ *(R and E)	↓ (R and E)	↓ HR*(R) ↓ ischemia† (E)	↑ in patients with angina; ↓ or ↔ in patients without angina
II. Nitrates	↑ (R) ↑ or ↔ (E)	↓ (R) ↓ or ↔ (E)	↑ HR (R) ↑ or ↔ HR (E) ↓ ischemia† (E)	↑ in patients with angina; ↔ in patients without angina; ↑ or ↔ in patients with congestive heart failure (CHF)
III. Calcium channel blockers Amlodipine Felodipine Isradipine Nicardipine Nifedipine Nimodipine Nisoldipine	↑ or ↔ (R and E)	↓ (R and E)	↑ or ↔ HR (R and E) ↓ ischemia† (E)	↑ in patients with angina; ↔ in patients without angina
Bepridil Diltiazem Verapamil	↓ (R and E)		↓ HR (R and E) ↓ ischemia† (E)	
IV. Digitalis	↓ in patients with atrial fibrillation and possibly CHF Not significantly altered in patients with sinus rhythm	↔ (R and E)	May produce nonspecific ST-T wave changes (R) May produce ST segment depression (E)	Improved only in patients with atrial fibrillation or in patients with CHF
V. Diuretics	↔ (R and E)	↔ or ↓ (R and E)	↔ or PVCs (R) May cause PVCs and "false positive" test results if hypokalemia occurs May cause PVCs if hypomagnesemia occurs (E)	↔, except possibly in patients with CHF
VI. Vasodilators, nonadrenergic	↑ or ↔ (R and E)	↓ (R and E)	↑ or ↔ HR (R and E)	↔, except ↑ or ↔ in patients with CHF
ACE inhibitors	↔ (R and E)	↓ (R and E)	↔ (R and E)	↔, except ↑ or ↔ in patients with CHF
α-Adrenergic blockers	↔ (R and E)	↓ (R and E)	↔ (R and E)	↔
Antiadrenergic agents without selective blockade	↓ or ↔ (R and E)	↓ (R and E)	↓ or ↔ HR (R and E)	↔

Table 9.3 (continued) – Effects of Medications on Heart Rate, Blood Pressure, the Electrocardiogram (ECG), and Exercise Capacity

Medications	Heart Rate	Blood Pressure	ECG	Exercise Capacity
VII. Antiarrhythmic agents	All antiarrhythmic agents may cause new or worsened arrhythmias (proarrhythmic effect)			
Class I				
Quinidine	↑ or ↔ (R and E)	↓ or ↔ (R)	↑ or ↔ HR (R)	↔
Disopyramide		↔ (E)	May prolong QRS and QT intervals (R)	
			Quinidine may result in "false negative" test results (E)	
Procainamide	↔ (R and E)	↔ (R and E)	May prolong QRS and QT intervals (R)	↔
			May result in "false positive" test results (E)	
Phenytoin	↔ (R and E)	↔ (R and E)	↔ (R and E)	↔
Tocainide				
Mexiletine				
Flecainide	↔ (R and E)	↔ (R and E)	May prolong QRS and QT intervals (R)	↔
Moricizine			↔ (E)	
Propafenone	↓ (R)	↔ (R and E)	↓ HR (R)	↔
	↓ or ↔ (E)		↓ or ↔ HR (E)	
Class II				
β-Blockers (see I.)				
Class III				
Amiodarone	↓ (R and E)	↔ (R and E)	↓ HR (R)	↔
			↔ (E)	
Class IV				
Calcium channel blockers (see III.)				
VIII. Bronchodilators	↔ (R and E)	↔ (R and E)	↔ (R and E)	Bronchodilators ↑ exercise capacity in patients limited by bronchospasm
Anticholinergic agents	↑ or ↔ (R and E)	↔	↑ or ↔ HR	
Methylxanthines			May produce PVCs (R and E)	
Sympathomimetic agents	↑ or ↔ (R and E)	↑, ↔, or ↓ (R and E)	↑ or ↔ HR (R and E)	↔
Cromolyn sodium	↔ (R and E)	↔ (R and E)	↔ (R and E)	↔
Corticosteroids	↔ (R and E)	↔ (R and E)	↔ (R and E)	↔
IX. Antihyperlipidemic agents	Clofibrate may provoke arrhythmias, angina in patients with prior myocardial infarction Nicotinic acid may ↓ BP All other antihyperlipidemic agents have no effect on HR, BP, and ECG			↔
X. Psychotropic medications				
Minor tranquilizers	May ↓ HR and BP by controlling anxiety; no other effects			
Antidepressants	↑ or ↔ (R and E)	↓ or ↔ (R and E)	Variable (R)	
			May result in "false positive" test results (E)	
Major tranquilizers	↑ or ↔ (R and E)	↓ or ↔ (R and E)	Variable (R)	
			May result in "false positive" or "false negative" test results (E)	
Lithium	↔ (R and E)	↔ (R and E)	May result in T wave changes and arrhythmias (R and E)	
XI. Nicotine	↑ or ↔ (R and E)	↑ (R and E)	↑ or ↔ HR	↔, except ↓ or ↔ in patients with angina
			May provoke ischemia, arrhythmias (R and E)	
XII. Antihistamines	↔ (R and E)	↔ (R and E)	↔ (R and E)	↔
XIII. Cold medications with sympathomimetic agents	Effects similar to those described in sympathomimetic agents, although magnitude of effects is usually smaller			↔
XIV. Thyroid medications	↑ (R and E)	↑ (R and E)	↑ HR	↔, unless angina worsened
			May provoke arrhythmias	
Only levothyroxine			↑ ischemia (R and E)	
XV. Alcohol	↔ (R and E)	Chronic use may have role in ↑ BP (R and E)	May provoke arrhythmias (R and E)	↔
XVI. Hypoglycemic agents Insulin and oral agents	↔ (R and E)	↔ (R and E)	↔ (R and E)	↔

Table 9.3 (continued) – Effects of Medications on Heart Rate, Blood Pressure, the Electrocardiogram (ECG), and Exercise Capacity

Medications	Heart Rate	Blood Pressure	ECG	Exercise Capacity
XI. Nicotine	↑ or ↔ (R and E)	↑ (R and E)	↑ or ↔ HR May provoke ischemia, arrhythmias (R and E)	↔, except ↓ or ↔ in patients with angina
XII. Antihistamines	↔ (R and E)	↔ (R and E)	↔ (R and E)	↔
XIII. Cold medications with sympathomimetic agents	Effects similar to those described in sympathomimetic agents, although magnitude of effects is usually smaller			↔
XIV. Thyroid medications Only levothyroxine	↑ (R and E)	↑ (R and E)	↑ HR May provoke arrhythmias ↑ ischemia (R and E)	↔, unless angina worsened
XV. Alcohol	↔ (R and E)	Chronic use may have role in ↑ BP	May provoke arrhythmias (R and E)	↔
XXI. Pentoxifylline	↔ (R and E)	↔ (R and E)	↔ (R and E)	↑ or ↔ in patients limited by intermittent claudication
XXII. Caffeine	Variable effects depending upon previous use Variable effects on exercise capacity May provoke arrhythmias			
XXIII. Anorexiants/diet pills	↑ or ↔ (R and E)	↑ or ↔ (R and E)	↑ or ↔ HR (R and E)	

Key: ↑ = increase; ↔ = no effect; ↓ = decrease; R = rest; E = exercise; HR = heart rate; PVCs = premature ventricular contractions.

*β-Blockers with ISA lower resting HR only slightly.

†May prevent or delay myocardial ischemia (see text).

References

1. World Health Report 1997. Geneva: World Health Organization, 1997.1. World Health Report 1997. Geneva: World Health Organization, 1997.
2. American Heart Association. Heart and Stroke Facts: 1994 Statistical Supplement. Dallas: American Heart Association, 1994.
3. Miller M, Vogel RA. The practice of coronary artery disease prevention. 1st ed. Baltimore: Williams & Wilkins, 1996:2.
4. Kannel WB, Dawber TR, Kagan A, et al. Factors of risk in the development of coronary heart disease: Six-year follow-up experience. Ann Intern Med 55:33–50, 1961.
5. McGinnis JM, Foege WH. Actual causes of death in the United States. JAMA 270:2207–2212, 1993.
6. McGill HC Jr. The cardiovascular pathology of smoking. Am Heart J 115:250–257, 1988.
7. Willett WC, Green A, Stampfe MJ, et al. Relative and absolute excess risk of coronary heart disease among women who smoke cigarettes. N Engl J Med 317:1303–1309, 1987.
8. Daly LE, Mulcahy R, Graham IM, Hickey M. Long term effect on mortality of stopping smoking after unstable angina and myocardial infarction. BMJ 287:324–326, 1983.
9. Glantz SA, Parmley WW. Passive smoking and heart disease: Epidemiology, physiology and biochemistry. Circulation 83:1–12, 1991.
10. He J, Vupputuri S, Allen K, et al. Passive smoking and the risk of coronary heart disease—a meta-analysis of epidemiologic studies. N Engl J Med 340:920–926, 1999.
11. American Heart Association, National Heart, Lung and Blood Institute. The cholesterol facts: A summary of the evidence relating to dietary fat, serum cholesterol and coronary heart disease. Circulation 81:1721–1733, 1990.
12. Expert Panel on Detection, Evaluation and Treatment of High Blood Cholesterol in Adults. Summary of the Second Report of the National Cholesteral Education Program (NCEP) Expert Panel on Detection, Evaluation, and Treatment of High Blood Cholesterol in Adults (Adult Treatment Panel II). JAMA 269: 3015–3023, 1993.
13. Stamler J, Wentworth D, Neaton JD. Is relationship between serum cholesterol and risk of premature death from coronary heart disease continuous and graded? JAMA 256:2823–2828, 1986.
14. Wilson PWF, D'Agostino RB, Levy D, et al. Prediction of coronary heart disease using risk factor categories. Circulation 97:1837–1847, 1998.
15. Sacks F, Pfeffer M, Moye L, et al. Effect of pravastatin oncoronary events after myocardial infarction in patients with average cholesterol levels. N Engl J Med 335:1001-1009, 1996.
16. Tonkin AM. Management of the long term intervention with pravastatin in ischemic heart disease study. Am J Cardiol 76:107C-112C, 1995.
17. Scandinavian Simvaastatin Survival Study Group. Baseline serum cholesterol and treatment effect in the Scandanavian Simvastatin Survival Study. Lancet 345:1274-1275, 1995.
18. Shepherd J. The Western Scotland Coronary Prevention Study: a trial of cholesterol reduction in Scottish men. Am J Cardiol 76:113C-117C, 1995.
19. Bowns JR, Clearfield M, Weiss S, et al. Primary prevention of acute coronary events with lovastatin in men and women with average cholesterol levels. Results of AFCAPS/TEXCAPS. JAMA 279:1615-1622, 1998.
20. Harper CR, Jacobson TA. New prospective on the management of low levels of high density lipoprotein cholesterol. Arch Intern Med 159:1049–1057, 1999.
21. Gordon T, Castelli WP, Hjortland MC, et al. High density lipoprotein as a protective factor against coronary heart disease. Am J Med 62:707–714, 1997.
22. Tall AR. Plasma high density lipoproteins. J Clin Invest 86:379–384, 1990.
23. Maier JA, Barcengi HL, Pagan IF, et al. The protective role of high density lipoprotein on oxidized low density lipoprotein induced U937/endothelial cell interactions. Eur J Biochem 221:35–41, 1994.
24. Rubins HB, Robins SJ, Collins D, et al. Gemfibrozil for the secondary prevention of coronary heart disease in men with low levels of HDL cholesterol. N Engl J Med 341:410, 1999.
25. The Sixth Report of the Joint National Committee on Prevention, Detection, Evaluation and Treatment of High Blood Pressure. National High Blood Pressure Education Program. National Institutes of Health. National Heart, Lung, and Blood Institute. NIH Publication 98-4080, 1997.
26. Stamler J, Neaton J, Wentworth D. Blood pressure and risk of fatal coronary heart disease. Hypertension 13:2–12, 1993.
27. Collins R, Petor, MacMahon S, et al. Blood pressure stroke and coronary heart disease. Lancet 335:827–838, 1990.

28. Mulrow CD, Cornell JA, Herrera CR, et al. Hypertension in the elderly: Implications and generalized ability of randomized trials. JAMA 272:1932–1938, 1994.

29. Butler WJ, Ostrander LD, Carman WJ, Lamphiear DE. Mortality from coronary heart disease in the Tecumseh Study: Long term effects of diabetes mellitus, glucose intolerance and other risk factors. Am J Epidemiol 1985 121:541–547.

30. Report of the Expert Committee on the Diagnosis and Complications of Diabetes Mellitus. Diabetes Care 20:1183–1197, 1997.

31. Bierman EL. George Lyman Duff Memorial Lecture. Atherogenesis in diabetes. Arterioscler Thromb 12:647–656, 1992.

32. Haffner SM, Lehto S, Ronnemaa T, et al. Mortality from coronary heart disease in subjects with type II diabetes and nondiabetic subjects with and without prior myocardial infarction. N Engl J Med 339:229–234, 1998.

33. Kullo IJ, Gau GT, Tajik AJ. Novel risk factors for atherosclerosis. Mayo Clin Proc 75:369–380, 2000.

34. Nygar DO, Nordrehaug JE, Refsum H, et al. Plasma homocysteine levels and mortality in patients with coronary artery disease. N Engl J Med 337:230–236, 1997.

35. Yang XC, Jing TY, Resnick LM, et al. Relation of hemostatic risk factors to other risk factors for coronary heart disease and to sex hormones in men. Arterioscler Thromb Vasc Biol 13:467–471, 1993.

36. Ridker PM. Evaluating novel cardiovascular risk factors. Ann Intern Med 130:1933–1937, 1999.

37. Kuezmarski RJ, Flegal KM, Campbell SM, et al. Increasing prevalence of overweight among US adults. JAMA 272:205–211, 1994.

38. Pi-Sunyer FX. Medical hazards of obesity. Ann Intern Med 110:655–660, 1993.

39. Hubert HB, Feineib M, McNamara PM, et al. Obesity as an independent risk factor for cardiovascular disease: A 26-year follow-up of participants in the Framingham Heart Study. Circulation 67:968–977, 1983.

40. Blackburn GL, Rosofsky W. Making the connection between weight loss, dieting, and health: The 10% solution. Weight Control Dig 2:121–127, 1992.

41. National Task Force on the Prevention and Treatment of Obesity. Long-term pharmacotherapy in the management of obesity. JAMA 276:1907–1915, 1996.

42. Fletcher GF, Balady G, Blair SN, et al. Statement on Exercise: Benefits and recommendations for physical activity programs for all Americans: A statement for health professionals by the Committee on Exercise and Cardiac Rehabilitation of the Council on Clinical Cardiology, American Heart Association. Circulation 94:857–862, 1996.

43. Pate RR, Pratt M, Blair SN, et al. Physical activity and public health: A recommendation from the Centers for Disease Control and Prevention and the American College of Sports Medicine. JAMA 273:402–407, 1995.

44. Caspersen CJ, Heath GW. The risk factor concept of coronary heart disease. In: ACSM's Resource Manual for Guidelines for Exercise Testing and Prescription. 2nd ed. Philadelphia: Lea & Febiger, 1993:151–167.

45. Pasternak RC, Grundy SM, Levy D, et al. Task Force 3. Spectrum of risk factors for coronary heart disease. J Am Coll Cardiol 27:978–990, 1996.

46. Writing Group for the PEPI Trial. Effects of estrogen and estrogen-progesterone regimen on heart disease risk factors in post-menopausal women. JAMA 273:199–208, 1995.

47. Hulley S, Grady D, Bush T, et al. Randomized trial of estrogen plus progestin for secondary prevention of coronary heart disease in postmenopausal women. JAMA 280:605–613, 1998.

48. Fuster V, Pearson TA. 27th Bethesda Conference. Matching the intensity of risk factor management with the hazard for coronary disease events. J Am Coll Cardiol 27:957–1047, 1996.

49. American Thoracic Society. Standards for the diagnosis and care of patients with chronic obstructive pulmonary disease. Am J Resp Crit Care Med 152:S77–S120, 1995.

50. Robins AG. Pathophysiology of emphysema. Clin Chest Med 4:413–420, 1983 (review).

51. Faling LJ. Pulmonary rehabilitation: physical modalities. Clin Chest Med 7:599–618, 1986 (review).

52. Pardy RL, Rivington RN, Despas PJ, et al. The effects of inspiratory muscle training on exercise performance in chronic airflow limitation. Am Rev Respir Dis 123:426–433, 1981.

53. Tattersfield AE. The site of the defect in asthma. Neurohumoral, mediator or smooth muscle? Chest 91(6 Suppl):184S–189S, 1987 (review).

54. Hargreave FE, Dolovich J, O'Byrne PM, et al. The origin of airway hyperresponsiveness. J Allergy Clin Immunol 78(5 Pt 1):825–832, 1986 (review).

55. McFadden ER Jr. Exercise-induced asthma. Assessment of current etiologic concepts. Chest 91(6 Suppl):151S–157S, 1987 (review).

56. Chrischilles C, Sherman T, Wallace R. Cost and health effects of osteoporotic fractures. Bone 15:377–386, 1994.

57. Salkeld G, Cameron ID, Cumming RG, et al. Quality of life related to fear of falling and hip fracture in older women: A time trade off study. BMJ 320:341–346, 2000.

58. Fuchs RK, Snow CM. Jumping improves femoral neck bone mass in children. Med Sci Sports Exerc 31:S83, 1999.

59. Winters KM, Snow CM. Detraining reverses positive effects of exercise on the musculoskeletal system in premenopausal women. J Bone Miner Res 15:2495–2503, 2000.

60. Shaw JM, Snow C. Weighted vest exercise improves indices of fall risk in older women. J Gerontol A Biol Sci Med Sci 53:M53–M58, 1998.

61. Bassey EJ, Rothwell MC, Littlewood JJ, Pye DW. Pre- and post-menopausal women have different bone mineral density responses to the same high-impact exercise. J Bone Miner Res 13:1805–1813, 1998.

62. Snow CM, Shaw JM, Winters KM, Witzke KA. Long-term exercise using weighted vests prevents hip bone loss in post-menopausal women. J Gerontol A Biol Sci Med Sci 55:M489–492, 2000.

63. Bassey EJ, Fiatarone MA, O'Neill EF, et al. Leg extensor power and functional performance in very old men and women. Clin Sci 82:321–327, 1992.

64. Jozsi AC, Campbell WW, Joseph L, et al. Changes in power with resistance training in older and younger men and women. J Gerontol A Biol Sci Med Sci 54:M591–596, 1999.

65. Brill PA, Probst JC, Greenhouse DL, et al. Clinical feasibility of a free-weight strength-training program for older adults. J Am Board Fam Pract 11:445–451, 1998.

66. Joakimsen RM, Magnus JH, Fonnebo V. Physical activity and predisposition for hip fractures: A review. Osteoporos Int 7:503–513, 1997.

67. Recker RR, Davies KM, Hinders SM, et al. Bone gain in young adult women. JAMA 268:2403–2408, 1992.

68. Videman T, Sarna S, Crites-Battie M, et al. The long term effects of physical loading and exercise lifestyles on back-related symptoms, disability, and spinal pathology among men. Spine 20(b):669–709, 1995.

69. Videman T. Experimental models of osteoarthritis: The role of immobilization. Clin Biomech 2:223–229, 1987.

70. Holm S, Nachemson A. Variations in the nutrition of the canine intervertebral disc induced by motion. Spine 8:866–874, 1983.

71. Richardson C, Jull G, Hodges P, Hides J. Therapeutic Exercise for Spinal Segmental Stabilization in Low Back Pain. Edinburgh: Churchill Livingstone, 1999.

72. Saal JA, Saal JS. Nonoperative treatment of herniated lumbar intervertebral disc with radiculopathy: An outcome study. Spine 14:431–437, 1989.

73. McArdle WD, Katch F, Katch V. Exercise Physiology: Energy, Nutrition and Human Performance. 4th ed. Baltimore: Williams & Wilkins, 1996.

74. Soukup JT, Maynard TS, Kovaleski JE. Resistance training guidelines for individuals with diabetes mellitus. Diabetes Educ 20:129–137, 1994.

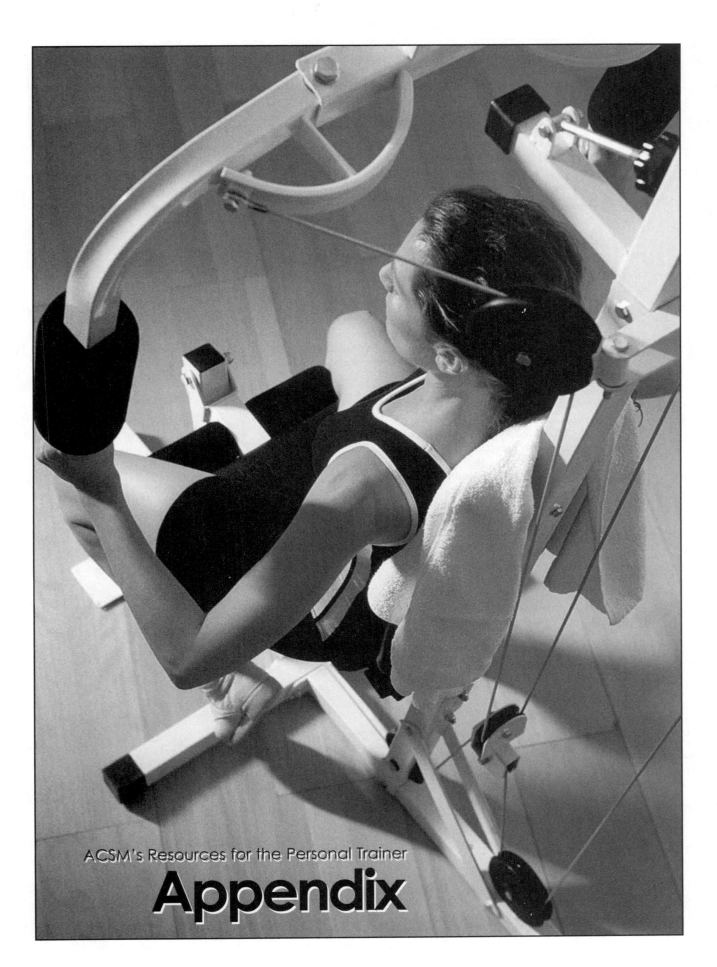

ACSM's Resources for the Personal Trainer

Appendix

ACSM certified Personal Trainer™

Scope of Practice

The ACSM certified Personal Trainer™ is a fitness professional involved in developing and implementing an individualized approach to exercise leadership in healthy populations and/or those individuals with medical clearance to exercise. Using a variety of teaching techniques, the Personal Trainer is proficient in leading and demonstrating safe and effective methods of exercise by applying the fundamental principles of exercise science. The ACSM certified Personal Trainer™ is familiar with forms of exercise used to improve, maintain, and/or optimize health-related components of physical fitness and performance. The ACSM certified Personal Trainer™ is proficient in writing appropriate exercise recommendations, leading and demonstrating safe and effective methods of exercise, and motivating individuals to begin and to continue with their healthy behaviors."

The written exam is delivered in a computer-based testing format (in English), at a Pearson VUE authorized testing center worldwide. The exam contains approximately 125-150 multiple-choice questions based on KSAs (knowledge, skills, and abilities) distributed across the following content areas. The table below lists the **approximate** percentage of questions from each content area, based on these KSAs:

CONTENT AREAS	Percentage
Exercise Physiology and Related Exercise Science	24%
Exercise Prescription (Training) and Programming	28%
Human Behavior	4%
Health Appraisal and Fitness Exercise Testing	13%
Safety, Injury Prevention, and Emergency Procedures	8%
Nutrition and Weight Management	9%
Clinical and Medical Considerations	10%
Program Administration, Quality Assurance, and Outcome Assessment	4%
Total	100%

Knowledge, Skills, and Abilities (KSAs)

I. EXERCISE PHYSIOLOGY AND RELATED EXERCISE SCIENCE
- Knowledge of the basic structures of bone, skeletal muscle, and connective tissues.
- Knowledge of the basic anatomy of the cardiovascular system and respiratory system.
- Knowledge of the definition of the following terms: inferior, superior, medial, lateral, supination, pronation, flexion, extension, adduction, abduction, hyperextension, rotation, circumduction, agonist, antagonist, and stabilizer.
- Knowledge of the plane in which each muscle action occurs.
- Knowledge of the interrelationships among center of gravity, base of support, balance, stability, and proper spinal alignment.
- Knowledge of the following curvatures of the spine: lordosis, scoliosis, and kyphosis.
- Knowledge to describe the myotatic stretch reflex.
- Knowledge of the biomechanical principles for the performance of the following activities: walking, jogging, running, swimming, cycling, weight lifting, and carrying or moving objects.
- Ability to define aerobic and anaerobic metabolism.
- Knowledge to describe the normal acute responses to cardiovascular exercise.
- Knowledge to describe the normal acute responses to resistance training.
- Knowledge of the normal chronic physiological adaptations associated with cardiovascular exercise.
- Knowledge of the normal chronic physiological adaptations associated with resistance training.
- Knowledge of the physiological principles related to warm-up and cool-down.
- Knowledge of the common theories of muscle fatigue and delayed onset muscle soreness (DOMS).
- Knowledge of the physiological adaptations that occur at rest and during submaximal and maximal exercise following chronic aerobic and anaerobic exercise training.
- Knowledge of the physiological principles involved in promoting gains in muscular strength and endurance.
- Knowledge of blood pressure responses associated with acute exercise, including changes in body position.
- Knowledge of how the principle of specificity relates to the components of fitness.
- Knowledge of the concept of detraining or reversibility of conditioning and its implications in fitness programs.
- Knowledge of the physical and psychological signs of overtraining and to provide recommendations for these problems.
- Knowledge of the following terms: progressive resistance, isotonic/isometric, concentric, eccentric, atrophy, hypertrophy, sets, repetitions, plyometrics, Valsalva maneuver.
- Ability to identify the major bones and muscles. Major muscles include, but are not limited to, the following: trapezius, pectoralis major, latissimus dorsi, biceps, triceps, rectus abdominis, internal and external obliques, erector spinae, gluteus maximus, quadriceps, hamstrings, adductors, abductors, and gastrocnemius.
- Ability to identify the major bones. Major bones include, but are not limited to the clavicle, scapula, strernum, humerus, carpals, ulna, radius, femur, fibia, tibia, and tarsals.
- Ability to identify the joints of the body.
- Knowledge of the primary action and joint range of motion for each major muscle group.
- Ability to locate the anatomic landmarks for palpation of peripheral pulses.

II. HEALTH APPRAISAL AND FITNESS EXERCISE TESTING
- Knowledge of and ability to discuss the physiological basis of the major components of physical fitness: flexibility, cardiovascular fitness, muscular strength, muscular endurance, and body composition.
- Knowledge of the importance of a health/medical history.
- Knowledge of the value of a medical clearance prior to exercise participation.
- Knowledge of the categories of participants who should receive medical clearance prior to administration of an exercise test or participation in an exercise program.
- Knowledge of relative and absolute contraindications to exercise testing or participation.
- Knowledge of the limitations of informed consent and medical clearance prior to exercise testing.
- Knowledge of the advantages/disadvantages and limitations of the various body composition techniques including, but not limited to: air displacement, plethysmography, hydrostatic weighing, Bod Pod, bioelectrical impedence.
- Skill in accurately measuring heart rate, and obtaining rating of perceived exertion (RPE) at rest

and during exercise according to established guidelines.
- Ability to locate common sites for measurement of skinfold thicknesses and circumferences (for determination of body composition and waist-hip ratio).
- Ability to obtain a basic health history and risk appraisal and to stratify risk in accordance with ACSM Guidelines.
- Ability to explain and obtain informed consent.
- Ability to instruct participants in the use of equipment and test procedures.
- Knowledge of the purpose and implementation of pre-activity fitness testing, including assessments of cardiovascular fitness, muscular strength, muscular endurance, and flexibility, and body composition.
- Ability to identify appropriate criteria for terminating a fitness evaluation and demonstrate proper procedures to be followed after discontinuing such a test.

III. EXERCISE PRESCRIPTION (TRAINING) AND PROGRAMMING

- Knowledge of the benefits and risks associated with exercise training in prepubescent and postpubescent youth.
- Knowledge of the benefits and precautions associated with resistance and endurance training in older adults.
- Knowledge of specific leadership techniques appropriate for working with participants of all ages.
- Knowledge of how to modify cardiovascular and resistance exercises based on age and physical condition.
- Knowledge of and ability to describe the unique adaptations to exercise training with regard to strength, functional capacity, and motor skills.
- Knowledge of common orthopedic and cardiovascular considerations for older participants and the ability to describe modifications in exercise prescription that are indicated.
- Knowledge of selecting appropriate testing and training modalities according to the age and functional capacity of the individual.
- Knowledge of the recommended intensity, duration, frequency, and type of physical activity necessary for development of cardiorespiratory fitness in an apparently healthy population.
- Knowledge to describe, and the ability to demonstrate (such as technique and breathing), exercises designed to enhance muscular strength and/or endurance of specific major muscle groups.
- Knowledge of the principles of overload, specificity, and progression and how they relate to exercise programming.
- Knowledge of the components incorporated into an exercise session and the proper sequence (i.e., preexercise evaluation, warm-up, aerobic stimulus phase, cool-down, muscular strength and/or endurance, and flexibility).
- Knowledge of special precautions and modifications of exercise programming for participation at altitude, different ambient temperatures, humidity, and environmental pollution.
- Knowledge of the importance and ability to record exercise sessions and performing periodic evaluations to assess changes in fitness status.
- Knowledge of the advantages and disadvantages of implementation of interval, continuous, and circuit training programs.
- Knowledge of the concept of "Activities of Daily Living" (ADLs) and its importance in the overall health of the individual.
- Knowledge of Progressive Adaptation in resistance training and it's implications on program design and periodization.
- Understanding of personal training client's "personal space" and how it plays into a trainer's interaction with their client.
- Skill to teach and demonstrate the components of an exercise session (*i.e.,* warm-up, aerobic stimulus phase, cool-down, muscular strength/endurance, flexibility).
- Skill to teach and demonstrate appropriate modifications in specific exercises for the following groups: older adults, pregnant and postnatal women, obese persons, and persons with low back pain.
- Skill to teach and demonstrate appropriate exercises for improving range of motion of all major joints.
- Skill in the use of various methods for establishing and monitoring levels of exercise intensity, including heart rate, RPE, and METs.
- Knowledge of and ability to apply methods used to monitor exercise intensity, including heart rate and rating of perceived exertion.
- Ability to describe modifications in exercise prescriptions for individuals with functional disabilities and musculoskeletal injuries.